MADE WHOLE
Made Simple

Learn to Heal Yourself Through Real Food & Healthy Habits

CRISTINA CURP, NTP
from *The Castaway Kitchen*

Victory Belt Publishing Inc.
Las Vegas

First published in 2020 by Victory Belt Publishing Inc.

ISBN-13: 978-1-628604-03-0

The author is not a licensed practitioner, physician, or medical professional and offers no medical diagnoses, treatments, suggestions, or counseling. The information presented herein has not been evaluated by the U.S. Food and Drug Administration, and it is not intended to diagnose, treat, cure, or prevent any disease. Full medical clearance from a licensed physician should be obtained before beginning or modifying any diet, exercise, or lifestyle program, and physicians should be informed of all nutritional changes.

The author/owner claims no responsibility to any person or entity for any liability, loss, or damage caused or alleged to be caused directly or indirectly as a result of the use, application, or interpretation of the information presented herein.

Cover photography and author portraits by Becca Borge

Cover design by Charisse Reyes and Justin-Aaron Velasco

Interior design by Yordan Terziev and Boryana Yordanova

Interior illustrations by Joanna Albright

TC 0120

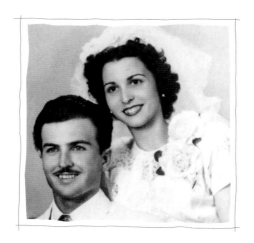

For my abuela,

Victoria Alfonso,

who taught me the power
of connecting with nature
and the importance of tradition.

You were such a constant
source of love, wisdom, and
nurturing in my life.

I know you're at peace and
happy with Abuelo in your
big garden in the sky.

CONTENTS

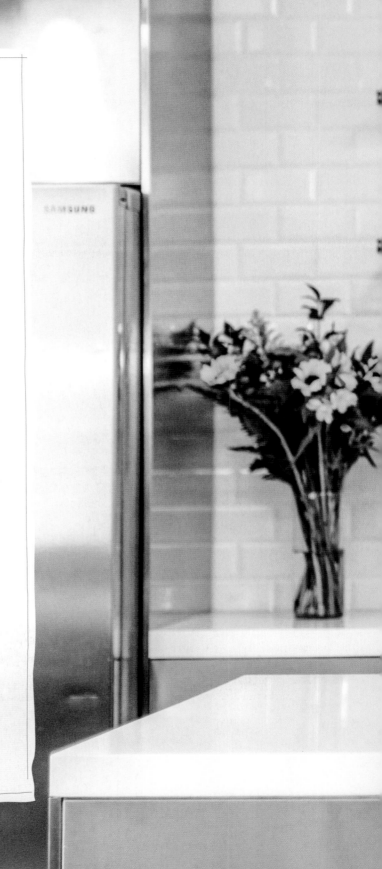

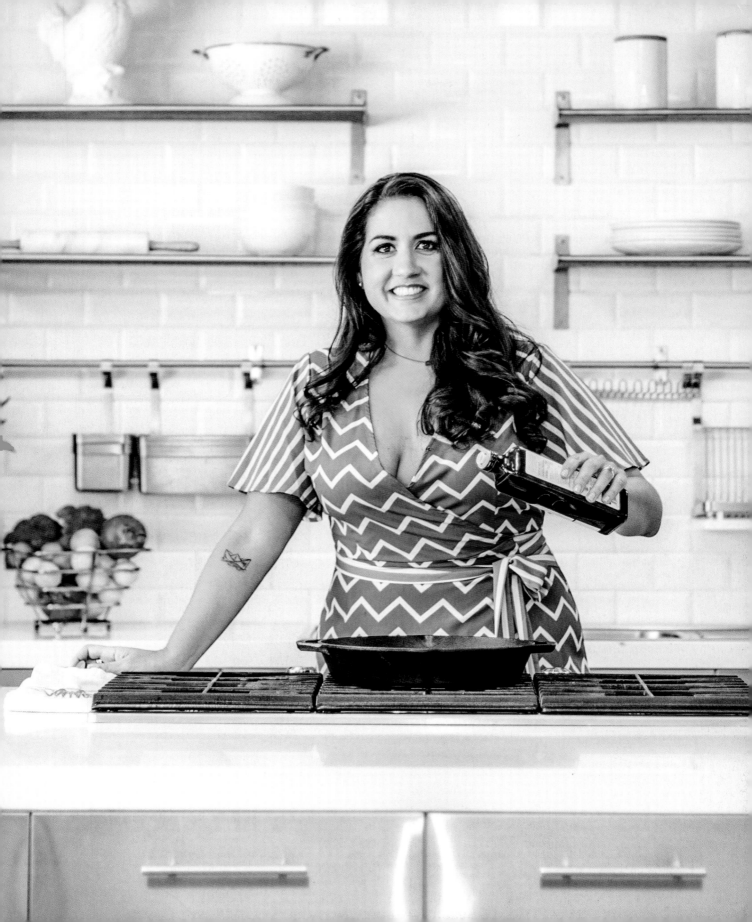

Foreword

Twenty years after my own struggle with chronic illness began, and after over ten years in clinical practice working with patients suffering from complex chronic illnesses, the sad truth is chronic illness is more prevalent than ever.

Chronic illness causes one out of ten deaths in America. One in six Americans has an autoimmune condition, nearly one in three has either prediabetes or diabetes, and one in two Americans is affected by some kind of chronic disease.

Among the causes of this epidemic are gut disorders, nutrient deficiencies, blood sugar imbalance, and food intolerances—all of which can frequently be addressed by relatively simple dietary changes.

Unfortunately, those of us who are voicing the empowering message of healing through nutrition and lifestyle change still struggle to be heard over messages that normalize chronic illness. People have started to accept acid reflux, chronic pain, autoimmune disease, and insulin resistance, for example, as part of life or "getting old."

We're surrounded by messages that promote addictive foodlike substances devoid of nutrition and promise easy solutions through pharmaceuticals that only address the symptoms—and often cause new symptoms that require more drugs to treat.

In my book *Unconventional Medicine,* I propose a new approach that involves collaboration between doctors and allied providers like nurse practitioners, nutritionists, and health coaches to provide a higher level of care with the potential to prevent and even reverse disease rather than just manage it.

Even with this collaborative, patient-centered approach, changing your diet and lifestyle is difficult. Most of us know a lot of the things we could do, but we still struggle with actually doing them.

To successfully prevent and reverse chronic illness, it's essential to have the support of not only medical experts but also health coaches—experts in behavior change—along with evidence-based, practical diet and lifestyle information and tools, as you'll find in this book.

Made Whole Made Simple takes a functional approach to nutrition that is applicable to anyone looking to live a healthy life. Instead of laying out another diet plan or set of rules for you to follow, Cristina explains the foundations of health and how to support the systems in your body using real, whole foods. She applies an ancestral template in a nondogmatic, bioindividual way so that you can customize your diet to fit your body's specific needs.

This book provides an excellent template, a springboard from which patterns in your eating, sleeping, and movement can take shape to support your body for better digestion, better blood sugar regulation, lowered inflammation, and more energy.

Going beyond the plate, this book provides valuable guidance for important lifestyle factors that are vital for healing, like stress management, movement, and the power of positive thought. *Made Whole Made Simple* is like having a health coach and a personal chef in your kitchen. Cristina strikes a beautiful balance between the science of food as medicine and how to apply it in the kitchen with easy recipes that are truly satisfying.

Chris Kresser, MS, LAc

Founder of KresserInstitute.com and author of *The Paleo Cure*

Park City, Utah

January 2020

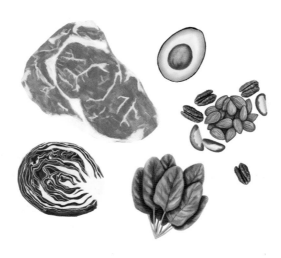

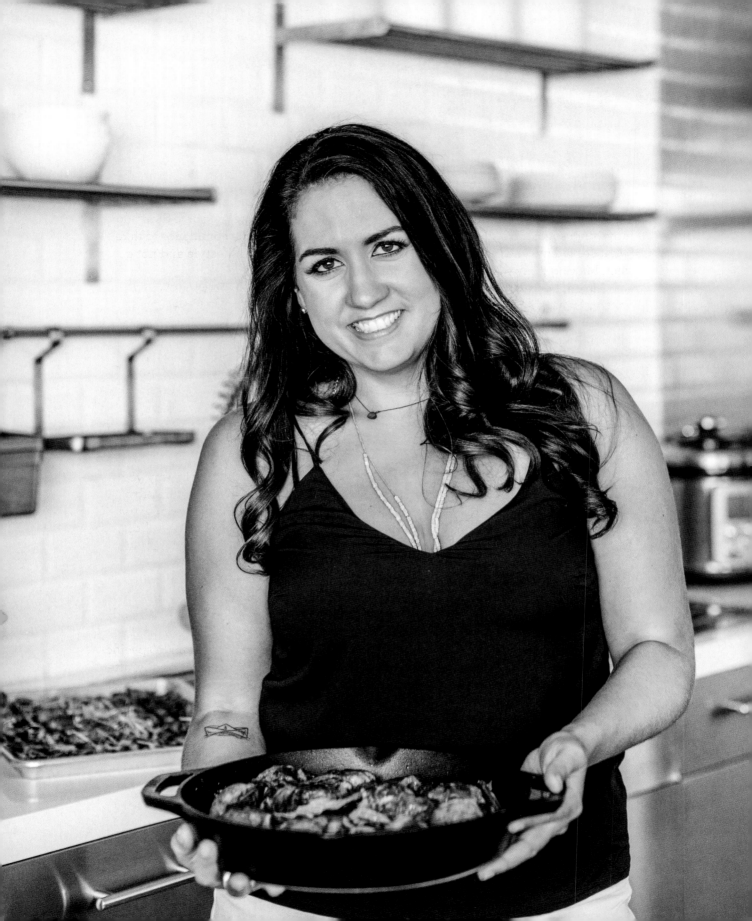

Introduction

I've been on every diet imaginable. Go ahead, think of a diet. Yup, I did it. Weight Watchers, South Beach Diet, low fat, juice cleanse, veganism, Whole30, Paleo, keto, Specific Carbohydrate Diet, the autoimmune protocol—I've done them all. Some I did to heal; some I did to lose weight. Some changed my life forever; some didn't do anything; some made things worse. Ultimately, it was having the confidence to take what served me and leave what didn't that made the way I eat a lifestyle and not a diet. Making it my own is what made it work.

Listen, I get it: there is a ton of conflicting information out there about how to eat, and it can be confusing. There is a lot of dogma. There are a lot of rules. And the online health and wellness space has been overrun by diet culture that often is disguised as wellness. While I totally support well-placed and healthy weight-loss goals, I can't support disordered eating, food fear, or eating frankenfoods as long as they fit your macros, because none of that supports long-lasting wellness—and wellness should be the goal, not weight loss. As someone who has battled both chronic illness and obesity, I can tell you that being in pain is worse than being overweight, and despite what society has been telling you all your life, your weight is not the reason for your symptoms or conditions; it's more likely a result of them. True health starts from the inside out!

Now, I'm not saying that you don't need to change anything about the way you eat. What you eat has a profound effect on how you feel, and you can't get healthy eating the same way that got you sick in the first place. But once you know how the food you eat interacts with your body and how your body works (yes, grade-school biology, here we come), you get a really cool view of nutrition—one that isn't about a set of rules but about how that information applies to *you*.

Knowing how it works is the first step in knowing how it works for you. I'm going to teach you the steps in digestion and what can go wrong, why hydration and blood sugar regulation are so important, and why a balanced intake of omega-6 and omega-3 fatty acids plays a huge role in a healthy inflammatory response. With that solid foundation of knowledge, you can layer on habits for success and tackle specific health issues, like hormone balance or autoimmunity—I'll show you how. Finally, after all that, I'll give you a ton of mouthwatering recipes that nourish your entire body for optimal system function. This is your baseline.

You can add ingredients to the recipes or omit ingredients from the recipes—and your life—as you see fit, but the recipes were designed to accompany the nutritional information in this book. They're chock-full of ingredients from the Farmacy (my collective name for real, whole, nutrient-rich foods; the term comes from *farm + pharmacy*—see what I did there?). This way, you stop looking at food as calories or grams of fat or carbs and start looking at it like, "Dayum, look at that delicious bowl of selenium-, zinc-, and B vitamin–rich goodness!"

Not only does each informational section feature lovely graphics showing which foods in the Farmacy contain which therapeutic nutrients, but the entire book is full of little nuggets of nutrient density trivia. I've always been a fan of nutrient density because nourishing foods are so much more satisfying. When your body gets what it needs, you can say goodbye to cravings!

The way you eat will change over time. Our needs change with the seasons of life (and the actual seasons too!). Knowing what's going on under the hood will allow you to navigate these changes with peace of mind and clarity. My goal with this book is to empower you to build a solid foundation of health with your food choices. I want you to be the leading expert in you! It's not about rules—no one likes living by other people's rules and being told what to do, not even (or, I should say, especially) my little boy. If you wouldn't live by someone else's rules, why would you eat that way?

It's your body and your life—you're in charge! Curating a healthy lifestyle that will stand the test of time is the goal, and I'm giving you the tools to do it in a way that works for you.

Burn the Wagon

Framing a healthy lifestyle as "on the wagon"—as the "other," the thing that's not "normal"—makes it oh-so-easy to feel like it's a prison sentence or like you're always one cookie away from falling off this wagon of healthy eating.

If you eat the cookie, you didn't fall off anything. You ate a cookie; life went on. Reframe your perspective on what it's like to lead a healthy lifestyle. Diets don't work, so why live on (and off) one forever? Every "off-the-wagon" bite etches guilt into your brain. That's no way to live.

What if you find that eating Paleo, keto, or a mix of both makes you feel great? Cool, then do that, but with enough know-how and wiggle room that you can live your life without feeling like you're failing or going off-plan if you eat [insert a food that you avoid out of guilt].

So let's reframe the way we think about foods. No more "yes foods" or "no foods." Instead, I like to think of foods as "feel good," "worth it," and "hard no."

Feel-good foods: These are the foods that I eat all the time—my usual suspects. I love these foods, and they love me right back. They make up the majority of my diet.

Worth-it foods: These foods don't make me feel my best, but I like how they taste or they have cultural significance for me (like gluten-free birthday cake or *buñuelos* at Christmas). I can eat them in small amounts without causing an autoimmune flare-up, inflammation, a skin reaction, or digestive distress. These are foods that I enjoy on occasion because the side effects are mild enough to make it worth it, but they're not mild enough that I want to live with them on a regular basis.

Hard-no foods: This list is short for me: gluten, nightshades, most dairy, and some grains. These foods cause very, very unwanted symptoms in my body, so I never eat them on purpose. Your list might be longer right now, but hopefully as you heal it will get shorter!

I live on my feel-good foods, and when the occasion arises, I enjoy my worth-it foods. I avoid my hard-no foods like a ninja dodging punches.

This is a lot less complicated for folks without food intolerances or allergies, but if I've learned one thing from working as a nutritional therapy practitioner and from the online health and wellness space, it's that most people have at least one symptom that they think is normal but isn't, and it's caused by a food or foods they're eating. After all, everything we eat is either feeding disease or fighting it.

Right now, I have a lit match and a crappy ol' guilt-infested wagon. Let's light it up. We do that by having a little chat with ourselves. It goes like this:

I deserve to feel good.

I choose foods that make me feel good.

Food is not good or bad; it's just food.

Some food makes me feel good, and some doesn't.

I am an adult, and I can make conscious choices regarding food and consequences.

I am in control of my life and my health.

Eating a certain way because it makes you feel your best, but making it sustainable by being flexible and knowing your personal dietary and emotional boundaries—that's food freedom.

Eating a certain way because it makes you feel your best, but white-knuckling your way through social situations and travel, overrestricting, and then bingeing on processed foods and running four miles or fasting to get "back on track"—that's diet culture (aka the wagon).

Needing the occasional reset or support to lead a healthy lifestyle—that's just human.

When you truly understand how your food choices affect your body, you can be clear on what are your feel-good foods, worth-it foods, and hard-no foods. And with that information in hand, you can make conscious choices that lead to a lifetime of health and vitality. It will become second nature, an intuitive process.

I look forward to the day when chemical-laden frankenfoods are no longer considered normal and organic produce and humanely raised animal proteins aren't considered specialty items. We need to normalize real food, which seems absurd, but it's our reality. Eating the way that humans did for thousands of years is somehow now the aberration, while eating a highly processed, highly inflammatory diet that humans adopted only a hundred years ago is standard. That's just not right.

The game is rigged, my friends. We have been sold the idea that we need to control ourselves around foods that are calorie rich and nutrient deficient, so they leave us hungry for more—not to mention full of chemicals that mess with our hormones. You don't get cravings because you lack willpower; you get cravings because your body is trying to tell you that it needs nutrients.

Ditch the wagon. Ditch the diets. Eat real food. Tap into your intuition, your hunger signals, and your body's amazing ability to heal so that you can enjoy a long and happy life (keyword: *enjoy*).

Got that? Cool. So let's go talk about how to find out which foods love you and which don't, and how to tell the difference. That way, you can make decisions based on your needs, not someone else's rules.

Before that, though, let me tell you a little bit about myself.

My Food-as-Medicine Journey

I'm Cristina Maria Curp, first-generation American, Miami born and raised, made with Cuban parts. My mom is a foodie, chef, and restaurant owner. My dad is a butcher—actually, it's the family trade—and back in Cuba they were farmers. Love of food is in my blood. I'm also a left-handed Gemini, I'm fluent in Spanish, and I wear size 11 shoes. I like to dance while I cook, and I never skimp on flavor.

As I write this, I live with my husband, son, and Schnauzer in Alexandria, Virginia. When I wrote my first book, *Made Whole,* we were living in Hawaii! Justin, my husband, is active-duty U.S. Navy, and because of that we move every few years. There are pros and cons to all that moving, but a major pro was that it prompted me to start my blog, *The Castaway Kitchen.*

I created *The Castaway Kitchen* five years ago, when we had just arrived in Hawaii. I was two years postpartum, twenty-nine years old, and so sick that I wasn't sure I would make it to forty. I have always, and I mean since year one, been overweight. I also struggled with ADHD, and at the age of thirteen I began getting painful boils on my skin, which turned out to be an autoinflammatory skin condition known as hidradenitis suppurativa. I was sick all the time as a child with sinus infections, bronchitis, and strep throat. I suffered from pain in my legs and chronic constipation. I struggled with binge eating and depression. Then, as a teen and young adult, I developed horrible self-esteem due to my weight and skin condition. I abused drugs and alcohol to cope. Have you heard the term *hot mess*? Well, it applied.

At twenty-nine, my weight had hit an all-time high, and I was dealing with inflammation, pain, fatigue, brain fog, and of course hidradenitis suppurativa. It was the pits. Something needed to change. So I did.

I began to pay attention to what I ate and how it affected my symptoms. I did a ton of research, and then I changed the way I cooked. I'd been working as an executive chef in a restaurant when I met my husband, and I used my culinary prowess to navigate the world of ancestral health, autoimmunity, and self-love. I began to share my adventures and recipes online, and folks began to pay attention. That's how *The Castaway Kitchen* was born.

I want to drive home the point that the change in me was vast and took several years, and in many ways, it still continues. The information that we have now about gut health and autoimmunity wasn't around when I was younger, so it took me a long time to connect the dots between what I ate and the way I felt. But now I no longer live with any of the problems that plagued me for so long: no ADHD, no digestive distress, no fatigue, pain, depression, or inflammation. I don't have addiction issues or binge-eating habits, and I feel better now than I did as a teen or in my twenties. I never knew that I was living my life at half capacity. Now that I'm finally operating at 100 percent, a whole new world has opened up to me, and my passion for food as medicine prompted me to enroll in the Nutritional Therapy Association program. Through the NTA I was certified as a nutritional therapy practitioner. It's a nine-month program that teaches a functional and ancestral approach to health (which complemented my BA in anthropology well). I chose this program because many registered dietitians and wellness experts I admire have done this program too or contribute to the curriculum. Sharing my story and my journey helped a lot of people, but what I learned in my training gave me the tools to help people write their own journeys to healing, not just mimic my own.

When I dove into the world of healing through food, I went all-out: six rounds of Whole30, six months of the autoimmune protocol (elimination phase and later the reintroductions), a few months of layering on the Specific Carbohydrate Diet, and later finding my way to keto, but with a Paleo approach and without my autoimmune trigger foods. I am you. I am the person who has tried it all in the pursuit of health. I am the person who read all of the health and wellness books and bought a million different meal plans and programs. I was the person who got really into food rules and even became a little annoying about it, a self-proclaimed enforcer of said rules.

I think everyone goes through that phase when they find a new way of eating. It's a coping mechanism—we need to hold on tight to the rules and draw a line in the sand because we don't trust ourselves. I get it, and if you're in that place right now, there is no judgment here, just understanding. But I do want you to know that it won't last forever, because forever is a really long time!

I healed my body, and I've maintained this thriving, healthy state *without* being restrictive or locked into food rules. I learned that to make this a true lifestyle, I needed to make it my own. It was uncharted territory, and I have felt moments of doubt, but I always go back to *bioindividuality*. No one else lives in my body; no one knows it like me. Same goes for you.

We need to stop asking, "Is that keto?" or "Is that compliant?" and start asking, "How does this make me feel?" Get away from diet dogma and diet identity and explore your unique needs.

While the changes in me go way beyond food, my food choices were the catalyst to an overhaul of my whole life. You're probably thinking, *Well, Cristina, I'm not THAT messed up!* You're probably not—I had a lot of healing to do. My point is, if I can do it, anyone can do it, with some education, empowerment, dedication, and self-care. True change doesn't happen overnight or in a week, but consistency always brings about lasting, sustainable, healing changes.

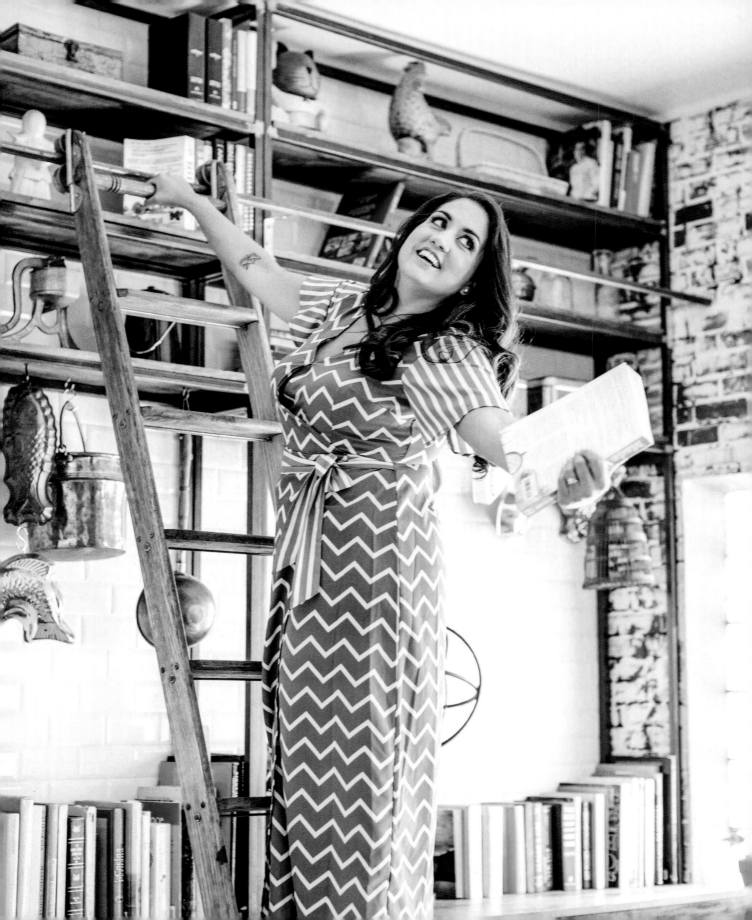

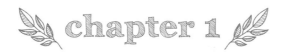

chapter 1

The House Won't Fall If the Bones Are Good

Pretty sure those are lyrics to a country song, but it's true: if you have strong foundational health, you get to experience something awesome: *resiliency*.

Too often, we go about playing whack-a-mole with symptoms, jumping from one diet to the next, focusing on the what instead of the why. I like to find the root cause of issues and tackle those, letting the symptoms subside on their own. That way, when life happens, like a crazy week of work, a stomach bug, or unexpected travel, you can bounce back instead of being out of commission for days.

Eating whole, unprocessed food most (if not all) of the time, managing stress, and prioritizing sleep are nonnegotiable when it comes to leading a healthy lifestyle. But broad recommendations like those can feel too vague, so let's break down some of the foundations of health so that you can figure out your own unique path to lasting wellness.

The foundations of health (the bones in my house metaphor) are digestion, hydration and mineral balance, blood sugar regulation, and fatty acid balance. Optimizing these factors through diet and lifestyle changes can dramatically improve your overall health. It really works!

I'm going to show you the why and the how of these foundations and tell you which foods and habits support them optimally. Then you can apply them to your life as you see fit.

Digestion

Proper digestion is imperative because what you eat fuels your body and makes up the cells, tissues, and organs that you're made of. If there's a problem with your digestion, you're not getting all of the nutrients in your food, and it can damage your gut lining.

Digestion begins before you even touch your food, when you feel hungry and start thinking about food, or see and smell it. That's when your salivary glands begin to secrete saliva. Ever drool just thinking of something yummy? You're not alone! The amylase in saliva starts the breakdown of carbohydrates, and chewing begins the mechanical breakdown of food (so chew slowly). Then, after you swallow, the muscles of the stomach churn the food and mix it with digestive enzymes and gastric juices (like pepsin and hydrochloric acid) secreted by the stomach and pancreas. It's important to have sufficient enzymes so food particles are broken down into smaller molecules, which is how your gut likes it.

This broken-down food makes a pit stop in the duodenum, the first part of the small intestine, where it returns to an alkaline state and fats are broken down by bile, which is secreted by the liver and gallbladder. Now the food is ready to travel through the small intestine, which is where nutrients are absorbed into the body.

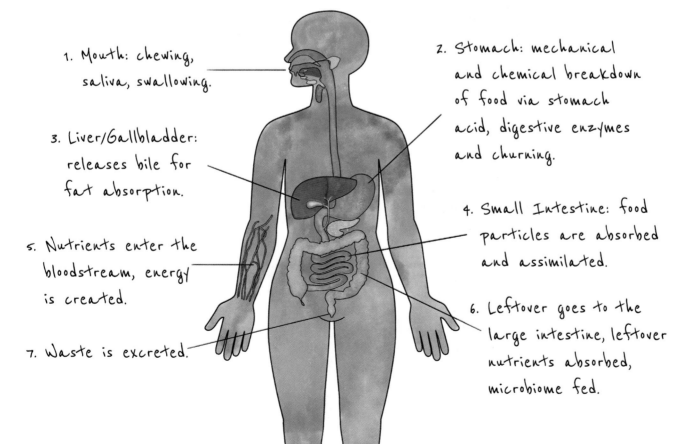

1. Mouth: chewing, saliva, swallowing.

2. Stomach: mechanical and chemical breakdown of food via stomach acid, digestive enzymes and churning.

3. Liver/Gallbladder: releases bile for fat absorption.

4. Small Intestine: food particles are absorbed and assimilated.

5. Nutrients enter the bloodstream, energy is created.

6. Leftover goes to the large intestine, leftover nutrients absorbed, microbiome fed.

7. Waste is excreted.

Microvilli, little hairlike protrusions, cover the inside of your small intestine and absorb small molecules, which then pass into interstitial fluid and then the bloodstream or lymph (the fluid of the lymphatic system, which is like a drainage system that removes toxins and waste products). *This is how nutrients circulate to all the cells in your body.*

It's also how we get energy: macronutrients enter the bloodstream from the small intestine and ultimately travel to cells, where mitochondria use them to create energy. The leftovers, like indigestible fiber, bile, and other waste, go to the large intestine, where water and other waste materials are recycled and the gut microbiota—the beneficial bacteria that thrive in your gut and have a symbiotic relationship with your body—take a second pass at extracting nutrients. Then waste is formed and expelled (fancy talk for poop).

This is a wonderful cascade of reactions, each one triggered by the step before it. Unfortunately, making sure this process can happen optimally is not a priority in health care. But doesn't it make sense that a lot of issues we face today occur because we throw a wrench in it? Have lots of burping, belching, or reflux after meals? Feel bloated and uncomfortable? Super reactive to so many foods? That's not optimal, and the most common source of this kind of disruption is stress. To understand why, let's start with what it means to be under stress.

The body has two baseline states: sympathetic, also called "fight or flight," and parasympathetic, also called "rest and digest." It's kind of obvious which one is better for digestion! Your body can't tell the difference between a nasty email from your boss and a tiger trying to eat you; both trigger a stress reaction, and since that reaction was initially developed to deal with the tiger, its goal is to make you capable of running or fighting—survival is the priority over digestion. So when you get that nasty email from your boss, your body enters a sympathetic, fight-or-flight state and decreases blood flow to the digestive system, which pumps the brakes on hydrochloric acid production and other important functions.

When there isn't enough hydrochloric acid to break down all the food in the stomach into small molecules, the cascade of chemical reactions that is digestion is interrupted. Bile production isn't stimulated, and when fats are not emulsified by bile, it wreaks havoc on the digestive system. Incompletely digested foods damage the epithelial cells and microvilli along the intestinal wall, which can cause the lining of the intestines to become leaky and allow large food particles and pathogens into the bloodstream and lymph. These particles and pathogens trigger an immune response and cause inflammation. At the same time, maldigested foods degenerate in your large intestine, causing an imbalance in your gut microbiome, which can lead to more inflammation and bloating. Leaky gut, as this condition is known, is associated with a ton of health problems, including, as the authors of one study noted, "autoimmune diseases such as inflammatory bowel disease, celiac disease, autoimmune hepatitis, type 1 diabetes (T1D), multiple sclerosis, and systemic lupus erythematosus."[1]

Healing the Damage from a Low-Fat Diet

Decades of low-fat diets have left many of us with stagnant bile. That's right, the bile secreted by the gallbladder and liver can become thick and less effective when you don't eat enough fat. This can cause gallbladder attacks, sharp pains in the upper right part of the abdomen.

Supporting your liver is a great way to support bile production. Foods like celery, radishes, bitter greens, fresh ginger, and beets support bile production.

In other words, you can eat all the feel-good foods in the world, but if you're not digesting them properly, they can still cause you harm. Gut health begins farther north.

Stress isn't the only thing that can disrupt digestion, of course. Eating too fast is a common mistake. Stop to enjoy your food, and aim to chew each bite for at least twenty seconds. Drinking too many liquids with your meals can dilute your gastric juices, so avoid chugging water with or around your meals. Certain medications, specifically proton pump inhibitors, stop stomach acid production and can lead to malnutrition. Eating too many processed foods, which are difficult to digest, can cause discomfort. All of these contribute to kinks in the digestive system that result in undigested foods and pathogens making it to your small intestine. But sitting down to a meal in a calm state instead of eating at your desk, during your commute, or while standing in the kitchen can make a big difference.

How to Optimize Digestion

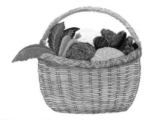

· Eat mostly whole, unprocessed foods.

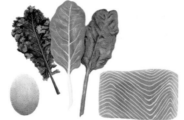

· Eat high-quality foods that have nutrients our bodies recognize and can absorb and assimilate. If it comes from the earth or roams on it, you're good.

· Try slow cooking, braising, pressure cooking, fermenting, and sprouting—all preparations that make foods easier to digest.

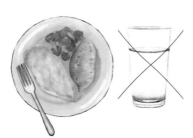

· Don't drink a lot of liquid with your meals—it waters down the gastric juices, so they're less effective in breaking down food.

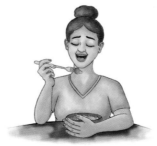

· Chew slowly to break down your food mechanically before it reaches your stomach.

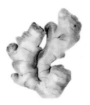

· Take digestive bitters and/or eat ginger or fennel seeds. By stimulating the bitter receptors on your tongue, they get the gastric juices flowing.

Hydration and Mineral Balance

While drinking lots of water with meals is not recommended, drinking plenty of water overall is a must! We need plenty of fluids for adequate blood volume and to help nutrients get where they need to go. Water's other critical functions include lubricating joints and organs, regulating body temperature, and even facilitating weight management.

Common signs of dehydration are dizziness, headaches, nausea, and light-headedness. Being dehydrated negatively affects not only physical performance, as you probably already know, but also cognitive performance.[2] If you're dehydrated, just by becoming properly hydrated you will experience many cognitive improvements, such as better mood and concentration, faster reaction time, and improved short-term memory.

I recommend aiming for 80 ounces of water a day, or more if you are working out. If you carry a 32-ounce reusable water bottle around with you and fill it up a few times a day, you're set. Water needs vary by person, but make sure you're getting enough to feel good.

It's also crucial to make sure you're not just drinking water, but absorbing it! The body absorbs water by osmosis in the small intestine, and that absorption depends on solutes, primarily sodium. This is where minerals come into play. The minerals calcium, chloride, magnesium, phosphorus, potassium, and sodium are all

Dehydration

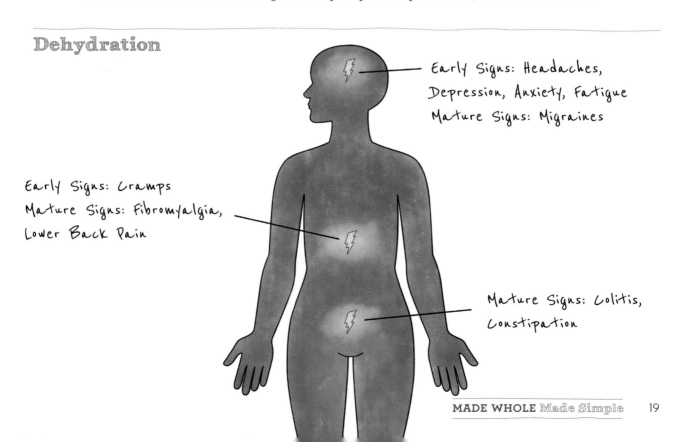

Early Signs: Headaches, Depression, Anxiety, Fatigue
Mature Signs: Migraines

Early Signs: Cramps
Mature Signs: Fibromyalgia, Lower Back Pain

Mature Signs: Colitis, Constipation

electrolytes. Electrolytes conduct electricity when dissolved in water, which is why they are essential for many processes in the body. They're important cofactors in almost every enzyme function, and we lose them when we sweat. Muscle weakness or cramps can be a sign of electrolyte depletion and/or dehydration.

We must consume minerals because our bodies do not make them. Minerals come from the earth, and when plants and animals (including us) burn, what remains is ash, which contains minerals! It's all very circle of life: what comes from the earth ultimately returns to it. Unfortunately, industrial farming has depleted the soil of minerals and other nutrients, so it's harder than ever to get enough in your diet.

Minerals are necessary cofactors for hormone function, and they're important for several functions in the body: contracting and relaxing muscles, transporting nutrients, maintaining a healthy pH balance, and more. The big ones are calcium, phosphorus, magnesium, sulfur, sodium, and chloride. Other important minerals include zinc, iron, boron, iodine, manganese, and selenium.

Zinc doesn't get enough attention. It's a constituent of over two hundred enzymes and is needed for cell replication, tissue repair, and growth. Low energy, impaired immune system, skin rashes, and abnormal hair loss are all symptoms of zinc deficiency. Zinc and copper need to remain in balance, and you don't want zinc toxicity or copper toxicity.[3] Getting your zinc from whole foods like oysters and red meat is best.

Food Sources of Electrolytes

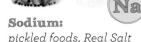 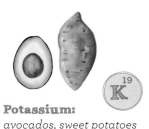 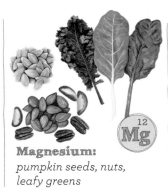 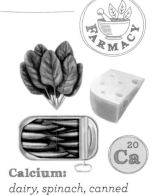

Sodium:
pickled foods, Real Salt

Potassium:
avocados, sweet potatoes

Magnesium:
pumpkin seeds, nuts, leafy greens

Calcium:
dairy, spinach, canned sardines

Fatty Acid Balance

Polyunsaturated fatty acids (PUFAs) are essential, which means that we need them but our bodies can't make them, so we must consume them. Vegetable oils, seed oils, and hydrogenated cooking oils are high in polyunsaturated fatty acids, but they are made in a complex process involving extreme heat and strong chemicals, which makes them highly unstable and prone to oxidation when heated. Here's why that's bad: Oxidation causes the formation of free radicals, highly reactive molecules that cause cell damage—essentially, free radicals make the oil carcinogenic. Our system counters free radicals with antioxidants, which is good, but also with inflammation, which can be problematic, especially when it's chronic.[4] Low-grade, chronic inflammation is associated with obesity, chronic pain, depression, vascular disease, and dementia. No surprise, studies have shown that processed cooking oils are like poison to our bodies.[5] Safe sources of PUFAs are small oily fish (sardines, mackerel), wild-caught salmon, grass-fed beef, chia seeds, and hemp hearts (yum!).

The two forms of PUFAs are omega-3 and omega-6. While both are essential, keeping them in balance is key for a healthy inflammatory response.

Our bodies use omega-3 and omega-6 fatty acids from our food to make prostaglandins, a type of hormone. Pro-inflammatory prostaglandins are made from omega-6 , while anti-inflammatory prostaglandins are made from omega-3. This is why it's important to have an optimal fatty acid balance; the ratio of omega-6 to omega-3 in your diet should be 1:1, but even 4:1 is great. These two essential fatty acids cannot be created in the body and must be consumed, so consuming them in proper ratios is key to avoiding too much or too little inflammation.

The problem is that many foods we consume in high amounts, like hydrogenated vegetable oils, nuts, and seeds, are much higher in omega-6 than omega-3, and it's omega-3 that helps keep inflammation in check. To keep the right balance of omega-6 and omega-3, you must be very intentional about your omega-3 fatty acid intake.

NSAIDs

Nonsteroidal anti-inflammatory drugs (NSAIDs) are commonly used (read: overused) to suppress chronic inflammatory symptoms. The problem is that they block the production of *all* prostaglandins, suppressing not only the body's inflammatory response but also its *anti*-inflammatory response.

When you get hurt, the damaged tissue releases prostaglandins, which cause swelling and communicate pain to the central nervous system. So when NSAIDs block the production of prostaglandins, you get less pain and less swelling—but they're not treating the injury. In fact, because they block important communication pathways in your body, they're masking symptoms without fixing the root cause of the pain.

James DiNicolantonio, a cardiovascular researcher and author of *The Salt Fix*, suggested that eating more omega-3 can inhibit inflammation just as NSAIDs do and can prevent chronic low-grade inflammation, which is a factor in many chronic diseases, including rheumatoid arthritis, atherosclerosis, diabetes, and heart disease.[6] How powerful is the magical fatty acid balance of omega-6 and omega-3, you ask? It's "I have an autoinflammatory disease and I haven't taken ibuprofen to reduce inflammation in five years" powerful.

Don't be afraid of omega-6, though. Not all inflammation is bad, and omega-6 is essential for a healthy, healing inflammatory response, like when you sprain your ankle and it swells. That's your body limiting mobility in order to protect the damaged tissue from further injury.

Chronic inflammation, however, is something else. This can be caused by leaky gut or by an overconsumption of inflammatory foods and rancid oils high in omega-6.

Most Americans today consume a lot of unhealthy oils like canola oil, soybean oil, rapeseed oil, and grape seed oil, which are unstable and prone to oxidation. By omitting these inflammatory processed oils from your diet and instead using saturated fats (such as ghee, grass-fed butter, or coconut oil) or monounsaturated fats (such as high-quality extra-virgin olive oil or avocado oil), as well as consuming whole foods rich in omega-3, you can keep your inflammatory response optimal!

Extra-Virgin Olive Oil

Despite what you may have heard, extra-virgin olive oil is great for cooking.

Olive oil is a monounsaturated fat, and like polyunsaturated fats, monounsaturated fats can become oxidized when they're exposed to high heat (although they don't oxidize as easily as polyunsaturated fats). So for a time, it was thought that olive oil was better for cold dishes than for cooking. However, that hypothesis has been debunked! Apparently the extremely high antioxidant content of olive oil counteracts any oxidation that may occur during the cooking process. It's even beneficial to cook meats rich in omega-3, like salmon and grass-fed beef, in olive oil to protect their delicate PUFAs from oxidation! It's just another great example of how, if we stick with traditional cooking methods, we can't go wrong. In many parts of Europe and the Middle East, people have been cooking with olive oil for centuries!

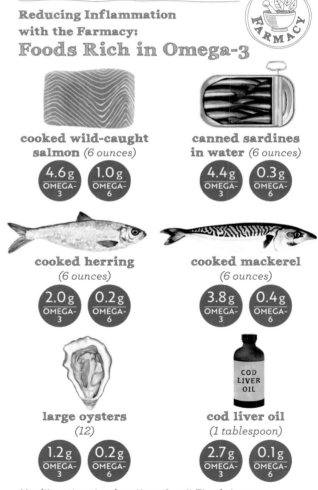

Reducing Inflammation with the Farmacy:
Foods Rich in Omega-3

cooked wild-caught salmon (6 ounces)
4.6 g OMEGA-3   1.0 g OMEGA-6

canned sardines in water (6 ounces)
4.4 g OMEGA-3   0.3 g OMEGA-6

cooked herring (6 ounces)
2.0 g OMEGA-3   0.2 g OMEGA-6

cooked mackerel (6 ounces)
3.8 g OMEGA-3   0.4 g OMEGA-6

large oysters (12)
1.2 g OMEGA-3   0.2 g OMEGA-6

cod liver oil (1 tablespoon)
2.7 g OMEGA-3   0.1 g OMEGA-6

You'll notice they're all seafood! That's because seafood is the best source of bioavailable omega-3 with the lowest omega-6.

Blood Sugar Regulation

Blood sugar regulation is important for everyone, not only those with metabolic disorders—it's inextricably linked to hormone health and stress management. Unfortunately, if you are on the standard American diet, you are more likely to have unstable blood sugar and even may be at risk for metabolic syndrome and type 2 diabetes. Let's first tackle how our bodies regulate blood sugar, and then we can dive into how dysfunction happens and what we can do and eat to remedy it!

When we refer to "blood sugar," what we really mean is the amount of glucose in the bloodstream, which by and large comes from carbohydrates in the diet. Glucose is a quick-burning fuel, and one that our bodies very tightly regulate. Even if you never ate any carbohydrates, you'd still have about 4 grams of glucose circulating in your bloodstream—your body would make it from dietary protein or even break down muscle to make it. Your body is really good at keeping you alive (thanks, body!).

Your blood sugar level fluctuates based on a lot of factors: what you're eating, how long it's been since you've eaten, whether you're in the middle of a workout, or whether you're super stressed. Ideally you would have pretty steady blood sugar that rises only after meals and promptly returns to an optimal range. There is a lot of debate on what the optimal range is, but I think 60 to 90 mg/dL is great. So blood sugar fluctuations are normal, but how drastic they are matters a lot. You want rolling hills, not peaks and valleys—high blood sugar and low blood sugar both sound the alarm in your body.

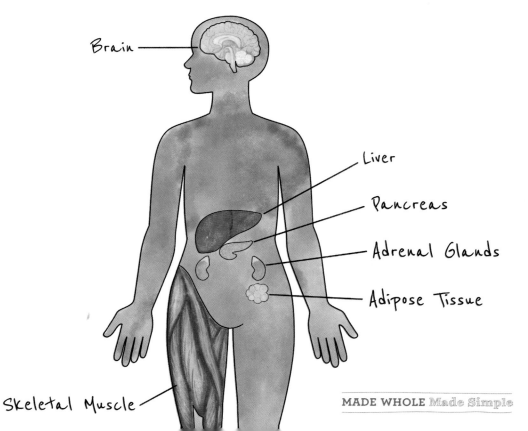

Brain

Liver

Pancreas

Adrenal Glands

Adipose Tissue

Skeletal Muscle

A lot of organs, tissues, and systems are involved in making sure blood sugar doesn't get too high or too low. The central nervous system is the mastermind, controlling the organs and tissues that in turn control blood sugar levels. The players are the pancreas, the adrenal glands, adipose tissue, the liver, and skeletal muscle.

- **The pancreas** secretes the hormones insulin and glucagon. Insulin stores energy in cells—which lowers blood sugar—while glucagon extracts energy from cells, raising blood sugar. Think of glucagon as a key that releases energy for cells and insulin as a lock that stores energy away in your cells.

- **The adrenal glands** release the hormones adrenaline, noradrenaline, and cortisol, which tell the pancreas to secrete glucagon or insulin.

- **Adipose tissue** houses energy in the form of triglycerides, which can be released (by glucagon) and used for fuel when blood sugar (and stored glucose) is low. In addition, adipose tissue is responsible for the secretion of several hormones, including leptin, which makes you feel hungry, and ghrelin, which makes you feel full.

- **The liver,** the great transformer, turns glucose from the bloodstream into glycogen, the storable form of glucose. It also transforms fatty acids into ketones, an alternative fuel that the body uses in the absence of glucose, and turns protein into glucose when needed.

- **Skeletal muscle**—that's right, the muscles on your body, your lean body mass— plays a part in blood sugar regulation by housing excess glucose (as glycogen) and providing protein that the liver can turn into glucose as needed.

Ideally, when you eat, it causes a mild immediate rise in blood sugar, which causes an increase in insulin. Your body uses the glucose it needs for energy, and what's left over is stored in the liver and muscles. When storage in the liver and muscles is used up, glucose is stored in adipose tissue as triglycerides, a kind of fat. The next time your body needs energy—like when you want to crush it at the gym or you need to run for your life—and there's not enough in your bloodstream, it will access what's in storage.

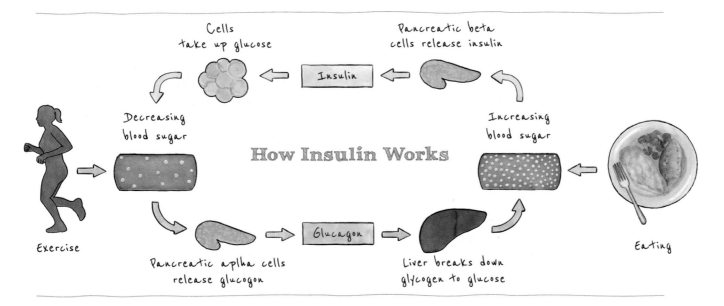

Cells take up glucose

Pancreatic beta cells release insulin

Insulin

Decreasing blood sugar

Increasing blood sugar

How Insulin Works

Exercise

Eating

Pancreatic aplha cells release glucogon

Glucagon

Liver breaks down glycogen to glucose

Glucose is a fast-burning fuel, and when it's available in your bloodstream or stored in your liver or muscles, it's your body's first choice for energy. When glucose isn't available, your body will metabolize fat for fuel: first fat from foods, and then the triglycerides stored in adipose tissue. Fat burns slower than glucose, and some body processes require glucose, so if the body needs glucose and there isn't any left in the liver or muscles, the liver can convert protein (from food or from skeletal muscle) into glucose.

When our bodies are working optimally, they're like hybrid cars: they can switch easily and smoothly between different types of fuel. This is called *metabolic flexibility*, and it lets you tap into your body's fat-burning abilities and stay sensitive to insulin. Unfortunately, most Americans today overconsume refined carbohydrates, eat rancid fats that cause inflammation, and lead increasingly sedentary lives, so there are no energy demands for all that fuel. This is a lethal combination.

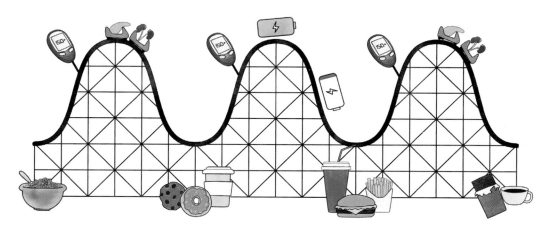

Refined carbohydrates are notorious for spiking blood glucose. Insulin rises in response to high blood sugar, and the spike in insulin means a lot of glucose is quickly moved out of the bloodstream, so within a few hours after eating refined carbs, we go from high blood sugar to low blood sugar, and the cycle starts again. When we ride that blood sugar roller coaster over and over again, our cells become resistant to insulin's message to accept glucose, so glucose stays in the bloodstream longer and blood glucose levels stay higher than they should. This is insulin resistance. The pancreas pumps out more and more insulin, frantically trying to lower blood sugar without success, and it eventually becomes exhausted. This is type 2 diabetes.

Even before the pancreas is exhausted, chronically high insulin and blood sugar can cause many health problems, like inflammation, polycystic ovary syndrome, and an impaired immune system. Studies show that chronically high insulin, leptin, and glucose cause inflammation on a cellular level, the kind of inflammation that causes illness.[7] And of course, inflammation is worse when we eat refined, rancid oils.

Waking up in the middle of the night regularly, or getting light-headed between meals, or getting angry or upset ("hangry") if you don't eat frequently could be symptoms of blood sugar dysregulation. If you have a lot of visceral fat (fat around your internal organs), this can lead to insulin resistance. While having a larger waist is often correlated with more visceral fat, thin people can have unhealthy amounts of visceral fat too. The most accurate way to find out how much visceral fat you have is with a CT scan or DEXA scan. Discuss this with your doctor if you feel you are more likely to develop insulin resistance.

So what's the best way to eat to have stable blood sugar? There's really no one-size-fits-all answer; how someone responds to a food, and particularly carbohydrates, is very contingent on their metabolic health, stress level, activity level, and overall eating patterns. While keeping blood glucose within a healthy range—just rolling hills, no peaks or valleys—is the goal, how you eat to get there is unique to you!

Experiment with the amount of carbohydrates on your plate and aim for whole-food sources of carbohydrates, like nuts, seeds, fruits, and vegetables, instead of refined carbs, like chips, bread, and pasta. All of the mouthwatering recipes in this book are designed not to spike your blood sugar. They are made with healthy fats and plenty of protein. The carbohydrates come in fiber-rich vegetable forms, ideal for those in healing or who thrive with a low-carb way of life. These recipes promote metabolic flexibility and energy balance.

Stress is another factor in blood sugar regulation. Both the central nervous system and the adrenal glands are involved in stress responses as well as blood sugar regulation, so it's easy to see that acute or chronic stress can disrupt blood sugar regulation. When your body is in fight-or-flight mode, it signals an energy dump into the bloodstream (so you have the energy you need to run from a tiger). This will usually cause a spike in blood sugar, even if you're on a low-carbohydrate diet. So while the foods you eat play an essential role in blood sugar regulation (and every other aspect of your health), so does stress.

Getting enough sleep and eating a nutrient-dense diet help your body cope with stress better, which in turn helps keep blood sugar stable. (Of course, there are also a lot of lifestyle factors involved in stress management, and I'll talk more about those later.)

You should feel a noticeable difference in your energy levels when you've optimized blood sugar regulation. With stable blood sugar, proper digestion, adequate hydration, and plenty of sleep and exercise, you will learn what it's like to operate at 100 percent capacity!

Checking Your Blood Sugar

If you feel unsure about how foods impact your blood sugar levels, get a blood glucose meter and check your levels for a few days. I also recommend reading *Wired to Eat* by Robb Wolf, in which he outlines a glucose tolerance test for very bioindividual data.

Fix Your Blood Sugar in 15 Minutes

Here's a super actionable quick tip for regulating blood sugar that you can implement today: go for a walk! Taking a brisk ten- to fifteen-minute walk after meals lowers blood glucose, especially after carbohydrate-heavy meals. Food is fuel, friends!

Nutrients That Support Healthy Blood Sugar Regulation

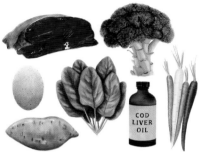

Vitamin A: *Supports the adrenal glands. Found in cod liver oil, eggs, beef liver, broccoli, sweet potatoes, carrots, and spinach.*

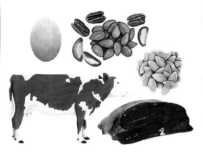

Thiamin (vitamin B1): *Needed to create an enzyme that metabolizes carbs. Abundant in beef, liver, eggs, nuts, and seeds.*

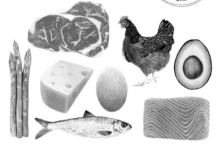

Riboflavin (vitamin B2): *Needed for the pancreas to secrete insulin; boosts metabolism and the immune system. Found in fish, meat, poultry, eggs, dairy, asparagus, and avocados.*

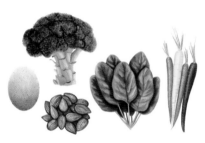

Biotin (vitamin B7): *Helps the body use glucose effectively, reducing hypoglycemia and sugar cravings. Mostly made in the gut by the microbiome but also found in spinach, carrots, broccoli, eggs, and almonds.*

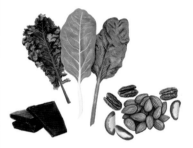

Manganese: *Needed for proper enzyme functions. Found in dark leafy greens, dark chocolate, and nuts.*

Ceylon cinnamon: *Contains a compound that improves insulin sensitivity.*

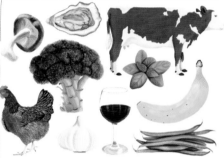

Chromium: *Needed to create glucose tolerance factor; low levels can result in insulin resistance. Found in oysters, broccoli, green beans, beef, poultry, mushrooms, bananas, basil, garlic, and red wine. (Note: You need adequate vitamin C and niacin to absorb chromium.)*

Berberine

Berberine is a derivative of an ancient Chinese herb, *Coptis chinesis*, which has been used to treat diabetes and gastrointestinal infections in China for many years. It's become popular because of its modulating effect on blood sugar—it's even said to be as effective as the prescription diabetes drug metformin. If you feel that you need blood sugar regulation support beyond stress management and dietary changes (please try those first), berberine could be a good supplement for you. But talk to your health-care provider before taking anything, especially if you're already undergoing treatment.

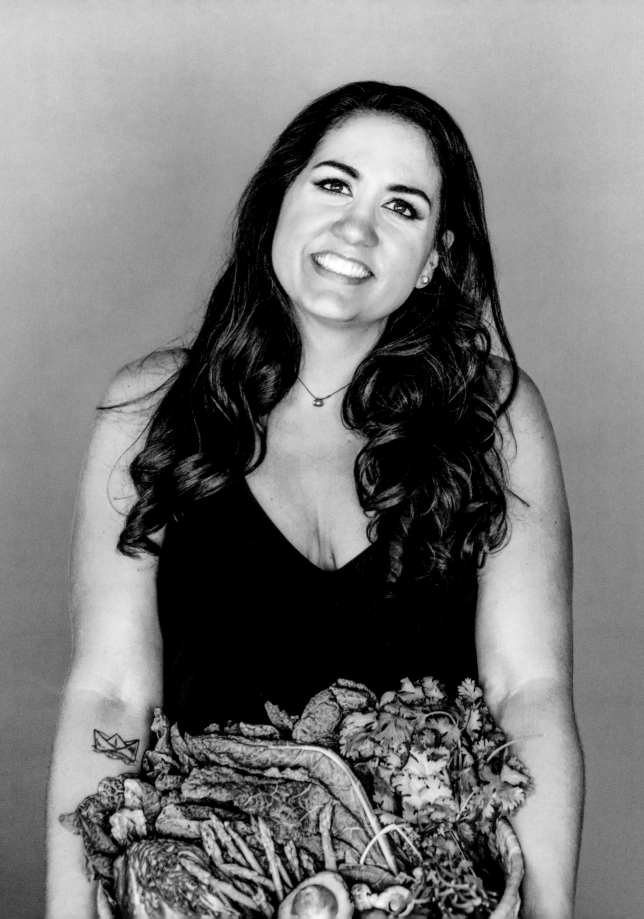

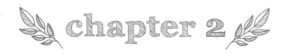

chapter 2

Where We Get Our Fuel

Cellular respiration is a bunch of really cool chemical reactions that convert the food we eat into energy. It's our mitochondria—the famous "powerhouses of the cells"—making magic happen. We literally create energy, and that's pretty cool.

There are three systems that create ATP, units of cellular energy:

- The creatine phosphate system creates ATP very quickly from phosphocreatine stored in striated muscle. This system is used for intense bursts of energy and does not require oxygen. This is what powers the save-your-life effort to climb up off a ledge or sprint for your life.

- The anaerobic glycolysis system uses glucose to create ATP. This system also creates energy rapidly, though not as fast as the creatine phosphate system. It's enough to power high-intensity interval training or heavy lifting beyond a few minutes. This burns through glycogen stores, and if you're an athlete or really active, you use this one a lot!

- The aerobic system generates sustained ATP through a process called the citric acid cycle. It uses carbs, fat, and protein to produce slow and steady fuel for the everyday functions of your body and normal activities. It's our endurance fuel. The citric acid cycle is the only pathway that burns fat for fuel.

While all three systems are always going and which is dominant depends on our energy needs, the aerobic system creates most of the energy we need. The aerobic system uses oxygen and your food to create ATP and creates carbon dioxide as waste, which you eliminate via breathing!

But remember, you don't need to do or eat anything special to create energy. Your body is an energy-creating machine! Humans are extremely adaptive omnivores, and we can produce energy from any of the macronutrients—carbs, fat, and protein.

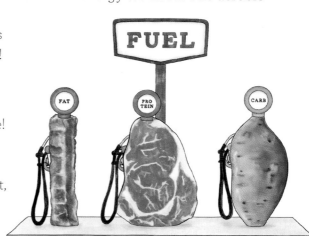

Carbs

In the digestive system, carbohydrates are broken down into simple sugars, which cross through the intestinal wall into the bloodstream and body tissues. After a pretty complex chemistry scenario within our cells, each molecule of glucose creates thirty-six molecules of ATP (energy).

It's a pretty straight shot from ingestion to energy, which is why carbs are useful for explosive movement and an active lifestyle. This is especially true for simple carbohydrates (monosaccharides)—they have a simpler molecular structure than complex carbohydrates (polysaccharides), so they break down faster, making them a very fast fuel that spikes blood sugar. Nuts, seeds, and some fruits (like berries) are considered complex carbohydrates, while simple carbohydrates include refined sweeteners (think table sugar, brown sugar, and high-fructose corn syrup), fruit juice concentrate, and refined grains. The added benefit of complex carbohydrates, in addition to their lesser effect on blood sugar, is that they contain micronutrients.

Considering Carbs

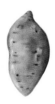

Sweet potatoes: *1 cup cooked has about 42 grams of carbohydrates, about 7 grams of which is fiber. They're a good source of vitamin C and also have manganese, potassium, vitamin A, niacin, magnesium, and phosphorus.*

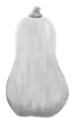

Butternut squash: *1 cup cooked has 21.5 grams of carbs, about 6 grams of which is fiber. They're a good source of vitamins A and C, and they also include vitamin E, calcium, potassium, and magnesium.*

Congee: *1 cup of this slow-cooked, bone broth–packed rice porridge has about 28 grams of carbohydrates and not much fiber—but it is a good source of resistant starch, which feeds good bacteria in the gut. The slow-cooking method breaks down the grains, making this traditional medicinal food easy to digest. If you're missing grains in your diet, I think this is a good option.*

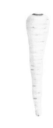

Parsnips: *1 cup cooked has about 17 grams of carbohydrates, 3.5 grams of which are fiber. Parsnips are a good source of vitamin C, folate, and manganese, and also have choline, potassium, and magnesium.*

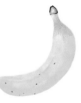

Bananas: *1 medium banana has 27 grams of carbs, and just over 3 grams of that is fiber. This tropical fruit is a decent source of potassium, vitamin C, and manganese.*

Apples: *1 apple with the skin has about 25 grams of carbohydrates, and 4.4 grams of that is fiber. Apple is a decent source of vitamin C and also has some potassium.*

Fat

Repeat after me: *Fat is my friend.* Fat became the enemy in the mid-twentieth century because large corporations had a lot to gain by selling margarine and other shelf-stable frankenfoods full of processed vegetable oils and refined sugar and lacking in natural fats. Fortunately, fat has since been reinstated as the wonderful, nutrient-dense, slow-burning fuel that it is.

Fat is essential for nutrient absorption and the production of hormones. Our bodies are good at storing fat: at any moment, even a lean person has over twenty thousand calories' worth of fat stored in their adipose tissue. Your stored body fat is what will keep you alive in times of famine.

Fats take longer to digest than carbohydrates. They're broken down into fatty acids and monoglycerides, which pass into the cells lining the small intestine and then are converted into triglycerides. The triglycerides bind to proteins, forming lipoproteins, and head to the bloodstream and lymphatic system. There the lipoproteins release fatty acids, which enter cells so the mitochondria can do their thing and use them to generate energy. Bibbidi-bobbidi-boo (lots of biochemistry), and we have 129 molecules of ATP from one fatty acid molecule. Fat takes longer to digest and to assimilate. It's a high-satiety food that creates lasting energy.

Don't Fear Cholesterol

In 2015, the *Dietary Guidelines for Americans* deemed cholesterol to be "no longer a nutrient of concern for overconsumption." This was a big step in undoing the decades-long smear campaign against this vital nutrient. However, a lot of misinformation lingers. In particular, dietary cholesterol is often still associated with heart disease.

It's true that cholesterol's presence in your arteries can be a sign of disease, but it's not the cause. Inflammation from sugar and processed oils is the culprit, and cholesterol is what the body uses to repair weak arterial walls. LDL cholesterol—which actually consists of a lipoprotein carrying a cholesterol molecule—transports the cholesterol "medics" to the scene, and HDL cholesterol—again, a lipoprotein carrying a cholesterol molecule—takes them back to the liver, where they are broken down or released as waste.

So instead of worrying about cholesterol, we need to take a closer look at what's truly causing inflammation in our bodies. Some common factors: processed vegetable oils, high insulin levels, and leaky gut.

Cholesterol is necessary for many functions, including the production of sex hormones, vitamin D, and bile. It's brain food, literally! In fact, it's so vital that our liver produces most of the cholesterol the body needs. So don't fear cholesterol!

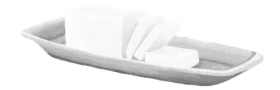

Protein

If I had to choose, I'd say protein is my favorite macronutrient. Not only does protein pack really important micronutrients, but foods that are primarily protein usually come packaged with healthy fats too—think of a delicious grass-fed steak!

During digestion, protein is broken down into peptides and amino acids, which go through the walls of the small intestine and into the bloodstream. From there, the peptides and amino acids travel to the liver and to cells all over the body, where they build and repair tissues and are used to create hormones.

But while those are protein's primary tasks, protein can also be used to create glucose when the need arises. The process of forming glucose from protein is called gluconeogenesis, which means "new sugar creation": *gluco* (sugar) + *neo* (new) + *genesis* (creation). However, this is a purely on-demand process; it happens only when glucose is needed and there's none available.

Gluconeogenesis requires the hormone glucagon, which is the liberator of energy. While insulin moves energy into your cells, glucagon does the opposite—it extracts energy from cells. Glucagon helps us survive. Let's say we've burned through all of our stored glycogen—in that case, this little hormone is going to stimulate gluconeogenesis. Even if you never ate an ounce of carbohydrates again, glucagon would ensure that your body created the glucose you needed to survive, either from the protein you consumed or, if need be, from your muscles.

Sourcing Protein

If you want to be a responsible omnivore, the conversation on sourcing protein needs to happen—not only for the quality of life of the animals you are eating but also for the health of the planet. Regenerative agriculture, which restores our rich topsoil, depends on grazing animals and is imperative for the future of the earth. I know grass-fed, grass-finished beef; pastured chicken; and humanely raised pork can be expensive, but do the best you can.

If you do buy conventionally raised meat, stick to leaner cuts. Like us, animals store toxins in their fat tissue, so fattier cuts will carry more of the toxins that conventionally raised animals are exposed to (like pesticides, hormones, and more). We're not just what we eat; we're what our food eats too!

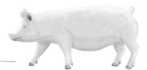

Staying Flexible

Metabolic flexibility is the body's capacity to adapt to use whatever fuel is available. This means that the body can switch seamlessly between burning primarily fat and burning primarily sugar. This adaptation keeps us sensitive to insulin and very resilient when it comes to energy demands and food choices. This ability is one reason humans have thrived all over the world. We are opportunistic eaters, and we can digest and live on whatever's available in our environment!

Depleting glycogen stores and dipping into a fat-burning state seems to be a natural cycle for humans. Yes, it's cyclical. While staying in a fat-burning state all the time works for many people, historically, humans have cycled in and out of fat-burning. It's how we survived on whatever was available, whether that was fresh fish or fresh fruit.

But today, most folks have lost their metabolic flexibility. That doesn't mean it's impossible to switch between burning sugar and burning fat—the ability is still there, deep down—but for most of us, it is difficult and takes time, when it should be quick and easy. The overconsumption of processed foods and sedentary lifestyles have locked us into a sugar-burning state. So what's the secret to tapping into the primal metabolic state in a modern world?

What Your Fuel Could Look Like

Energy requirements vary greatly from person to person, and your primary fuel source will vary depending on the types of activities you prefer, your metabolic health, your body type, and your own preferences. I can't give you a definitive answer here because this book isn't about one-size-fits-all recommendations. What I can do is give you examples from my life that show you don't need to be locked into a fat-burning state or a glucose-burning state. You can enjoy your feel-good foods and all fuel sources to your advantage—you can be metabolically flexible!

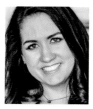 **Cristina** has a history of insulin resistance and chronic inflammation. Feels best on a high-fat, high-protein diet with moderate carbohydrates. Likes heavy lifting, long walks, and the occasional HIIT class. Eats mostly low-carb, high-fat, but adds in starchy carbohydrates around HIIT workouts. Is mostly in a fat-burning state, but uses glucose to her advantage around workouts or on certain days of her cycle.

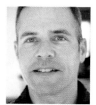 **Justin** has always been active and fit. No chronic illness. Avid cyclist, active-duty military. Eats whatever his wife makes him (meat and vegetables), but adds carbs like white rice, fruit, and the occasional ice cream cone. Intuitively fasts sometimes, usually on the weekends. Uses added carbohydrates around bike rides. Is mostly in a glucose-burning state, but dips into fat-burning after long bike rides or during fasts.

Becoming Fat Adapted

There are many roads to metabolic flexibility, but essentially, the trick is to get your body used to burning fat. While becoming "fat adapted" is an idea embraced by the ketogenic community, you don't necessarily have to follow a very-low-carb, high-fat ketogenic diet to be able to burn fat for fuel. Remember from page 29 that the three systems that create ATP use different fuels for different kinds of activities: for example, if you're doing HIIT workouts, you'll be using more glucose, and that glucose is drawn from both the food you eat and your glycogen stores. If you match your fuel to your activity level, you can set yourself up to burn through your glycogen stores, and that's when your body defaults to fat burning. Do that enough times, or stay in the glycogen-depleted state long enough, and your body will start to prefer fat as fuel. This is being fat adapted, and it means that even in the presence of a glucose spill, the body will still prefer fat oxidation. You will be able to stay in a fat-burning state even when you consume more carbohydrates; exactly how much will vary depending on the person.

You can deplete glycogen stores by eating less than 50 grams of carbs per day for several weeks, paired with light activity. You can also deplete glycogen stores by eating about 150 grams of carbs a day while taking part in high-intensity exercise, like CrossFit or endurance cycling. You can also deplete glycogen stores by fasting for sixteen hours a few times a week, paired with moderate physical activity.

Eating a low-carb diet may not be right for everyone, but neither is the overconsumption of carbohydrates, especially refined and processed sugars and grains, which have been proven to cause metabolic disorders, inflammation, and other conditions. If you feel best using glucose as your primary fuel, focus on whole-food carbohydrates, and stay active so you dip into a fat-burning state occasionally and keep up your ability to be metabolically flexible. People like to put labels on things to explain their way of eating, but it all boils down to how you can fuel your body best for the way you need it to perform. Stable blood sugar, plenty of energy, and good sleep—that's the goal no matter what you eat!

The ability to efficiently switch between fat-burning and sugar-burning appears only in a balanced body—you need to get your foundational ducks in a row first. There's no sense in messing with your macronutrient ratios if you have not addressed proper digestion, hydration, mineral balance, fatty acid balance, and blood sugar regulation—all of which were covered in the previous chapter. The cool thing is that working on that last one, blood sugar regulation, will naturally get you to a place where you're metabolically flexible, especially when you throw physical activity into the mix.

Keeping a Flexible Mentality

While you embark on this quest to become metabolically flexible, I would like to remind you that it's not about restriction or being on a diet; it's about finding what works for you. The most important thing is to stick to whole foods and tap into your body's natural hunger signals: eat when you're hungry, stop when you're not. With proper digestion, stable blood sugar, and healthy hormones, those signals from leptin and ghrelin should be loud and clear.

Living this way is about freedom, flexibility, and bioindividuality. I like to think about how our ancestors ate. If Jane and Joe were out hunting large game forty thousand years ago and stumbled upon a tree of ripe pears, do you think that they would say, "Pass, that doesn't fit into my macros"? I don't think so.

Try to picture life before agriculture, before food was readily available. Going after big game was an endurance sport played with handmade tools—not quite as chill as stopping by Whole Foods to pick up a steak. You need to wake up and find food, and it's at least a few hours before you kill and cook a rabbit (and boy, did you have to sprint for it!), but maybe you found a few berries along the way to tide you over. Then your tribe decides to do a little migrating. You walk for several hours before you find a river and decide to hang out there for the rest of the night. Fishing is a bust, so you dig up some root vegetables and have those before it gets dark. The next morning you have better luck with fishing and eat your fill before you keep walking. This is all hypothetical, of course, but you get the point. Eating times varied and the type and quantity of food varied, but our ancestors didn't just survive, they thrived.

Flexibility is what lets you stay with a way of eating for the long term. When you focus on real food and the foundations of good health, and when you find your feel-good foods and worth-it foods and learn to dodge your hard-no foods, your body will be healthy and resilient, and you will enjoy metabolic flexibility. I know you might not feel that way right now, but you will get there. Once you ditch the standard American diet and the idea that hyperpalatable processed foods are meant to be moderated (diet culture), and once you're no longer addicted to sugar, there is a freedom in truly enjoying foods that make you feel great.

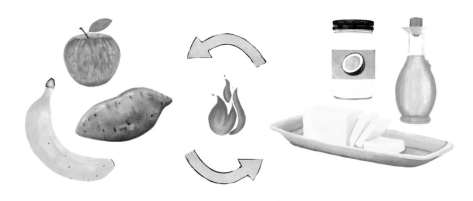

Consider the Ancestral Template

As we think about what foods are best to nourish our bodies, let's talk a little more about what humans were eating over forty thousand years ago—before farming, before we got hip to domesticating animals or knew how to season food—and why it matters.

Why Should We Eat Like Our Ancestors?

We have good evidence that an ancestral way of eating is simply better for our bodies than the standard American diet, starting with the work of Weston A. Price. Price was a dentist who studied several cultures all over the world in the early 1930s. In his book *Nutrition and Physical Degeneration*, he explains that everywhere he went, the people who consumed traditional diets from their area, as opposed to westernized diets, had better dental health and cranial formation. He also noted that the healthiest communities were those that consumed animal fats.

On top of that, studies show that before agriculture, people were generally free of many of the chronic illnesses that plague us today, particularly cardiovascular disease and metabolic disorders.[8] I wonder when animal protein and fats got all the blame for chronic illness? Oh yeah, it was about the time the processed food industry boomed. Bad science and politics led to a decades-long smear campaign on foods that were historically the cornerstone of our diets.

How People Ate 40,000 Years Ago

There's a lot of speculation about what Jane and Joe were noshing on in the Paleolithic days, but one thing seems certain: there was no single way of eating back then. There was no corner store or Instacart, and people had to eat what they could hunt and find, what was within walking distance and in season (and I'm not talking about just walking down to the farmers market).

While folks ate different things all over the world more than forty thousand years ago, the one thing they all had in common was the absence of refined carbohydrates and processed oils. Yup, no Twinkies back then. It's also pretty clear that animal protein was a significant part of the diet in every region, and there is an evolutionary explanation for that: essentially, because fat has more calories per gram than carbohydrates or protein, the high amount of fat in meat gave us more energy, which allowed us to develop such large brains. We still expend a lot of energy on brain metabolism, which is why we thrive on energy-rich (calorie-dense) diets.[9]

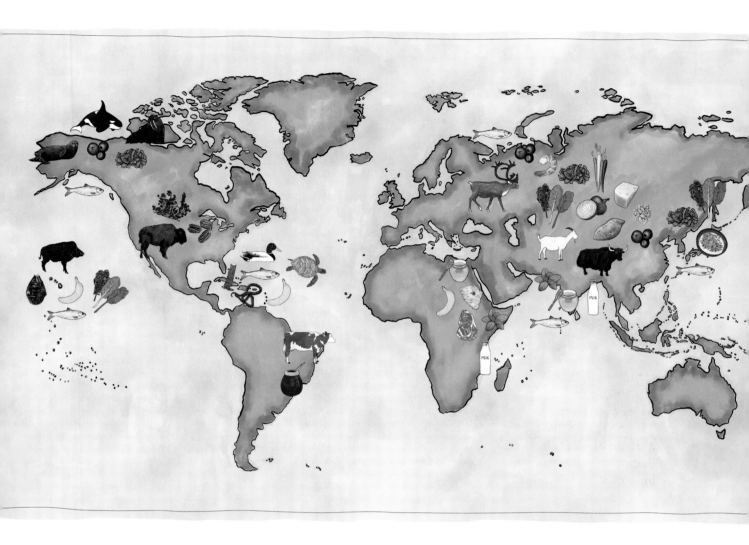

"These ethnographic and anthropological studies tell us that there was no single, uniform diet which typified the nutritional patterns of all pre-agricultural humans. Humans were masters of flexibility, with the ability to live in a rain forest or near the polar ice caps."

—Janette Brand-Miller, Neil Mann, and Loren Cordain,
"Paleolithic Nutrition: What Did Our Ancestors Eat?"

In *Meat in the Human Diet: An Anthropological Perspective*, Neil Mann states:

> The gut is the only organ which can vary in size sufficiently to offset the metabolic cost of the larger brain. Diets high in bulky food of low digestibility require relatively enlarged gut size with voluminous fermenting chambers (rumen and caecum). Diets consisting of high-quality foods are associated with relatively small gut size, with simple stomachs, reduced colon size, but proportionately long small intestine, as seen in carnivores. With the relatively poor macronutrient density of wild plant foods, particularly in the open grassland areas, the obvious solution for our ancestors was to include increasingly large amounts of animal-derived food in the diet. The increasing consumption of meat, rich in protein and fats (particularly unsaturated forms), would provide a basis for the threefold increase in human brain size in the last 4.5 million years, from the perspective of both energy supply and brain fatty acid substrate availability.[10]

While Mann definitely makes a case for a protein-centered diet, he acknowledges that plants have always been part of our diet. In fact, he makes the case that humans are "truly omnivores" because of our digestive system. We have highly acidic "simple stomachs" (compared to cows' multichambered stomachs, for example) and thin small intestines, like carnivorous animals. However, we also have large intestines, which makes us a hybrid of carnivore and frugivore (fruit-eating animal). While meat offers highly digestible and bioavailable nutrients, plant matter offers diversity, fiber, polyphenols, and vitamin C! They're a match made in heaven for us omnivores.

So what did an ancestral diet look like, broadly speaking? Here's what early humans ate for hundreds of thousands of years before the dawn of agriculture:

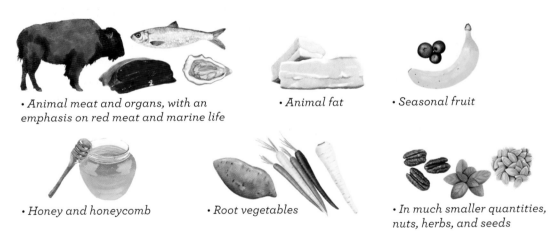

• *Animal meat and organs, with an emphasis on red meat and marine life*

• *Animal fat*

• *Seasonal fruit*

• *Honey and honeycomb*

• *Root vegetables*

• *In much smaller quantities, nuts, herbs, and seeds*

Anti-inflammatory and antioxidant compounds such as turmeric, tea, dark leafy greens, and sulfur-rich cruciferous vegetables probably weren't a big part of their diet, but we know that these foods support healthy detox.[11] Considering that our ancestors didn't deal with much of a toxic load, they probably didn't need these as much as we do today! I think including these foods in our modern-day approach to ancestral health is important, just as it's important to make modifications for blood sugar dysregulation and metabolic disorders, such as a low-carb approach. The ancestral template is just that, a template, one that we can learn from and adjust to fit our modern-day lives.

Applying the Ancestral Template Today

To be clear, I'm not suggesting that you go out and hunt and forage for food, unless you want to. Before the rise of agriculture, there was a transitional era when humans began to settle down more and migrate less, during which they practiced swidden cultivation, which is the practice of clearing a wooded area by fire to grow food for a few years before leaving it to regenerate. They began to combine foods and season them to make meals that sort of resemble how we cook today.

Today, we need to find a similar kind of happy medium, though in an entirely different world. True, agriculture gave rise to the population concentration and food availability that sprouted civilization as we now know it. But one pitfall of all of today's modern wonders is that we're completely disconnected with where our food comes from. We need to tap into our innate wisdom and common sense about what's good for us and makes us feel good—that's the true guidance we need. Fortunately, we evolved to these big brains of ours, and we can cook food that is good for us and make it taste damn good too.

You don't need to follow the list of foods our ancestors ate. The most important lessons from our ancestors are to keep it simple, to eat seasonally, to eat plenty of fish, and to move our bodies a lot! But knowing the foods our bodies evolved to handle is helpful. I like to think of the ancestral template as simply plants and animals. If you stick to those most of the time, you're good. It's when we get into Flamin' Hot Cheetos territory or "burgers" with twenty-five laboratory-made ingredients that we run into trouble. We're strange animals, architects of our own destruction.

Sometimes we focus too much on food rules, macronutrients, or what someone else is eating. There is an entire multibillion-dollar industry that thrives on perpetuating rules, confusion, and dogma around food. So please keep in mind that everything I have covered until now is just information intended to help you understand how your body works and the role food plays in it.

The power is yours. What you do with this information is your choice. My suggestion: focus on foundational health. Don't think about what not to eat, but do add foods from the farmacy to your plate. Focus on nutrient density. Keep your eyes on your own plate, and keep it super simple. We burned the wagon; don't build a new one.

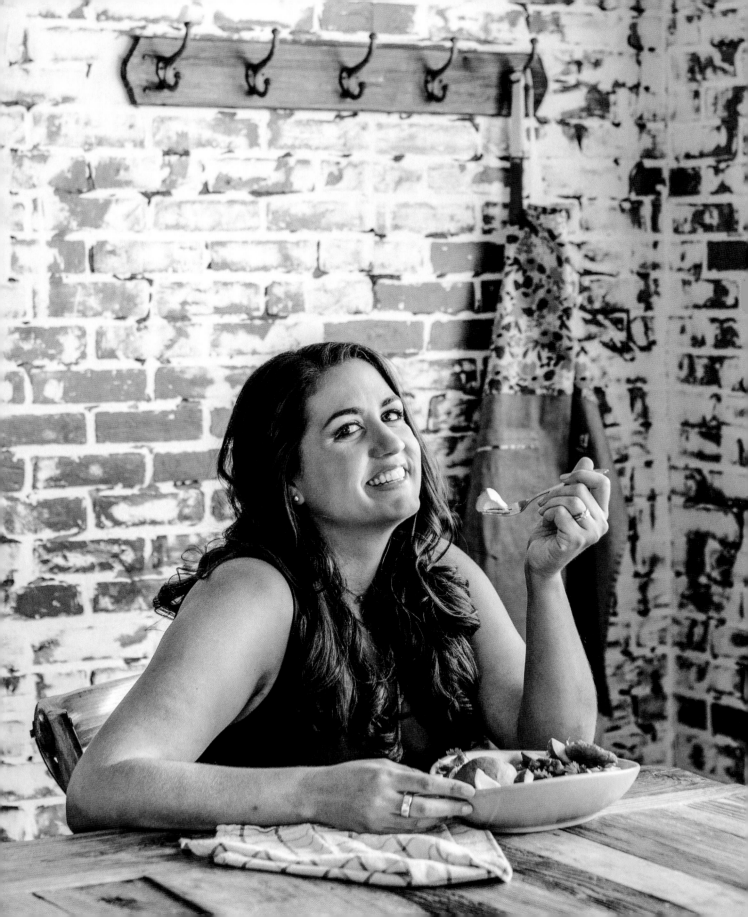

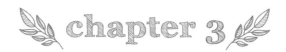

chapter 3

Eating for Healing

I did things a little backward in my healing journey. I went through all the elimination protocols and extreme focus on health issues before learning about the real foundations of health. It was a lot more work and a lot more restriction than most folks need to go through. When you address the foundations first and learn from the ancestral template, many if not all of your health concerns may resolve in a few weeks or months.

But sometimes you need to go the extra mile. In this chapter, I shine a light on some common health concerns, like hormone health and autoimmunity, and briefly cover some dietary protocols that can be effective in bringing relief of symptoms or help you discover your hard-no foods.

Hormone Health

There are so many endocrine disruptors in the environment today, and our bodies are dealing with such a heavy toxic load, that balancing hormones can feel like an uphill battle. But nourishing the endocrine system is less difficult than it might seem: it's all about stabilizing blood sugar, eating nutrient-dense foods, and managing stress.

Hormones fall into five categories:

- Steroid hormones (like sex hormones) are derived from cholesterol.
- Thyroid hormones are derived from iodine and the amino acid tyrosine.
- Amine hormones are derived from modified amino acids.
- Peptide hormones and protein hormones are derived from chains of amino acids.
- Eicosanoid hormones (like prostaglandins) are derived from omega-3 and omega-6 fatty acids.

Hormones regulate metabolism, reproduction, growth and development, the immune system, muscle contractions, gland secretions, and other functions.

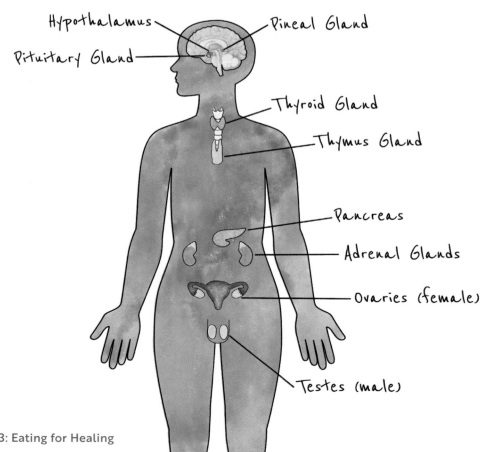

The pituitary gland is attached to the hypothalamus, which is a small part of your brain. The small but powerful pituitary gland secretes hormones that control the thyroid, reproductive organs, and adrenal glands. The pituitary and hypothalamus are like the control center for the endocrine system, affecting everything from growth hormone to thyroid-stimulating hormone and even prolactin (which helps breast milk production).

The thyroid, a little gland that lives by your throat, is the boss when it comes to cellular metabolism. It's the thermostat of the body! There are three main thyroid hormones: (1) thyroid-stimulating hormone, which is converted to (2) T4, which is converted to (3) the active thyroid hormone, T3, which acts as a modulator for cell functions in every organ in the body. Thyroid hormones also regulate oxygen use, stimulate protein synthesis, and increase glucose uptake during the creation of ATP. Low thyroid function can lead to high triglyceride levels, difficulty losing weight, hair loss, and fatigue. An overactive thyroid can cause anxiety, nausea, amenorrhea, and weight loss.

The thymus gland plays a major role in the immune system, but it still has a role to play in the endocrine system. It is responsible for secreting thymosin, a hormone that stimulates the development of immune T cells. T cells mature in the thymus before they join the immune system in the lymph nodes.

The adrenal glands are in charge of the flight-or-fight response. Located bilaterally just north of the belly button, these glands produce glucocorticoids, mineralocorticoids, and sex hormones—in fact, after menopause, when the ovaries no longer produce sex hormones, the adrenals take over. Glucocorticoids like cortisol regulate blood glucose and inflammation. Mineralocorticoids like aldosterone are in charge of the sodium-potassium balance, which regulates blood pressure. Sex hormones such as estrogen and testosterone are produced in the ovaries, testes, or adrenal cortex.

As we learned in the blood sugar regulation section, the central nervous system (which includes the hypothalamus and pituitary) and the adrenals signal the pancreas to release the hormones insulin or glucagon to respond to energy demands and blood sugar regulation. The HPA axis (hypothalamus, pituitary, and adrenals) is the central stress response system, and there's a beautiful dynamic between the nervous system and the endocrine system, which also affects blood sugar!

The endocrine system is a web, all interconnected, and you must support the whole as well as the parts! So how do you do that?

First, stable blood sugar is foundational for hormone balance. When you have blood sugar dysregulation—when you're on that blood sugar roller coaster—it puts stress on the adrenal glands, which in turn puts stress on the pituitary gland (and central nervous system), which impacts the thyroid and the production of sex hormones. For more on stabilizing blood sugar, see pages 23 to 27.

Second, as clichéd as it sounds, you have to manage stress (easier said than done, I know). Stress can come from overtraining, undereating, overworking, toxic relationships, or environmental toxins. Some stress, like what your body experiences during a workout, can be healthy, but there is a fine line between a healthy amount of stress, which strengthens the body, and chronic stress, which depletes the body. Remember that, in addition to

Reverse T3

Prolonged low-calorie diets increase reverse T3, the antithesis of T3. It pumps the brakes on your metabolism and stops fat burning. A nutrient-rich diet, along with stable blood sugar, movement, and plenty of sleep, is key for balancing thyroid hormones and achieving sustainable weight loss.

pushing it at the gym and crushing it at work, a nonstop lifestyle is also paired with a toxic load on your body, and your hormones can't tell the difference between real danger and perceived danger (tiger attack or nasty email).

Third, you need to be mindful of toxins in your diet as well as in household items and beauty products. I use cast-iron pans in my cooking, never nonstick, because of the chemicals in nonstick coating. I also recommend you reduce the use of plastic in your home and never store or reheat food in plastic containers. Information about nontoxic household cleaners and personal care products could fill an entire book on its own, but on my blog, I share my choices (visit https://thecastawaykitchen.com/2019/12/endocrine-disruptors/).

Of course, you have to focus on the foundations first; that's why they are called foundations. In addition to stable blood sugar, proper digestion is important for absorbing all the protein, fats, and minerals that hormones need to thrive. The proper fatty acid balance is important for reducing inflammation and supporting detox pathways. Almost any stage of inflammation is affected by hormone actions; insulin and glucocorticoids have direct effects of vascular reactivity and inflammatory responses.[12] Getting the right minerals and staying hydrated are essential for intercellular communications and enzyme production, which are important cofactors in hormone function. Chapter 1 covers how to build these necessary foundations.

Detox Support

Our bodies are really good at detoxification—we have kidneys, a liver, and several enzyme functions for the task. However, we are primal beings living in an industrial world, and we're surrounded by endocrine disruptors! Beyond focusing on whole foods and cleaning up your environment, there are a few easy and affordable holistic approaches to supporting detox. There's no need for harsh or expensive detox programs—your body is really good at cleaning house and is constantly working to keep you in fighting shape. These gentle methods will support your body in its work:

- **Warm Epsom salt baths.** Add high-quality essential oils like lavender, lemon, peppermint, and rosemary for a lovely spa-like experience. Magnesium sulfate plays several roles in the detoxification process, from helping glutathione production to reducing oxidative stress.

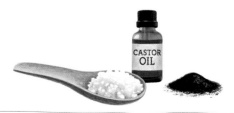

- **Castor oil liver pack.** Rub a small amount of castor oil on your skin on the right side of your abdomen, just below your ribs—right over your liver. Hold a warm piece of wool cloth over it for thirty minutes. This is an ancient and holistic method for stimulating the lymph and liver and reducing inflammation, used in Egypt, China, and India, and you can do it daily.

- **Dry brushing.** Use a coarse, natural bristle brush to gently brush your skin in a general upward motion and toward areas where your lymph nodes are (inner thighs, breasts, and underarms). This stimulates the lymphatic system, which carries waste and toxins from your glands and organs. Dry brushing also makes your skin soft!

- **Dandelion tea.** Made from the roots and greens of dandelions. Dandelion contains antioxidant phytochemicals and can act as a diuretic.

- **Binders.** Compounds such as activated charcoal, diatomaceous earth, and bentonite clay bind to pathogens in the gut so that they can be eliminated. These are best taken between meals and alone, as they can diminish the effects of any medication or supplement taken with them.

The Endocrine System and Minerals

Did you know that each organ and gland in the endocrine system has a mineral that it loves and needs most to function properly?

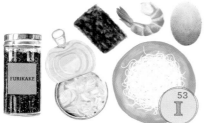

Iodine: *The thyroid converts iodine into thyroid hormones. Food sources include eggs, tuna, shrimp, kelp noodles, furikake, and nori.*

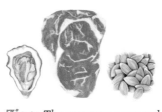

Zinc: *The prostate accumulates more zinc than any other organ or gland. It also helps produce testosterone and prolactin. Researchers have found that adequate levels of zinc suppress tumor growth in the prostate. Food sources include oysters, pumpkin seeds, and red meat.*

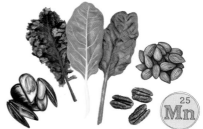

Manganese: *The pituitary gland oversees many hormone-secreting glands in the body and likes to store manganese for its antioxidant properties. Food sources include leafy greens, almonds, pecans, and mussels.*

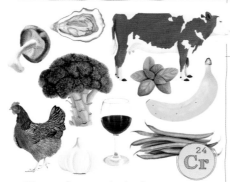

Chromium: *The body uses chromium to regulate carbohydrate metabolism; low levels can result in insulin resistance. Food sources include oysters, broccoli, green beans, beef, poultry, mushrooms, bananas, basil, garlic, and red wine. You need adequate vitamin C and niacin to absorb chromium.*

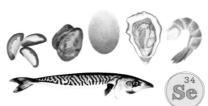

Selenium: *The ovaries and testicles actively take up and store selenium; it's essential for sperm development in men and ovarian follicle development in women. Food sources include Brazil nuts, oysters, chicken liver, mackerel, shrimp, and eggs.*

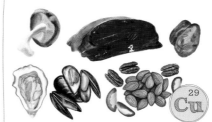

Copper: *Copper is critical for energy production and stimulates the production of epinephrine and norepinephrine in the adrenal glands. It's important to keep it in balance with zinc. Food sources include liver, oysters and other shellfish, nuts, and shiitake mushrooms.*

Why You Should Track Your Cycle

In women of reproductive age, menstrual cycles are like a vital sign. We can learn a lot about what is going on in our bodies when we track our cycles. Many hormone imbalances are born of a dietary imbalance or metabolic dysfunction. Use a tracking app, a moon mandala, or a basal body temperature chart to track your cycle. It's a wonderful step in connecting with your body. I love Dr. Jolene Brighten, author of *Beyond the Pill*, as a resource in female hormone wellness. My sister Laura Mar, podcast cohost and sexual health educator, has wonderful content for charting and body literacy on www.cyclescience.org.

Autoimmunity and Leaky Gut

When it comes to gut health and the immune system, it's all about removing the stressor and supporting the system. The digestive system works north to south, and it heals that way too. So if you're struggling with your gut despite removing potentially problematic foods from your diet, you need to start higher up the chain. Remember, digestion begins in the mind with the parasympathetic "rest-and-digest" state and continues to the mouth, then the stomach, and so on.

All day, every day, your immune system is distinguishing between you and the world around you. It's like the seagulls in *Finding Nemo*, but instead of saying, "Mine? Mine? Mine?" your immune system is asking every molecule it encounters, "Are you me? Are you me? Are you me?" When you have impaired digestion and large food particles and pathogens make it out of your intestine and into your bloodstream and lymph, it sets off the immune system's inflammatory response; the alarm bells ringing constantly: "THIS IS NOT ME!"

When that alarm goes off, the immune system responds with inflammation. If everything is working smoothly and you have the right balance of fatty acids in your diet, it eliminates the problem particles and clears up and repairs any damaged tissue. But when you have leaky gut and large particles and pathogens are escaping the gut regularly, then you have chronic inflammation and the stage is set for further health problems.

Many diseases are caused by or made worse by leaky gut, especially autoimmune diseases like Hashimoto's, lupus, rheumatoid arthritis, type 1 diabetes, and multiple sclerosis, and the foods we eat, in turn, can make leaky gut worse or better—foods have a huge impact on the maintenance or alteration of our microbiome and intestinal barrier function.[13] When autoimmunity is present, certain foods may cause the "this is not me" reaction, and the symptoms depend on your diagnosis. With rheumatoid arthritis, you get joint pain and swelling; with Hashimoto's, you can get fatigue, weight gain, or hair loss; and with Crohn's disease, you can get mouth sores, abdominal pain, or diarrhea.

When we heal the gastrointestinal tract from end to end, avoid inflammatory foods, and properly nourish our bodies and gut microbiomes, we can heal leaky gut, reverse symptoms of chronic illness, and even put diseases into remission. This is why it's imperative for those of us with autoimmunity to know, without a doubt, what our feel-good foods, worth-it foods, and hard-no foods are.

Supporting the immune system with proper nutrition is paramount, so our bodies' own antioxidants can do their job: cleaning house. We can further support them by consuming antioxidants in the form of foods rich in vitamin E, vitamin C, selenium, and plant polyphenols.

Nutrients That Support the Immune System

The following nutrients and corresponding foods are essential for a healthy immune response:

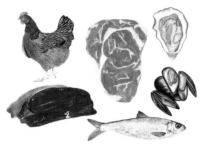

Amino acids: *grass-fed beef, free-range chicken, wild-caught fish, shellfish, offal*

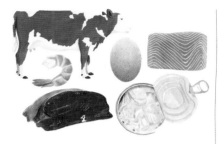

Vitamin A: *liver, eggs, grass-fed beef, shrimp, salmon, tuna*

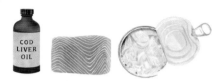

Vitamin D: *cod liver oil, salmon, bluefin tuna*

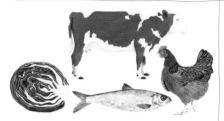

Glutamine: *beef, chicken, fish, cabbage*

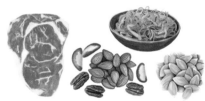

Arginine: *nuts and seeds, beef, seaweed*

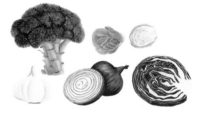

Glutathione: *milk thistle, garlic, onions, broccoli, Brussels sprouts, cabbage*

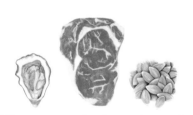

Zinc: *oysters, beef, pumpkin seeds*

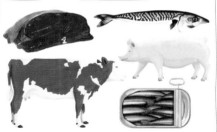

B vitamins: *organ meat, mackerel, sardines, pork, beef*

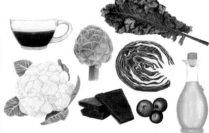

Antioxidants: *cauliflower, extra-virgin olive oil, blueberries, artichokes, red cabbage, kale, dark chocolate, coffee, black tea*

The Vagus Nerve and Autoimmunity

The vagus nerve runs from the brain, across the chest, through the upper body, and into the abdomen, with branches that reach into every major organ in the body. It's part of the autonomic nervous system, which controls functions like breathing, digesting food, and getting turned on—essentially things we do unconsciously!

This nerve is essentially in charge of the mind-body connection. Have you ever heard someone say, "The body remembers"? I believe it! I think the vagus nerve, which connects our conscious and subconscious minds as well as our entire nervous system, is responsible. Researchers have found that stimulating the vagus nerve with electrical implant can reduce the symptoms of rheumatoid arthritis, an autoimmune condition.[14] A study of over fifteen thousand participants showed a correlation between adverse childhood experiences and hospitalizations later in life for autoimmune disease. The study concluded that "childhood traumatic stress increased the likelihood of hospitalization with a diagnosed autoimmune disease decades into adulthood."[15]

Many people who live with autoimmune disease report that stress can induce major flareups. As one of these people, I can share with you that, for me, that is true. I believe that to find clinical remission, addressing trauma and managing stress are imperative.

The connection between the brain, body, and soul is one reason I believe in the power of affirmation. Through the vagus nerve, our bodies respond to our thoughts, so think positive, think healing, think self-love. Believe it and it will be true.

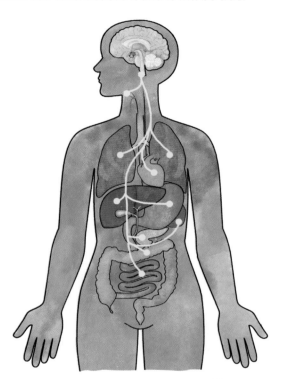

Healing Protocols: Useful but Not Forever

I mentioned earlier that healing the gut is all about removing the stressors (any food that is triggering inflammation in your body) and supporting the digestive system. Different ways of eating will help you identify and remove stressors; these ways of eating are commonly known as elimination protocols. But before I dive into these diets, I want to emphasize the importance of the information in Chapter 1. Study it, apply it to your body, and take note. Truly understand the cause-and-effect of proper digestion, hydration, fatty acid balance, and blood sugar regulation. Make the lifestyle changes. Get your mindset right. Without a strong foundation, your dietary endeavors will be for naught.

Also, remember why you're trying a new way of eating in the first place. Through my own journey and my work, I have seen more harm than good come from people making their food choices part of their identity. The goal of making deliberate choices about what to eat isn't to color within the lines, follow rules, or apply moral implications to ways of eating. The goal is to heal our minds and bodies, come hell or high water. That's why it's imperative to address the root cause. If you get bloated when you eat spinach and you just omit spinach from your diet, you're not addressing why it makes you bloated. If you have an adverse reaction to a long list of foods, it can seem like there is nothing left to eat, so the goal has to be to get back to a place where your system can handle more foods. This is why I think it's important to work on the bigger picture when trying an elimination protocol, which is why we address the foundation first.

What Is an Elimination Protocol?

Elimination protocols are just what they sound like: you eliminate potentially problematic foods from your diet for a given amount of time. They can be useful because they can bring about almost immediate relief of symptoms. When you stop eating a food that was like poison to your body, you have more energy and mental clarity and are able to tackle lasting lifestyle changes. But eliminating foods alone will not address the root cause. Think of an elimination protocol as a research study: you want to gain information about your body through this experiment.

The way these protocols work is that you adhere to a set of food parameters for a set amount of time. During this time, you eliminate foods and food groups that can potentially cause harm. Top allergens like gluten, wheat, soy, corn, nuts, and eggs are a good place to start. Dairy, nightshades, grains, legumes, and sweeteners may be other culprits. Trigger foods (foods that cause symptoms) are different for everyone, even for two people who have the same condition.

When you begin to feel better, you add foods back in one at a time, tracking your food intake, mood, and symptoms with each reintroduction. This should help you connect the dots between foods you eat and how you feel. Reintroductions are where the magic happens. If you stay in the elimination phase too long, you will find yourself in an on-and-off-the-wagon scenario at some point. Reintroductions show you which foods are causing symptoms, which is great, but they also tell you which are not, and that's awesome for eating a wide variety of foods and feeling like long-term change is sustainable! Symptoms to look for during reintroduction include autoimmune flareups, headaches, stomachaches, loose stools or constipation, bloating, hives, fatigue, and any kind of inflammation (achy joints, swollen gums, etc.).

Reintroducing Foods

Here's the proper way to reintroduce foods: Eat a small amount of one new food and wait twenty-four hours. If no reaction occurs, have a slightly larger portion and then wait another twenty-four hours. If that goes well, try again, this time with a hefty portion of that same food. Wait seventy-two hours. Write down any symptoms you experience, including digestive symptoms, skin irritations or breakouts, changes in energy and sleep quality, and so on. If all goes well, continue adding foods one at a time like this.

I'd like to stress that I don't believe any elimination protocol is meant to be followed forever. A rigid protocol is the opposite of flexible and enjoyable, and trying to adhere to one for a long time isn't a good way to make a sustainable lifestyle change. I know that once you find freedom from pain and debilitating symptoms by avoiding certain foods, it can be scary to reintroduce those foods. I get it, I've been there. Just work on feeling safe and strong, stay positive, and keep moving forward.

Popular Protocols

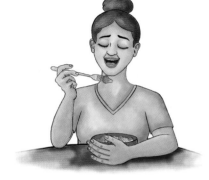

There are many elimination protocols, each of which focuses on eliminating different kinds of foods. They can also vary in how many foods are eliminated and how long they're meant to be followed. These are the four I think will work best to help you heal.

Autoimmune Paleo (AIP) has been studied as a treatment for conditions like irritable bowel syndrome and showed great results. Autoimmune Paleo omits all grains, legumes, nuts, seeds, seed-based spices, nightshades, eggs, dairy, gluten, additives, and refined sugars. I outlined AIP in detail in my first book, *Made Whole*, and on my blog, *The Castaway Kitchen*. Another great resource for AIP is *The Paleo Approach* by Dr. Sarah Ballantyne. Many of the recipes in this book are AIP compliant. This elimination protocol is ideal for those with autoimmune disease or food allergies, but again, it won't treat the root cause—it will just give you insight into which foods are currently triggers.

AIP keto combines AIP with a low-carb, high-fat approach. A low-carb, high-fat, ketogenic diet is anti-inflammatory in two ways: first, it lowers insulin levels, and high insulin levels can cause inflammation; and second, it generates molecules called ketones, which are anti-inflammatory. AIP keto is more restrictive than AIP, but it's very effective for those dealing with autoimmune disease paired with hormone imbalance or metabolic disorders. Most of the recipes in this book are well suited for a low-carb, high-fat diet and many of them are AIP compliant too, so you can use them for this protocol.

A **low-FODMAP diet** minimizes fermentable oligo-, di-, and monosaccharides and polyols (FODMAPs), which are short-chain carbohydrates that are not well digested in the small intestine. In some people, FODMAPs ferment in the gut, causing painful bloating and gas. Again, if we address the foundations and heal north to south, these foods should be safely reintroduced after being eliminated for a period to give the gut time to heal. You can find complete lists of high-FODMAP foods online. This elimination protocol omits onions and garlic, which would kill my soul, so I personally have never done it, nor have I needed to.

Paleo + Hard-No-Food-Free isn't really a protocol, but it works for a lot of people. It's based on a strict Paleo diet, which means no dairy, grains, or gluten. A Paleo diet also omits refined sugars and processed foods, so it works well as an elimination protocol. Most people who make it a lifestyle take an 80/20 approach, eating strict Paleo 80 percent of the time but being more flexible the other 20 percent. While eating strict Paleo, you can also remove any foods you suspect cause issues for you—for example, nuts, eggs, or nightshades. Because I feel this path is very doable for most people, the recipes in this book are all Paleo-friendly, nightshade-free, and dairy-free (save for a little butter on occasion), and most of them are nut-free. Some are also coconut-free and/or egg-free.

All of these protocols are helpful in finding out your feel-good foods, worth-it foods, and hard-no foods. I like to frame this as a mission to discover which foods your body loves! It's a wonderful thing to know without a doubt the foods that make you feel superhuman.

When you combine that knowledge with foundational health, you get a lifelong solution, a way of life and a way of eating that is just right for you. Bonus: as your needs change over time, you have the information and the power to meet those changes.

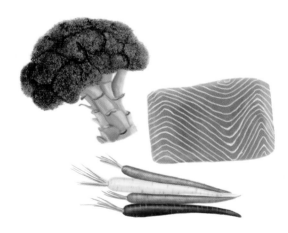

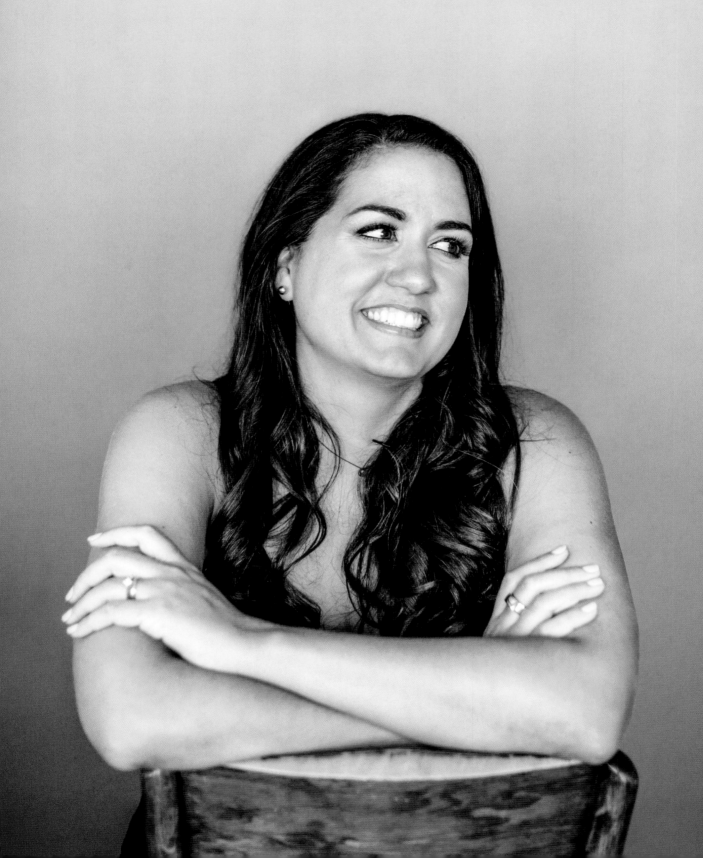

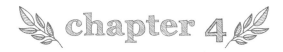

chapter 4

Habits for a Healthy Life

Remember when I said, "You can't get healthy eating the same way that got you sick in the first place"? By now, you might have taken a few notes and decided on where you're going to make those dietary changes. To support that decision, you're going to make some lifestyle adjustments too!

I'm not making the changes; *you are*. This is your show, baby! You don't want to continue the vicious cycle of overrestriction and bingeing, right? Food as medicine can't become another source of self-loathing. You can't make change from a place of hate—you have to honor your body and love yourself enough to commit to a lifestyle that will nourish and heal you.

If I was working with you as nutritional coaching client, we would have covered all of this material over the course of three months, so let's pause now, take a deep breath, and exhale slowly. There's no need to rush through all of these changes. Master one change before you layer on the next. Work on relaxing before you sit down to eat and give it a few weeks. If you feel better, then that's a sign you're on the right path and you can explore the next step.

Tackle the foundations one at a time and explore your dietary choices slowly. No pressure, no judgment. There are no wrong moves here. There are no rules. There is only food and how it makes you feel. Cook from this book—I promise the recipes are easy. Take another deep breath. Exhale slowly.

Okay, let's dive into some lifestyle factors that support the foundations, because although good health starts on your plate, it definitely doesn't end there.

Movement

If I had to recommend either walking for two hours a day or taking a forty-five-minute HIIT class, I would pick walking every time. Don't get me wrong, I love a good, hard, pool-of-sweat-on-the-floor workout as much as the next person. However, one hour of movement isn't going to combat a sedentary lifestyle. If you're new to working out, just focus on getting your steps in. Walk to the store, take the stairs, get up from your desk once an hour. Just move your body. If you're already a ten-thousand-steps-a-day kind of person, awesome! Try lifting some heavy weights. Strength training helps with insulin sensitivity, bone density, and metabolic rate. As we age, it's important to eat enough protein and keep lifting weights to avoid muscle loss and injury.

Sleep

Proper sleep is more important than movement. There, I said it. If you're not sleeping well, you need to make it a priority. Lack of sleep impairs cognitive function, ages you, messes with your hunger signals, and can impair your immune function. Go to bed early. Have a good nighttime routine so your body knows it's time to wind down. Take a bath, drink some tea, and dim the lights. Make sure you're getting at least seven hours of sleep a night. A cold, dark (yes, cavelike) room is ideal for quality sleep. I got some cheap blackout shades at Home Depot and installed them myself: *game changer*.

Mindfulness

It's loud, it's busy, it's nonstop out there. Our minds have never been more occupied or our attention more fragmented. It's a stark contrast to the decline in our physical activity. In the same way we need to move our bodies more, we desperately need to quiet our minds more. Whether it's prayer, meditation, coloring, knitting, or gardening, find an activity that lets you thoroughly unplug. Disconnect from your phone, email, deadlines, and stress. Spend time in nature as often as possible, from the beach to the mountaintops or even your neighborhood park. Get sun on your face and put your bare feet in the grass.

Affirmations

Positive thought is paramount in self-healing!

I am made
WHOLE.
My body is
STRONG,
RESILIENT,
THRIVING.
I feel
AMAZING
today.

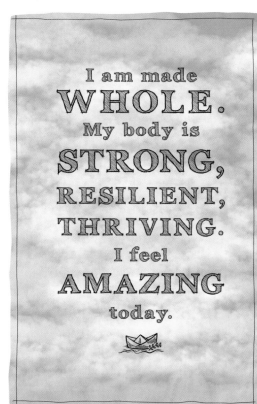

I love
MYSELF.
Today is going
to be a
GREAT DAY.

I am capable of
INCREDIBLE
things.

Right now,
in this
moment,
just as I am,
I am
ENOUGH.

I will
OVERCOME
this.

There is
NOTHING
that can hold
me down.

I am
POWERFUL.

Connection

Hugs heal, and no one can tell me otherwise. We're clan folk; we need human connection, and not just through a screen—we need to see, hear, and touch other people. Find your people. Make time for them. Join a fitness class, volunteer, or sign up for a community meetup! I move around a lot because of my husband's career, and during the times of transition, I lean on my online connections more and more for support, but they can never fill the void completely. The internet can be magical, but the best magic is when internet friends become friends in real life! Foster your relationships.

Stress Management

Often, the thing that causes us the most stress is something near and dear to us. Having healthy boundaries, even with family members, can be a great way to better manage stress. Think of your healthy boundaries as a glowing egg of light that surrounds you and filters everything you take in and everything you let out. The most sustainable way to manage stress is to practice healthy boundaries, which includes knowing when to say no.

All of the above habits will help with stress too! Our bodies need healthy levels of cortisol, which is part of blood sugar regulation and hormone health. We need to support our system with nutrient-dense foods so that it can handle life's demands, but we also need to prioritize and scrutinize what those demands are.

A great way to break the stress cycle at any moment of the day is through conscious breathing. The 4-7-8 breath is known to lower your heart rate almost immediately. Inhale for four seconds, hold your breath for seven seconds, and exhale for eight seconds, making a ssshhhh sound. Repeat this sequence four times.

Another effective breathing pattern is to inhale deeply for five seconds and then exhale deeply for five seconds. Repeat until you feel calm. Studies have found that people in a meditative state often fall into this breathing pattern.

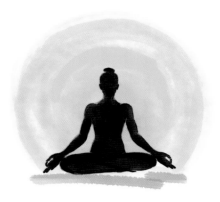

Fasting

Fasting has been around since the beginning of time. When food wasn't readily available, people had no choice but to fast. In several cultures, fasting is part of spiritual and healing ceremonies. While it's definitely become a trendy topic in recent years, there are indisputable benefits to fasting, the main one being that it's a hormetic stressor—a mild stress on the body that has positive benefits. Fasting enhances cells' ability to cope with stress and to resist disease. Plus, while you fast, your body isn't doing the very big and complex job of digesting food, so your mitochondria have time to clean house via autophagy, the process of breaking down and recycling old, worn-out parts of the cells.

It seems counterintuitive, but when you're not eating, your body seems to heal better. Biomarkers for disease improve, oxidative stress is reduced, and cognitive function gets a boost. However, regular intermittent fasting isn't about eating less; it's about eating during a specific window of time. Chronically undereating can downregulate your metabolism and suppress your immune system. Eat to fuel your needs; just do it during a specific window. Pick a window of eight to ten hours when you will have your meals—say, between 10 a.m. and 7 p.m. Outside of that window, don't eat. You'll sleep through most of the time you're not eating, so it's not as wild as it sounds. It's like having a late breakfast or an early dinner and cutting out nighttime snacking.

Fasting will probably happen organically at some point or another. Don't force it, but if you find your hunger changing once you've addressed the foundations, listen to your body—you might be surprised at how your eating patterns change. Remember, no white-knuckling here; if fasting doesn't feel right for you, don't do it. Exercise also stimulates autophagy, so fasting isn't your only option!

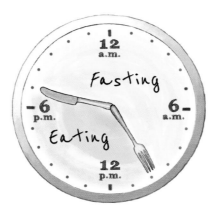

Batch Cooking / Meal Prep

Being prepared is essential when making dietary changes, especially when you are trying out a healing protocol. You don't want to get caught hangry with an empty fridge. This is why I like batch cooking—making double batches of a few recipes to have on hand. All of the recipes in this book were designed to be perfect for meal prep: they use just one or two sheet pans or one pot, or they're cooked in a slow cooker or pressure cooker, or there's no cooking involved at all. Pick one recipe in each cooking method category and you can whip them up practically at the same time. Choose recipes with overlapping ingredients. Start with the slow cooker or pressure cooker ingredient. Put the sheet pan meal in the oven and then start the one-pot dish. Finish with the no-cook dish. Boom, you have five different meals ready to go for the week! The following plans show this approach in action.

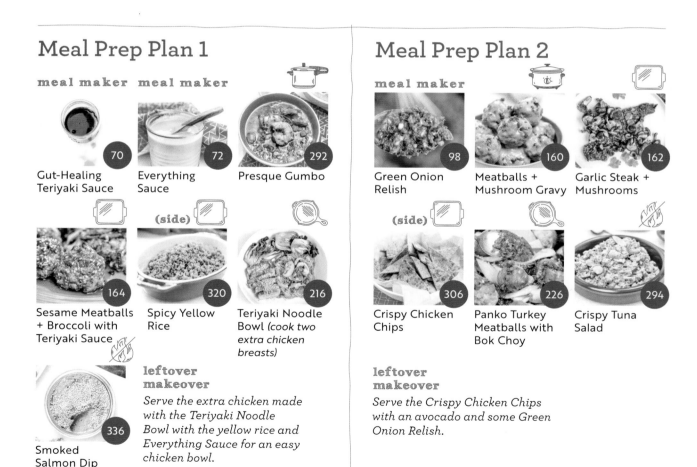

Meal Prep Plan 1

meal maker **meal maker**

70 Gut-Healing Teriyaki Sauce

72 Everything Sauce

292 Presque Gumbo

164 Sesame Meatballs + Broccoli with Teriyaki Sauce

320 Spicy Yellow Rice **(side)**

216 Teriyaki Noodle Bowl *(cook two extra chicken breasts)*

336 Smoked Salmon Dip

leftover makeover
Serve the extra chicken made with the Teriyaki Noodle Bowl with the yellow rice and Everything Sauce for an easy chicken bowl.

Meal Prep Plan 2

meal maker

98 Green Onion Relish

160 Meatballs + Mushroom Gravy

162 Garlic Steak + Mushrooms

(side)

306 Crispy Chicken Chips

226 Panko Turkey Meatballs with Bok Choy

294 Crispy Tuna Salad

leftover makeover
Serve the Crispy Chicken Chips with an avocado and some Green Onion Relish.

Meal Prep Plan 3

meal maker **meal maker** **meal maker**

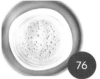
Salted Cashew Cream — 76

or Cauliflower Sour Cream — 74

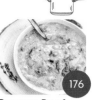
Horseradish Mayo — 94

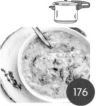
Creamy Beef + Bacon Soup — 176

Legend

 - Slow Cooker

- Pressure Cooker

- Sheet Pan

- One Pot

- No Cook

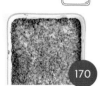
Kitchen Sink Casserole — 170

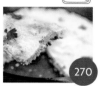
Salmon Herb Skillet Cake *(serve with Horseradish Mayo, from above)* — 270

(side)

Warm Garlic Herb Radish Salad — 298

Chia Seed Pudding Five Ways *(pick your favorite flavor)* — 350

leftover makeover
Make a quick salad with cocktail shrimp, arugula, avocado, and horseradish mayo.

Meal Prep Plan 4

meal maker

Onion + Bacon Spread — 88

Hail Mary Chicken — 258

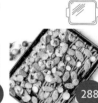
Shrimp + Sausage Sheet Pan — 288

(side)

Spicy Yellow Rice — 320

(side)
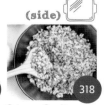
or Crispy Garlic Rice — 318

Burger Bar — 136

Pumpkin Pie Squares — 348

leftover makeover
Make taco bowls using the leftover chicken and rice along with some aioli, an avocado, and fresh cilantro.

Meal Prep Plan 5 AIP

meal maker **meal maker**

Cauliflower Sour Cream — 74

Frozen Herb Blocks — 109

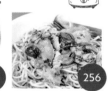
Garlic Chicken over Zoodles — 256

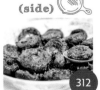
Mushroom Herb Meatballs with Cauliflower Steaks — 174

(side)
Herby Skillet Mushrooms — 312

Balsamic Braised Meatballs + Kale — 152

Herbed Yellowfin Tuna Steaks — 276

leftover makeover
Use leftover Frozen Herb Blocks to make the tuna steaks and serve with leftover Cauliflower Sour Cream.

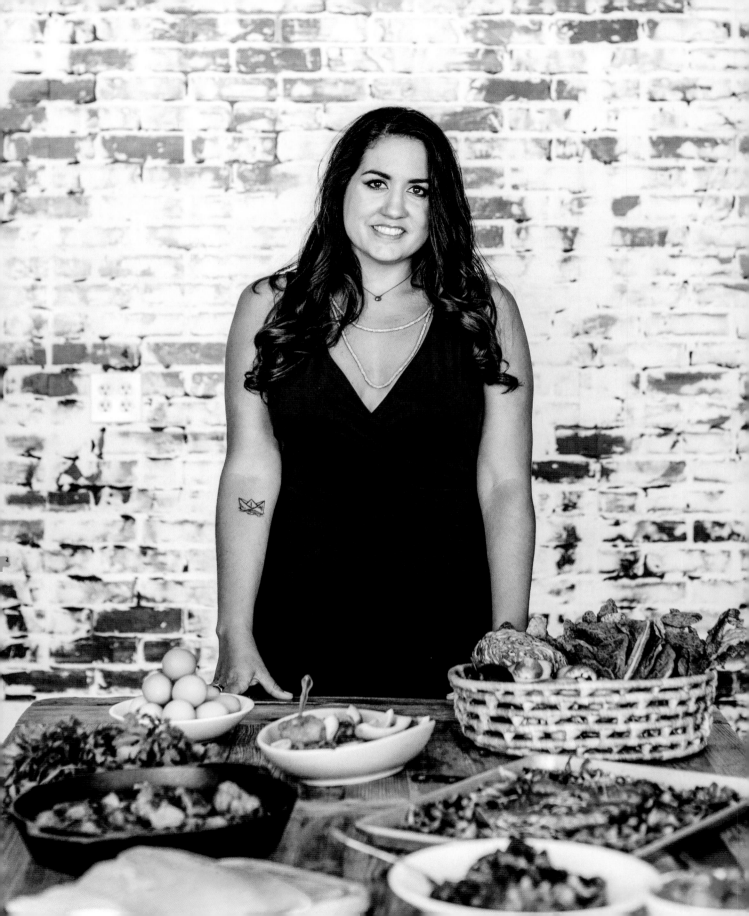

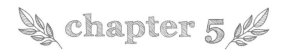

chapter 5

Kitchen Handbook

All of the recipes in this book are designed to be easy, even if you're new to cooking from scratch. Using fresh ingredients doesn't have to be complicated. I promise you that all of the cooking techniques are straightforward. There is nothing fancy here, and most of the longer ingredient lists are just a bunch of dried seasonings!

The ingredients are chosen carefully; they are all good for you and make dishes that will help you feel amazing. The ingredients in these recipes are just that—real *ingredients*, not food products parading as real food, just as it should be.

When you're at the store, feel free to buy precut vegetables, riced cauliflower, and high-quality bone broth—doing so can cut down on your time in the kitchen. Luckily, with the growth of the real food movement, there are now brands that you can trust for some foods, such as condiments. But of course, always check labels. I have included a list of preferred brands in the back of this book to make shopping easier (see page 359).

Almost all of the recipes in this book are made using one large skillet or one or two sheet pans; a smaller number use a saucepan or a heavy pot, like a Dutch oven. The vast majority fall into the one-pot/one-pan category because everyone has these tools. However, I did include a handful of delectable recipes for slow cookers and pressure cookers. These electric appliances have the ease of hands-off cooking, with very little cleanup.

With the recipes in this book, I want to show you that healing through food can be easy. After all, that's what *Made Whole Made Simple* means: healing made simple. Preparing real foods from scratch is something anyone can do, no matter their skill level.

Bone Broth

I use bone broth in my recipes—not vegetable stock, chicken stock, or water. There's a reason for that: bone broth is a simple addition to your diet that gives you a ton of health benefits. Bone broth is the original medicinal food! It improves gut health and is nutrient dense, anti-inflammatory, and delicious. Bone broth is as old as time, made in the nose-to-tail approach of our ancestors, who made use of all the goodness from the animals they hunted for food. Simmering bones for a long time extracts collagen, glycine, proline, and glutamine from them—all fantastic nutrients. By consuming bone broth, you're getting easy-to-digest, highly absorbable nutrients with every sip. Not to mention that using real bone broth adds wonderful flavor and texture to your food.

It's easy to make your own bone broth. Just get beef marrow bones or chicken feet and necks—really, any animal bones will work—and cook them in a slow cooker or in a stockpot with filtered water, bay leaves, and a splash of apple cider vinegar for forty-eight hours. (I included a wonderful bone broth recipe in my first book, *Made Whole*.) However, to save time, you can always buy premade broth. I use only Bonafide Provisions brand; it is sold in the freezer aisles of Target, Walmart, Whole Foods, and really any major grocer. I trust the company and know the owner, and their product passes the chill test: a true bone broth is thick and gelatinous when it's chilled. Many broths on the market are labeled as bone broth because they use "meat flavor," but they don't pass the chill test.

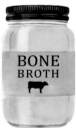

I am partial to beef broth or broth made with a mixture of various animal bones, but for the recipes in this book, you can use chicken bone broth or whichever variation you prefer.

Aw, Nuts! Why Raw?

As I discussed in the section on balancing fatty acids, polyunsaturated fats are very sensitive to heat. When you buy roasted nuts, you're getting nuts whose delicate healthy fats have been oxidized. The benefit of raw nuts is that you can protect these fats.

Soaking raw nuts reduces phytic acid, which blocks nutrient absorption. It also makes the nuts easier to digest and makes them better for you by keeping their fats intact. (It removes dust and tannins as well, which are difficult to digest.) Soak raw nuts in filtered water with a pinch of salt for several hours, then drain and air-dry or dehydrate them (at a low temperature).

Slow cooking, fermenting, and sprouting are all ancient ways of preparing foods, and our ancestors prepared foods in these ways for good reason!

Why Filtered Water?

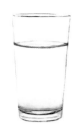

We're fortunate to live in an industrialized country where we can turn on the tap and get potable water any time of the day. However, tap water isn't as clean as you might think. Think of all of the miles and miles of pipeline it has gone through, which aren't sterile. Many city water plants use harsh ingredients like chlorine to disinfect it, and though it keeps us from getting sick, chlorine isn't an ingredient I want in my soup or my coffee.

I believe that using filtered water for cooking, making coffee, and more is important to our health. You don't want to undermine your efforts of healing and then consume water with pathogens in it.

There are several affordable and viable options for water filtration at home, from the kind you screw onto your faucet to portable systems like Berkey water filters, which is what I use.

A Note on Salt

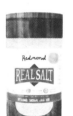

I like cooking with unrefined salt that contains many important trace minerals. Redmond Real Salt is my favorite brand. It contains essential minerals (in addition to sodium), and I find it to be less salty than other salts. I made every recipe in this book with finely ground Redmond Real Salt. If you use another salt, you might want to start with a little less than the recipe calls for and add more to taste.

Always taste your food as you go and salt as you go. This is the first step in becoming an intuitive cook!

Reading the Recipes

The recipes are marked with AIP and allergen icons for quick reference:

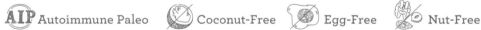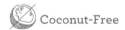 Autoimmune Paleo   Coconut-Free   Egg-Free   Nut-Free

You can also refer to the allergen index on pages 363 to 365.

There are icons indicating the cooking method as well:

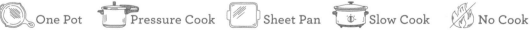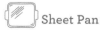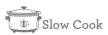 One Pot   Pressure Cook   Sheet Pan   Slow Cook   No Cook

Finally, these icons flag recipes that are quick to make or require very few ingredients:

 30 Minutes or Less   5 Ingredients or Fewer

Tools

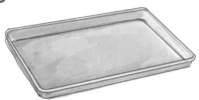

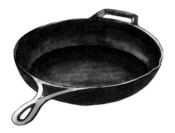

Sheet pans: I use the size that is most common in home kitchens: 18 by 13 inches with a 1-inch rim. In a professional kitchen, these are referred to as "half sheet pans." Having two of them is a good idea because overcrowding your pan will skew your results. Another bonus: having two pans enables you to cook different parts of a meal in stages; you can put a longer-cooking component in the oven first and later put a second sheet pan in the oven with a quicker-cooking part of the meal, like fish, and have everything ready at the same time. Finally, several of the recipes in this book require two sheet pans. For all these reasons, I highly recommend getting two of them. They are workhorses. I like Nordic Ware. They're made with aluminum, but you can always line them with parchment paper if you're worried about leaching, although from what I've read, that usually happens when food simmers.

Extra-large, 15- or 16-inch skillet: I use a 15-inch cast-iron skillet, which is large enough to make one-pan meals that will feed a family of four or five. If properly maintained, cast-iron cookware will last forever. Well-seasoned cast iron has the added benefit of being nonstick. I have a great YouTube video showing how to use, clean, and care for cast iron on The Castaway Kitchen YouTube channel (https://youtu.be/COWgQ9pDBzY), and I included cast-iron maintenance tips in my previous book, *Made Whole*.

For some people, large cast-iron skillets can be too heavy to handle; in that case, stainless-steel skillets are a good alternative. If you preheat a stainless-steel pan the same way you would cast iron, waiting until it comes to temperature over medium heat before adding the cooking fat, food shouldn't stick to it. Another good lighter-weight option that is nonstick yet nontoxic is Green Pan brand skillets. Seeking out nontoxic nonstick pans is important because traditional nonstick cookware uses hazardous materials that can leach into your food.

Always use the right size pan for the job. If you stir-fry a recipe that serves four in an 8-inch skillet, it won't cook properly—you will end up with soggy or undercooked food.

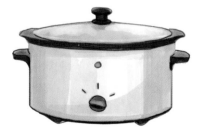

Slow cooker and/or pressure cooker: There are a few slow cooker and pressure cooker recipes in this book. My slow cooker and pressure cooker are both 6 quarts. I kept the instructions universal so that you can apply them to your appliance regardless of the brand.

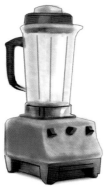

Blender: As a restaurant chef, I got used to working with high-powered blenders, and I continue to use one in my home. It is a workhorse in a from-scratch kitchen; from nut milks to soups, the results from a high-powered blender are smoother, creamier, and done much faster! However, a regular blender will work for every recipe in this book (though the Stir-In Coffee Creamer on page 107 will need to be strained if it's not made in a high-powered blender), and considering the cost, a high-powered blender is not a must-have. But if you're ready to invest in one, I love Vitamix and Blendtec blenders.

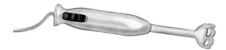

Immersion blender or stick blender: This tool is wonderful for one-pot recipes and for making mayo. It is perfect for smaller, lighter blending jobs that don't require the use of a full blender, and the cleanup is much easier too.

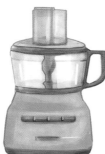

Food processor: If you're unsure about your knife skills or you simply want to save time in the kitchen, this tool is great for mincing, grating, and more. It makes ricing cauliflower a breeze and is wonderful for making sauces and nut butters.

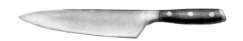

Chef's knife: I use only one knife in my kitchen, and it's a well-sharpened chef's knife. Instead of spending a lot of money on a nice set of knives, spend it on one really good chef's knife. It's a game changer for an avid cook. Remember, a sharp knife is safer than a dull knife.

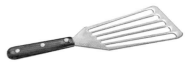

Fish spatula: This tool is great not only for fish but also for frying eggs, flipping pancakes, and more. A thin metal fish spatula is a cast-iron skillet's best friend. This duo will ensure that your food has perfect lift every time. It's also great for scraping up crispy bits on your sheet pan.

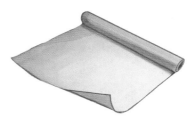

Unbleached parchment paper: This stuff makes cleanup really easy! Use it to line your sheet pans when roasting or baking or to line your workspace.

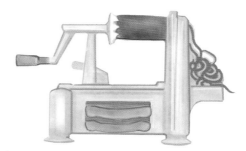

Spiral slicer: These days, you can buy spiralized zucchini at any grocer, but if you're into making your own zucchini noodles, popularly known as "zoodles," having a spiral slicer is a must. This inexpensive tool is available online and at most home goods and grocery stores.

Easy Swaps

This entire book is about making food that fits your needs. So if there are ingredients that I don't include but work for you, feel free to use them to make the recipes. In some recipes, I offer specific suggestions for ingredient swaps, such as using heavy cream instead of coconut cream or tomato paste instead of pumpkin puree. If you don't find the ingredient option you're looking for in a recipe, use this quick guide to ingredient substitutions. It will make customizing the recipes for your needs easy peasy!

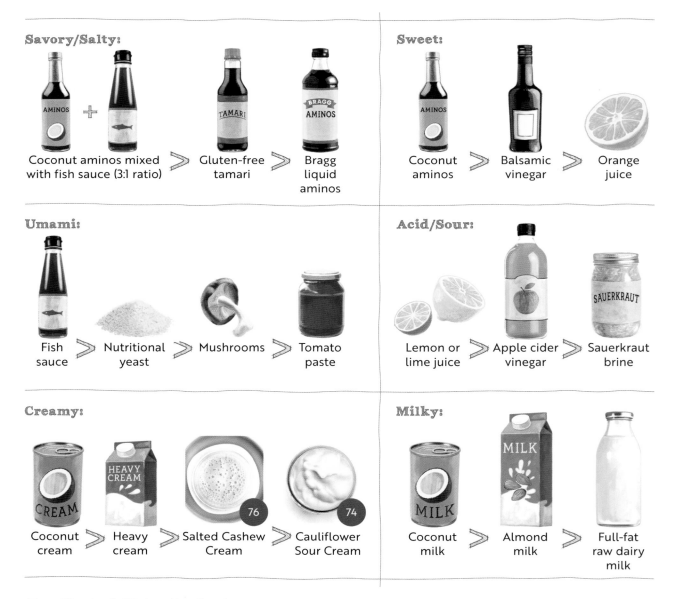

Savory/Salty:

Coconut aminos mixed with fish sauce (3:1 ratio) > Gluten-free tamari > Bragg liquid aminos

Sweet:

Coconut aminos > Balsamic vinegar > Orange juice

Umami:

Fish sauce > Nutritional yeast > Mushrooms > Tomato paste

Acid/Sour:

Lemon or lime juice > Apple cider vinegar > Sauerkraut brine

Creamy:

Coconut cream > Heavy cream > Salted Cashew Cream 76 > Cauliflower Sour Cream 74

Milky:

Coconut milk > Almond milk > Full-fat raw dairy milk

Noodles:

   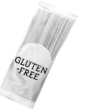

Shirataki noodles > Kelp noodles > Zucchini noodles > Gluten-free noodles

Spicy:

Black or white pepper > Wasabi > Cayenne

Cheesy:

Parmesan, mozzarella, goat cheese > Nutritional yeast > Nutritional yeast and mayo > Mozz Blocks 104

Nuts / Nut Butter:

Seeds/ Seed butter > Coconut flakes/ Coconut butter

Breadcrumbs:

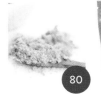   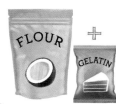

Pork panko, store-bought or homemade 80 > Flax meal > Almond meal or flour > Coconut flour + gelatin (4:1 ratio)

Binder:

Eggs > Flax egg > Gelatin

Saturated Fats:

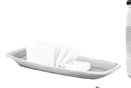   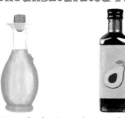

Butter > Ghee > Coconut oil > Lard > Tallow

Monounsaturated Fats:

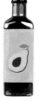 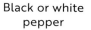

Extra-virgin olive oil > Avocado oil

MEAL MAKERS

Sauces, spreads, seasonings, and more! All the staples you need to make your meals pop with flavor and nutrients. I like to keep a few homemade sauces in the fridge and homemade seasoning blends in the pantry so it's easy to add great flavor to my cooking. If you're looking for ways to use the recipes in this chapter, see the index on page 361. The meal prep plans on pages 58 and 59 are written so that you reuse a sauce or other Meal Maker recipe that week. Waste not, want not!

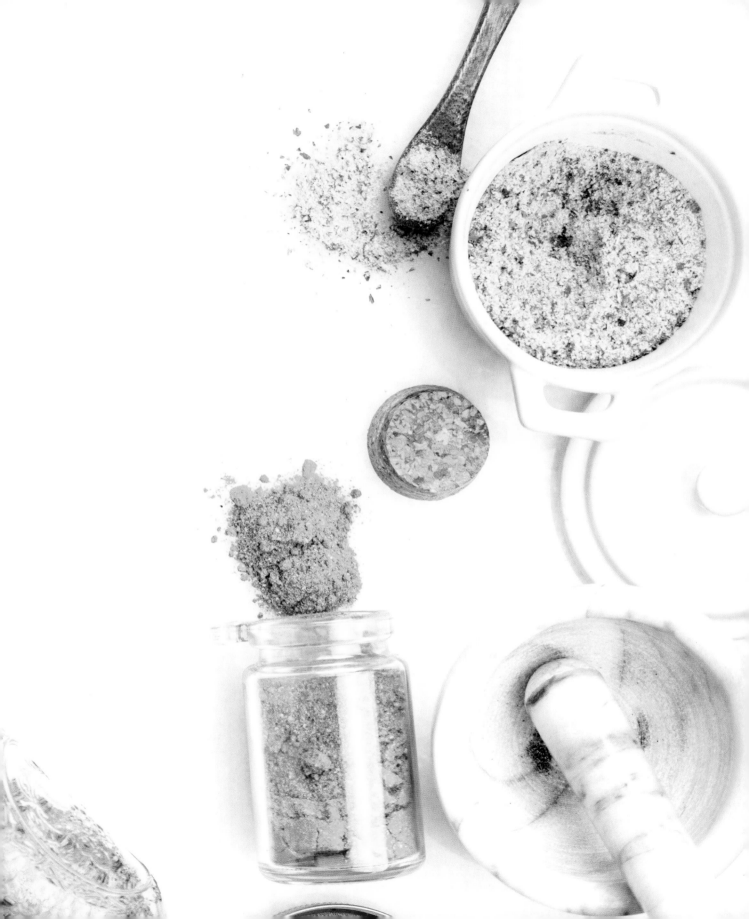

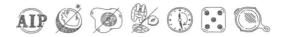

Gut-Healing Teriyaki Sauce

Makes 1 cup (1 tablespoon per serving) ◦ Prep Time: 5 minutes ◦ Cook Time: 15 minutes

This is the kind of food voodoo that makes my heart skip a beat. This glazy, sweet, and salty Asian-inspired condiment is made by reducing some bone broth and vinegar, blooming coconut aminos in gelatin, and then mixing the solid coconut amino mass into the bone broth reduction. Grass-fed gelatin is made from bones and connective tissue of pastured cows, and it strengthens the gut wall, making it less permeable. This sauce becomes solid when cold and liquid when hot. The magical part: it's thick and glazelike when it's lukewarm. It's soy-, flour-, starch-, and all-other-junk-free.

1 cup bone broth

¼ cup plus 2 tablespoons coconut aminos, divided

2 tablespoons red wine vinegar

1 tablespoon fish sauce

2 tablespoons unflavored grass-fed beef gelatin

◦ In a small saucepan over medium heat, combine the broth, ¼ cup of the coconut aminos, the vinegar, and fish sauce. Bring to a boil, then turn the heat down to medium-low and simmer for 10 minutes.

◦ While it simmers, put the remaining 2 tablespoons of coconut aminos in a small bowl or cup and sprinkle the gelatin over it. Let it sit for 1 minute, until a solid gelatinous mass forms.

◦ Remove the saucepan from the heat. Add the gelatinous mass to the broth mixture and whisk until smooth. Pour the sauce into a jar and let it cool for 20 minutes before using; it should be thick enough to coat the back of a spoon. Store in an airtight jar in the fridge for up to 3 weeks.

◦ Once the sauce cools completely, it will become solid. To make it liquid again, just run warm water over the jar or microwave it for 20 seconds, then spoon it over your dish.

modifications: *To make this sauce coconut-free, replace the coconut aminos with low-sodium gluten-free tamari.*

Per serving: Calories **14** · Fat **0g** · Total Carbs **1.1g** · Fiber **0g** · Protein **2.2g**

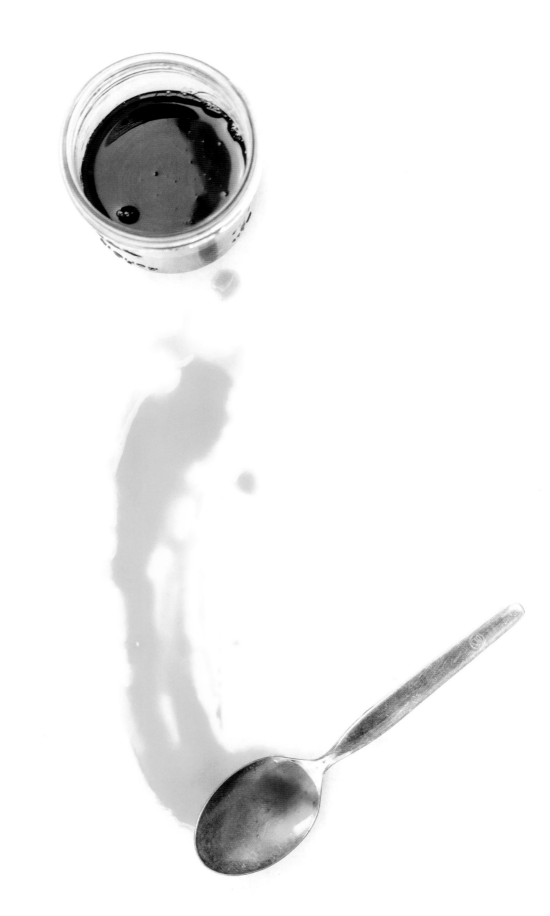

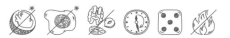

Everything Sauce

Makes 1 cup (1 tablespoon per serving) ◦ Prep Time: 5 minutes

I've been putting this sauce on everything for a long time. It's a combination so simple yet so delightful, you'll put it on everything too! I recommend using homemade mayo here; check out the Traditional Mayo variation of the Horseradish Mayo on page 94. Or you can use a high-quality store-bought mayo. Primal Kitchen is the brand I prefer.

½ cup avocado oil mayonnaise

¼ cup coconut aminos

¼ cup spicy brown or Dijon mustard

modifications: To make this sauce coconut-free, use 3 tablespoons low-sodium gluten-free tamari and 1 tablespoon honey in place of the coconut aminos. To make it egg-free, use any egg-free mayo substitute that you enjoy.

◦ Combine the ingredients in a glass jar and stir with a fork until fully mixed.

◦ Store the jar in the fridge with the lid tightly closed for up to 10 days. Always use a clean spoon to serve the sauce from the jar and promptly store it again so it lasts longer.

Per serving: Calories **59** · Fat **6g** · Total Carbs **1.5g** · Fiber **0g** · Protein **0g**

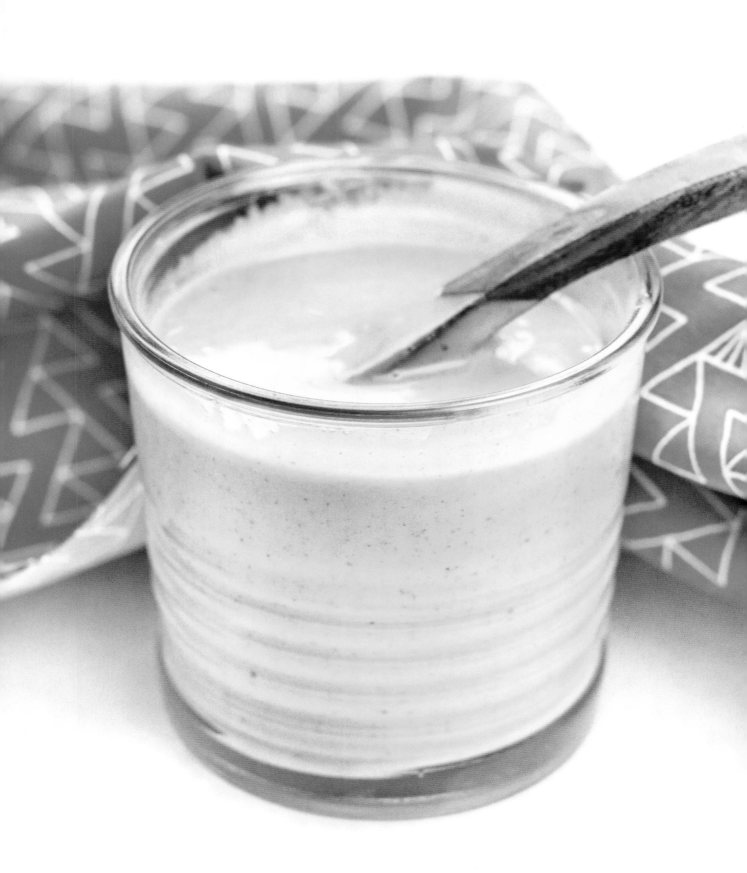

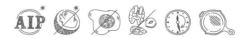

Cauliflower Sour Cream

Makes 3 cups (¼ cup per serving) ○ Prep Time: 5 minutes ○ Cook Time: 20 minutes

This smooth cream has a nice tang to it. It's the perfect sauce thickener or creamy topping for savory dishes, and it's an excellent veggie-based substitute for coconut cream and heavy cream. It makes an appearance in some of the pan sauces and dishes in this book; please refer to the Meal Makers index on page 361. Keep a jar of this cream in the fridge so you can quickly turn boring meals into delicious, creamy creations.

1 small head cauliflower (about 12 ounces), cored

1 medium parsnip (about 3½ ounces)

¾ cup filtered water

2 tablespoons ghee or coconut oil

1 tablespoon red wine vinegar

½ teaspoon fine salt

¼ teaspoon ground white pepper

○ Chop the cauliflower and peel and dice the parsnip.

○ Boil the vegetables in a large saucepan until tender, about 15 minutes. Drain the water and transfer the tender vegetables to a high-powered blender or food processor.

○ Add the water, ghee, vinegar, salt, and pepper. Blend on high until creamy and smooth, about 1 minute in a high-powered blender.

○ Transfer the cauliflower sour cream to a quart-sized jar or container with a tight-fitting lid. Store in the fridge for up to 8 days. You can also freeze it in silicone molds in ¼-cup portions to use for cooking when needed.

note: *If you don't do well with cauliflower, you may omit it and increase the number of parsnips to four or five (about 15 ounces total). The cream will have a slightly sweeter flavor and will be slightly starchy.*

modifications: *To make this cream AIP compliant, use coconut oil and omit the white pepper. To make it coconut-free, use ghee.*

variation: cauliflower alfredo sauce. *Add ½ cup bone broth, 2 teaspoons fish sauce, 1 teaspoon garlic powder, and ½ teaspoon ground black pepper to the blender. Fish sauce has a wonderful umami flavor that tricks your palate into thinking there's Parmesan in there.*

Per serving: Calories **31** · Fat **2.2g** · Total Carbs **2.5g** · Fiber **0.8g** · Protein **0.5g**

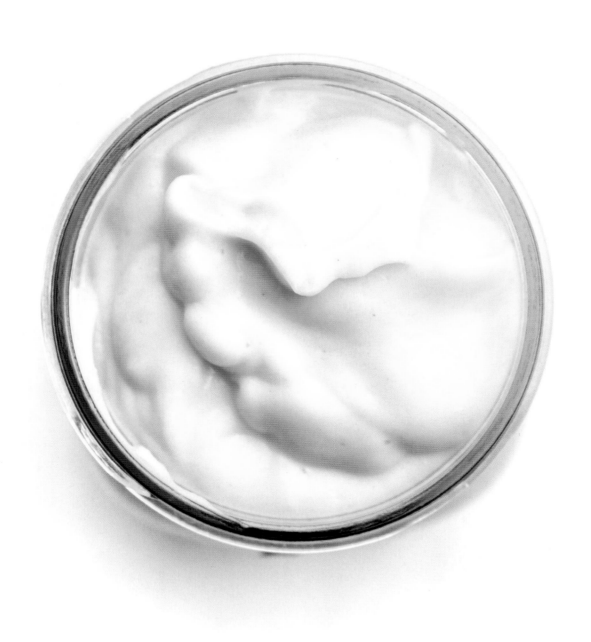

Salted Cashew Cream

Makes 3 cups (¼ cup per serving) ⊙ Prep Time: 2 minutes, plus 4 hours to soak

This is a wonderful cooking cream for those who tolerate cashews. It involves soaking the cashews first to reduce their phytic acid (which interferes with nutrient absorption) and make them easier to digest. The cashews are then blended into a silky heavy cream–like substance with a hit of lemon for acidity. This cream thickens when heated and is the perfect dairy alternative for baking and pan sauces.

12 ounces raw cashews

2 cups filtered water, plus more for soaking

½ teaspoon plus 1 pinch fine salt

Juice of 1 lemon

note: In a high-powered blender like a Blendtec or Vitamix, blending the cashews will take 60 to 90 seconds on high. If you don't have a high-powered blender, it will take longer, and you won't get a perfectly smooth texture; I recommend straining the cream through a fine-mesh sieve or nut milk bag.

variation: cashew alfredo sauce. Make it a cheese sauce! Add ½ cup bone broth, 2 teaspoons fish sauce, 1 teaspoon garlic powder, and ½ teaspoon ground black pepper for an Alfredo-like experience. Like aged Parmesan, fish sauce is umami— your taste buds won't know the difference!

⊙ Submerge the cashews in filtered water and add a pinch of salt. Soak for 4 hours.

⊙ Drain and rinse the cashews with fresh water, then put them in a blender with the 2 cups of water, the remaining ½ teaspoon of salt, and the lemon juice. Blend until smooth. Store in an airtight container in the fridge for up to 5 days.

Per serving: Calories **90** · Fat **7.1g** · Total Carbs **5.1g** · Fiber **0.5g** · Protein **3g**

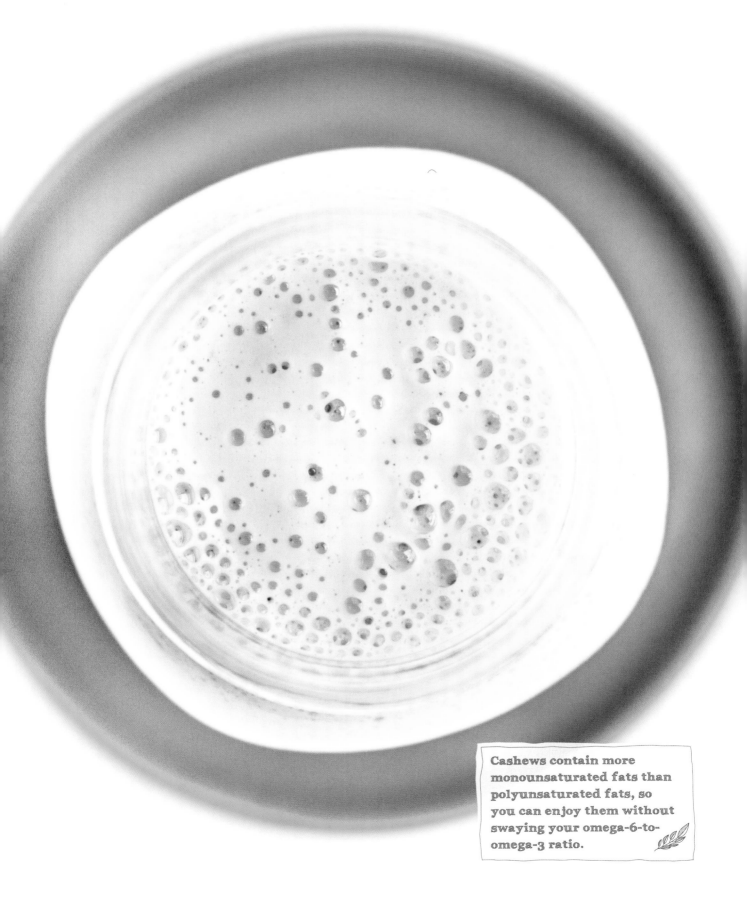

Cashews contain more monounsaturated fats than polyunsaturated fats, so you can enjoy them without swaying your omega-6-to-omega-3 ratio.

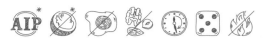

Asian Garlic Compound Butter

Makes 2 cups (2 tablespoons per serving) ● Prep Time: 10 minutes

You know those fancy Japanese restaurants where they cook your food at the table? The most popular chain is Benihana, and I grew up going there for special occasions. They cook everything in a blend of soy sauce, garlic, and butter, and it's amazing. I made a soy-free version at home with coconut aminos and grass-fed butter, and it's amazing too. (Soy sauce is not gluten-free unless you are specifically using gluten-free tamari.) Cook with this just as you would with butter—it works especially well in Asian-flavored dishes.

20 cloves garlic, peeled

½ cup coconut aminos

1 cup (2 sticks) salted grass-fed butter, ghee, or lard, softened

modifications: *To make this butter dairy-free and AIP compliant, use lard instead of butter or ghee. You can also use Navitas Butter-Flavored Coconut Oil if you would like a dairy-free compound butter with a classic "buttery" flavor. To make it coconut-free, use low-sodium gluten-free tamari.*

● Place the garlic and coconut aminos in a food processor and process until almost smooth. With the motor running, add the softened butter 2 tablespoons at a time and continue to process until a light-brown creamy butter has formed.

● Use a rubber spatula to transfer the mixture to a glass container with a tight-fitting lid. Store in the fridge for up to 10 days.

Per serving: Calories **118** · Fat **11.6g** · Total Carbs **2.8g** · Fiber **0.1g** · Protein **0.4g**

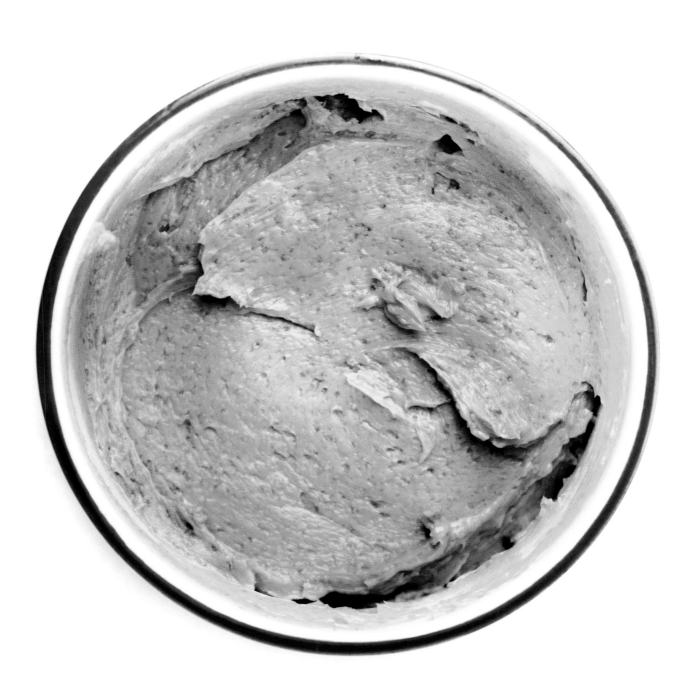

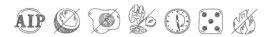

Homemade Pork Panko

Makes 1½ cups (¼ cup per serving) ○ Prep Time: 10 minutes

Pork panko—ground pork rinds—is a game changer for allergen-free cooking. It's wonderful for breading and as a flour substitute. I love Bacon's Heir brand, and I buy a one-pound bag a few times a year; it lasts a long time. However, if you can't get that product where you are, you can use this method to make your own pork panko at home! The most important thing here is to use high-quality pork rinds—the fluffy pork clouds that don't have the skin attached. Also, make sure they were fried in lard or another high-quality fat, not seed-based oils. If I can't get Bacon's Heir pork panko for any reason, I use EPIC Oven-Baked Pork Rinds with Pink Himalayan Salt, which are available almost everywhere these days.

---

5 cups pork rinds (about 5 ounces)

○ Put the pork rinds in a food processor and pulse until they are ground to a fine crumb but not mushy. Periodically stop and use a rubber spatula to work the larger pieces into the center of the bowl; this will help keep it from becoming mushy.

○ Transfer the ground pork rinds to a glass jar and store at room temperature for up to 10 days.

Per serving: Calories **324** · Fat **24.3g** · Total Carbs **0g** · Fiber **0g** · Protein **32.4g**

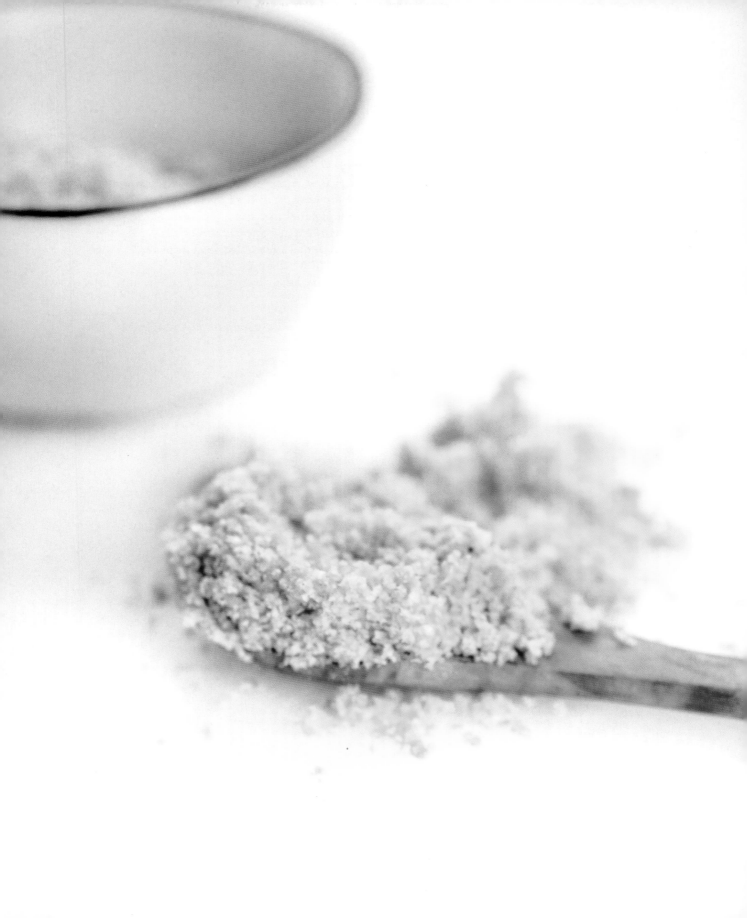

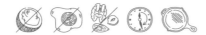 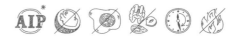

Castaway Seed Blend

Makes about ½ cup ◦ Prep Time: 10 minutes
Cook Time: 5 minutes

I love the nutty and earthy flavors that this toasted seed spice blend brings to food: it adds warmth without a lot of heat. Cumin seeds, sesame seeds, mustard seeds, and more come together in what is soon to be your go-to blend. It's perfect for jazzing up grilled chicken and taking steaks from good to great.

---

2 tablespoons cumin seeds

2 tablespoons garlic powder

2 tablespoons mustard seeds

2 tablespoons white peppercorns

1 tablespoon onion powder

1 tablespoon sesame seeds

2 teaspoons dried minced lemon peel (see note)

◦ Heat a small skillet over medium heat. Combine the spices in the skillet and toast until the seeds begin to crackle and pop and the sesame seeds smell toasted, about 5 minutes.

◦ Immediately transfer the seed blend to a spice grinder or coffee grinder; you may also use a high-powered blender. Let it cool for a few minutes, then grind the seed blend until it becomes a fine powder.

◦ Store in a glass jar with a tight-fitting lid in a cool, dry place for up to 2 weeks.

note: *I keep McCormick's dried minced lemon peel, called California Lemon Peel, in my spice cabinet. Another option is to mince strips of dried lemon peel. If you can't find dried lemon peel in any form— minced or in strips—you can use grated fresh lemon zest here as well; it will dry up nicely in the skillet.*

Citrus Curry Powder

Makes about ½ cup ◦ Prep Time: 5 minutes

When I learned nightshades were on my no-fly list, I thought curry powder was lost to me forever—until I realized that I could easily make my own version at home. This one might not have cayenne, but it makes up for it with spectacular flavor and heat from the white pepper.

---

2 tablespoons garlic powder

2 tablespoons turmeric powder

1 tablespoon dried minced lemon peel (see note)

1 tablespoon ground cumin

1 tablespoon onion powder

2 teaspoons ginger powder

2 teaspoons ground cinnamon

2 teaspoons ground mustard seeds

2 teaspoons ground white pepper

½ teaspoon ground black pepper

◦ Whisk together all of the ingredients until well combined. Transfer to a glass jar with a tight-fitting lid. Store in a cool, dry place for up to 2 weeks.

modifications: *To make this seasoning AIP compliant, omit the cumin, mustard seeds, and white and black pepper. Double the ginger powder and add ½ teaspoon ground cloves.*

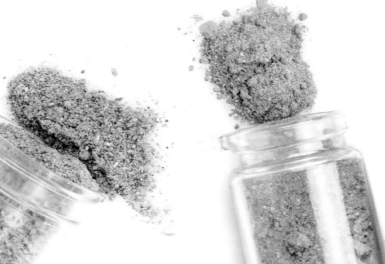

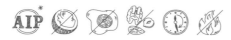 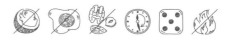

Cuban Sazón

Makes about ½ cup ◦ Prep Time: 5 minutes

This *sazón,* or seasoning blend, brings together some of my favorite flavors from my grandmother's kitchen, without the nightshades. Use it to add some Latin flair to any savory dish.

2 tablespoons garlic powder

2 tablespoons onion powder

1 tablespoon dried parsley

1 tablespoon ground cumin

1 teaspoon dried oregano leaves

1 teaspoon ground black pepper

◦ Mix all of the ingredients together and store in an airtight glass jar in a cool, dry place for up to 2 weeks.

modifications: *To make this seasoning AIP compliant, omit the cumin and black pepper. Add 2 teaspoons ginger powder, 2 teaspoons dried minced lemon peel (see note, opposite), and ½ teaspoon turmeric powder.*

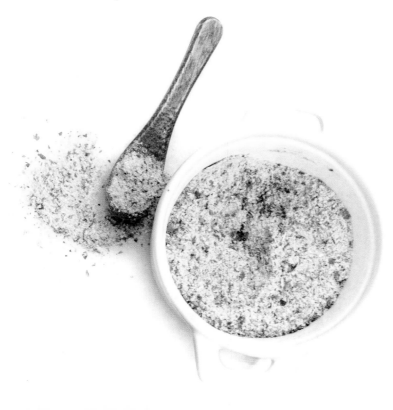

Turn Up the Heat Spice Blend

Makes about ¼ cup ◦ Prep Time: 5 minutes

This mix of spices gets its heat not from chili peppers but from white pepper, wasabi, and ginger. It isn't as spicy as a seasoning made with cayenne (which, as a nightshade, is on my hard-no list), but you can mix it into food to kick up the heat or sprinkle it on top as a finisher. Try it in my Legit Fried Chicken Tenders (page 228) or Presque Gumbo (page 292).

2 tablespoons ground white pepper

2 tablespoons wasabi powder (see note)

1 tablespoon ginger powder

1 tablespoon ground black pepper

◦ Mix all of the ingredients together and store in an airtight glass jar in a cool, dry place for up to 2 weeks.

note: *It's hard to find wasabi without junk in it. Granted, in the US it's impossible to find real wasabi, but we make do with horseradish concoctions. What you want to look for when shopping at your Asian market or the international aisle of your grocery store is a powder that doesn't contain sugar, food coloring, or maltodextrin. I like Asian Gourmet Japanese Wasabi, which is made from dehydrated horseradish root, mustard seed, spinach powder, and wasabi root power.*

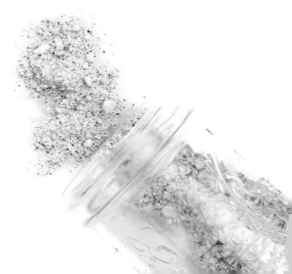

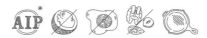

Pickled Asparagus + Pickled Radishes

1 jar pickled radishes + 1 jar pickled asparagus (6 servings per jar)
Prep Time: 5 minutes, plus 30 minutes to cool and 4 hours to pickle ○ Cook Time: 8 minutes

The pickled red onions in my first book, *Made Whole,* were so wildly popular, I knew I had to include more of my favorite pickled vegetables in this book. Radishes are spicy, crunchy little roots that are surprisingly low in carbs and packed with potassium and magnesium. Hello, electrolytes! Asparagus is high in glutathione, a powerful antioxidant. The beautiful colors make these pickled veggies the perfect addition to any meal. You will need two canning jars for this recipe: a widemouthed quart-sized jar and a 12-ounce jar.

2 cups filtered water

1½ cups apple cider vinegar

1 teaspoon fine salt (see note)

1 teaspoon black peppercorns

1 teaspoon stevia glycerite (optional)

2 cloves garlic, peeled

2 sprigs fresh rosemary

1½ cups thinly sliced radishes (about 2 bunches)

12 asparagus spears, trimmed to 6 inches

○ In a saucepan, combine the water, vinegar, salt, peppercorns, and stevia, if using. Bring to a simmer over medium heat.

○ While the brine comes to a simmer, clean a widemouthed quart-sized canning jar and a 12-ounce canning jar thoroughly with hot water and soap and dry with a clean kitchen towel.

○ Put a clove of garlic and a sprig of rosemary in each jar. Put the sliced radishes in the smaller jar and the asparagus in the larger one, trimming them more if necessary.

○ Once the salt has dissolved in the brine, pour it into the jars to cover the vegetables. Let the jars sit out at room temperature for 30 minutes, then cover them with tight-fitting lids and put them in the fridge to chill and develop flavor for at least 4 hours.

○ Store in the fridge for up to a month. Always use a clean fork or spoon to retrieve the pickled vegetables from the jars.

note: *For pickling, do not use a salt that contains iodine, such as table salt. An unrefined salt like Redmond Real Salt will work well here.*

modifications: *To make these veggies AIP compliant, replace the peppercorns in the brine with two ¼-inch pieces of peeled ginger; just make sure that each jar gets a knob when dividing the hot brine between them. Replace the stevia with 1 teaspoon yacón syrup.*

Per serving (2 spears asparagus): Calories **15** · Fat **0g** · Total Carbs **1.6g** · Fiber **0.7g** · Protein **0.7g**

Per serving (¼ cup radishes): Calories **13** · Fat **0g** · Total Carbs **14g** · Fiber **0.5g** · Protein **0.2g**

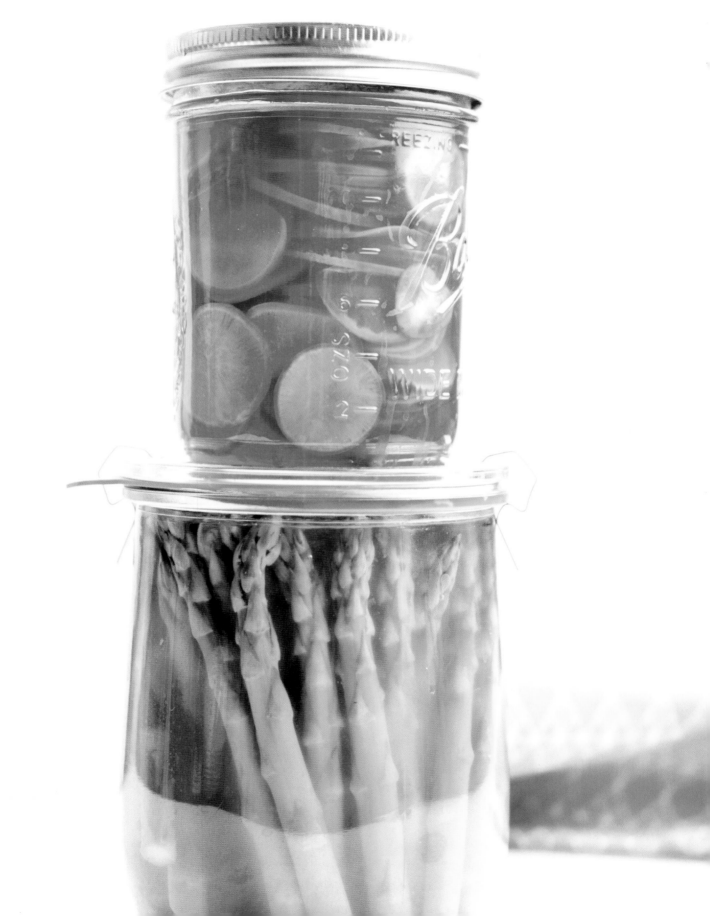

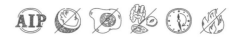

Gremolata with Olive Oil

Makes 1 cup (1 tablespoon per serving) ◦ Prep Time: 10 minutes

Traditional gremolata is a mixture of chopped herbs, garlic, and citrus zest. This wet rendition is reminiscent of chimichurri but forgoes the cilantro and vinegar. It's a deep green, nutrient-dense sauce that pairs perfectly with grilled meats and fried eggs.

2 cups roughly chopped fresh parsley

3 cloves garlic, peeled

Grated zest of 1 lemon

Juice of 3 lemons

¼ cup extra-virgin olive oil

½ teaspoon fine salt

◦ Put all of the ingredients in a food processor and pulse until minced.

◦ Store the gremolata in a glass jar in the fridge for up to a month. Always use a clean spoon to serve it from the jar.

Per serving: Calories **37** · Fat **3.6g** · Total Carbs **1.3g** · Fiber **0.3g** · Protein **0.3g**

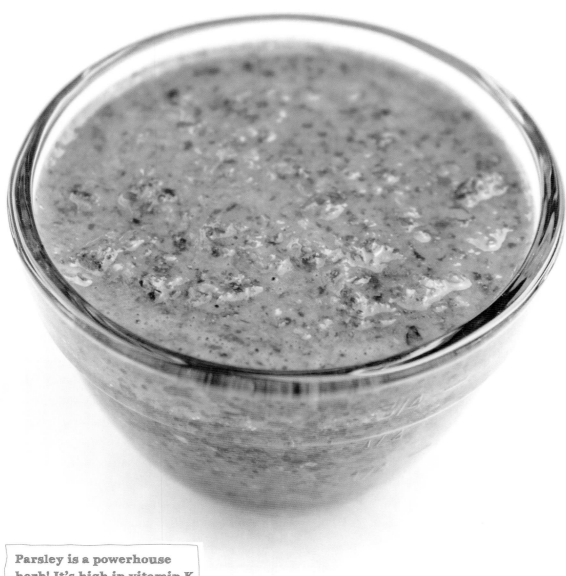

Parsley is a powerhouse herb! It's high in vitamin K and myricetin, which has anticancer effects.

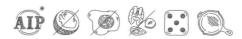

Onion + Bacon Spread

Makes 1 cup (1 tablespoon per serving) ◦ Prep Time: 10 minutes ◦ Cook Time: 50 minutes

If you're like me, you wish you could add bacon and caramelized onions to every meal. The delectable combination of sweet and salty is irresistible! However, frying up bacon and properly caramelizing onions takes way too long to do every day. Enter this spread: in an hour of your time, you'll have a jar of happiness sitting in your fridge, at the ready for all your bacon and onion needs, saving you time in the long run when it comes to dressing up your meals. A bit of mustard ups the creaminess and adds a little tang to balance the flavor. Slather this spread on burgers or steaks, or use it as a dip for roasted vegetables—you can't go wrong with bacon and onions.

7 slices thick-cut bacon (about 10 ounces)

1 large onion, thinly sliced

2 bay leaves

1 sprig fresh thyme

2 teaspoons spicy brown or Dijon mustard

◦ Heat a 15-inch skillet over medium heat. Line up the bacon in the skillet. Cook for 10 minutes, then flip the bacon over and cook for another 10 minutes, or until crispy.

◦ Use tongs to remove the bacon from the skillet, leaving all of the fat behind, and set the bacon aside. Add the onion, bay leaves, and thyme to the skillet. Cook, stirring occasionally, for 30 minutes, or until the onions are dark brown and very tender. Remove the bay leaves and thyme stem.

◦ Use a rubber spatula to transfer the onion mixture and all of the bacon fat to a quart-sized jar. Add the mustard and use an immersion blender to blend until creamy and mostly smooth, leaving some small chunks.

◦ Mince or crumble the crispy bacon and stir it into the onion mixture. Store the jar in the fridge for up to 2 weeks.

modifications: *To make this spread AIP compliant, replace the mustard with 2 teaspoons prepared horseradish.*

Per serving: Calories **29** · Fat **1.9g** · Total Carbs **1g** · Fiber **0.2g** · Protein **1.9g**

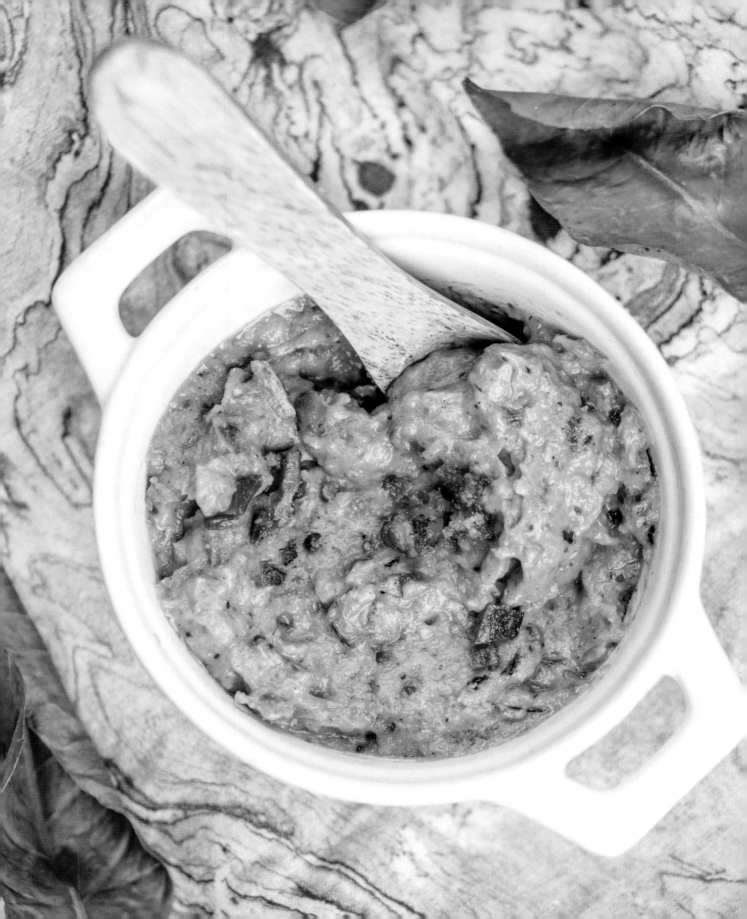

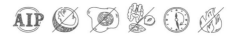

Briny Arugula Pesto

Makes 1½ cups (¼ cup per serving) ○ Prep Time: 15 minutes

I love a good herb sauce! Pesto is definitely in my top five, and I've always loved arugula pesto. The peppery green is absolutely divine and doubles well as an herb. This rendition uses green olives and a whole lot of garlic for a briny, tangy pesto without dairy or nuts. This versatile sauce is perfect on meats, eggs, greens, and noodles, and it pairs well with Mediterranean flavors—you even can use it as a tapenade. Perhaps it's not even a pesto at all, but to avoid overcomplicating things, we'll just run with it.

3 cups arugula

10 large green olives, pitted

8 cloves garlic, peeled

½ cup extra-virgin olive oil

1 tablespoon aged balsamic vinegar (see notes)

1 teaspoon prepared horseradish

½ teaspoon fine salt

○ Put all of the ingredients in a food processor and pulse until you have a slightly chunky but well-combined sauce. Store in a jar in the fridge for up to 3 weeks.

notes: *Instead of using plain green olives, you can use garlic-stuffed green olives to make this pesto even more garlicky.*

Not all aged balsamic vinegars are created equal. Grape must should not be the first ingredient. If it is, you're getting grape syrup instead of a truly aged vinegar, and your balsamic, while sweet and syrupy, isn't a true balsamic and will have way more carbs and sugar per serving.

variation: basil + arugula pesto. *For a more traditional pesto, omit the olives and add 2 cups fresh basil and ¼ cup whole raw cashews, pine nuts, or shelled hemp seeds (aka hemp hearts).*

Per serving: Calories **182** · Fat **19.1g** · Total Carbs **3g** · Fiber **0.6g** · Protein **0.7g**

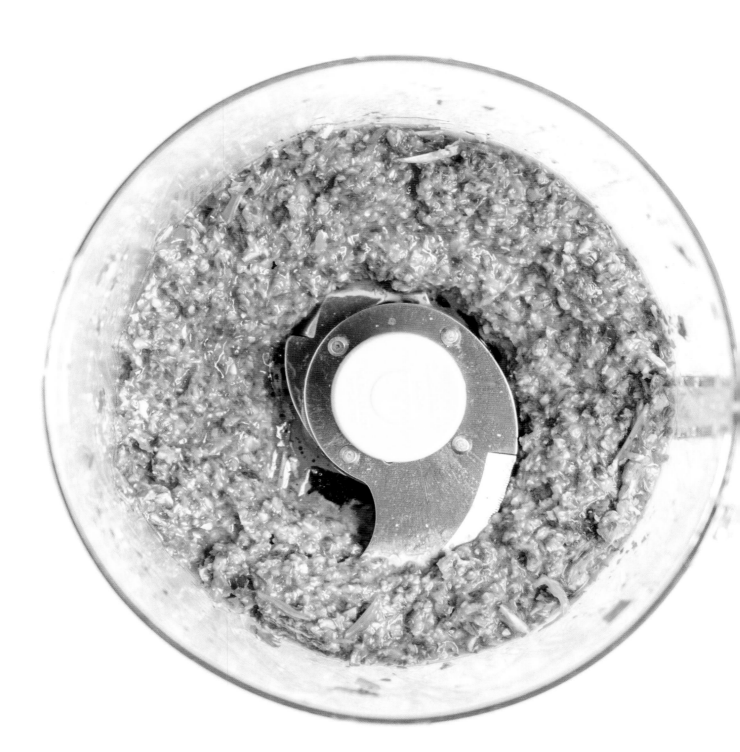

Balsamic Roasted Cashews

Serves 8 (2 tablespoons per serving) ◦ Prep Time: 10 minutes ◦ Cook Time: 20 minutes

These delightful roasted cashews are flavored with balsamic vinegar, vanilla, ginger, and cinnamon. They remind me of honey roasted nuts, but without the inflammatory oils and sugar. Note: The serving size is just 2 tablespoons because cashews, while high in monounsaturated fats, are also quite starchy. But 2 tablespoons is plenty for a delicious addition to a salad or snack plate—try adding them to a Crispy Chicken + Strawberry Balsamic Salad (page 222) or a charcuterie platter featuring Roasted Garlic "Hummus" (page 324).

1 cup whole raw cashews (see notes)

2 tablespoons aged balsamic vinegar (see notes, page 90)

1 tablespoon coconut aminos

1 teaspoon vanilla extract

½ teaspoon ginger powder

½ teaspoon ground cinnamon

Pinch of fine salt

◦ Place an oven rack in the middle position. Preheat the oven to 400°F. Line a sheet pan with parchment paper.

◦ Put the cashews on the prepared sheet pan and add the remaining ingredients. Toss to combine and coat the cashews, then spread them out over the parchment paper.

◦ Roast in the oven on the middle rack for 15 to 20 minutes, until the cashews are evenly browned all over and the liquid has dried up. Remove from the oven and let cool, then use a spatula to scrape up the cashews and mix them together.

◦ Store at room temperature for up to 5 days.

notes: *To reduce the phytic acid in nuts, soaking them is recommended: see page 62 for more information.*

For a lower-carb version, use macadamia nuts, which have half the carbs of cashews.

Per serving: Calories **97** · Fat **7.1g** · Total Carbs **6.2g** · Fiber **0.6g** · Protein **3g**

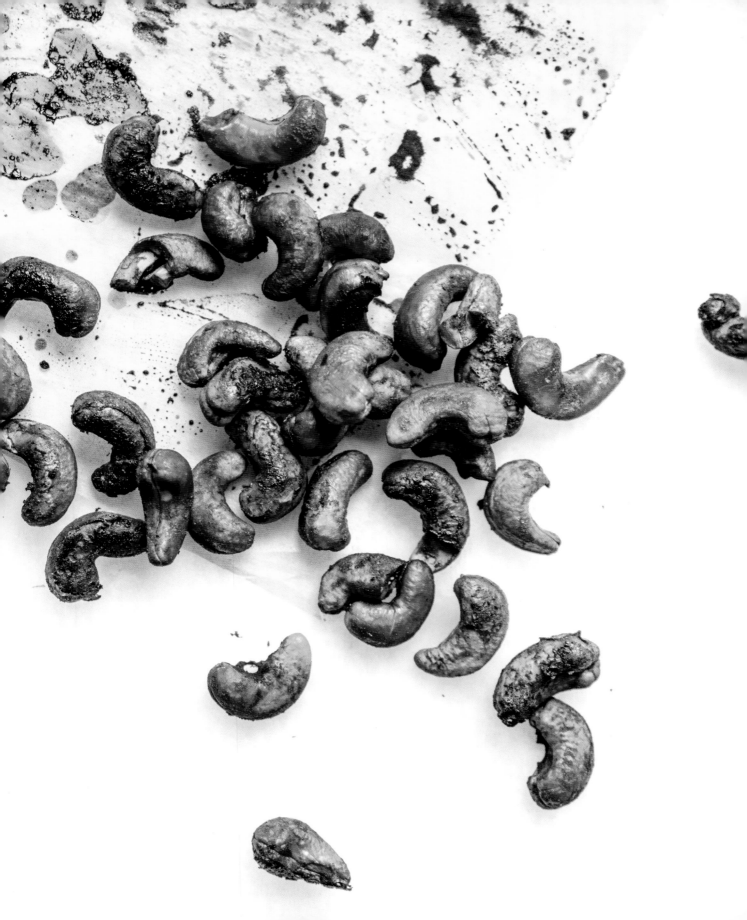

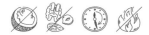

Horseradish Mayo

Makes 1½ cups (2 tablespoons per serving)　○　Prep Time: 3 minutes

Eating for better eyesight? Forget the carrots and reach for egg yolks! They are rich in lutein and zeaxanthin, which block blue light from reaching the retina. Blue light emitted from screens damages the retina's light-sensitive cells. This three-yolk mayo packs grated horseradish root, which gives it a tangy flavor, and is high in glucosinolates, sulfur-containing compounds said to have anticancer effects. Who knew mayo could have so many superpowers?

3 large egg yolks, room temperature

¾ cup avocado oil

2 tablespoons white wine vinegar

1 tablespoon prepared horseradish

1 tablespoon spicy brown or Dijon mustard

¼ teaspoon fine salt

○ Carefully place the egg yolks at the bottom of a widemouthed quart-sized jar so they don't break. Add the remaining ingredients. Insert an immersion blender into the jar, cupping the yolks with the end of the blender.

○ Turn on the blender and hold it still for 30 seconds, until you see the mixture becoming white and creamy, then slowly move the blender up and down in small motions until the entire mixture has become white, thick, and creamy.

○ Use a rubber spatula to scrape any mayo off the blender. Cover the jar with a tight-fitting lid and store it in the fridge for up to 10 days.

notes: *You can use any vinegar you have on hand, except balsamic.*

I have yet to figure out a homemade egg-free mayo, but there is a creamy, AIP-friendly egg-free sauce called Toum in my first book, Made Whole. *Chosen Foods also makes a good egg-free mayo. You can mix horseradish into that to get a similar condiment.*

variation: traditional aioli. *Replace the horseradish with 1 tablespoon minced garlic.*

variation: traditional mayo. *Leave out the horseradish.*

Per serving: Calories **137** · Fat **14.8g** · Total Carbs **0.4g** · Fiber **0.1g** · Protein **0.7g**

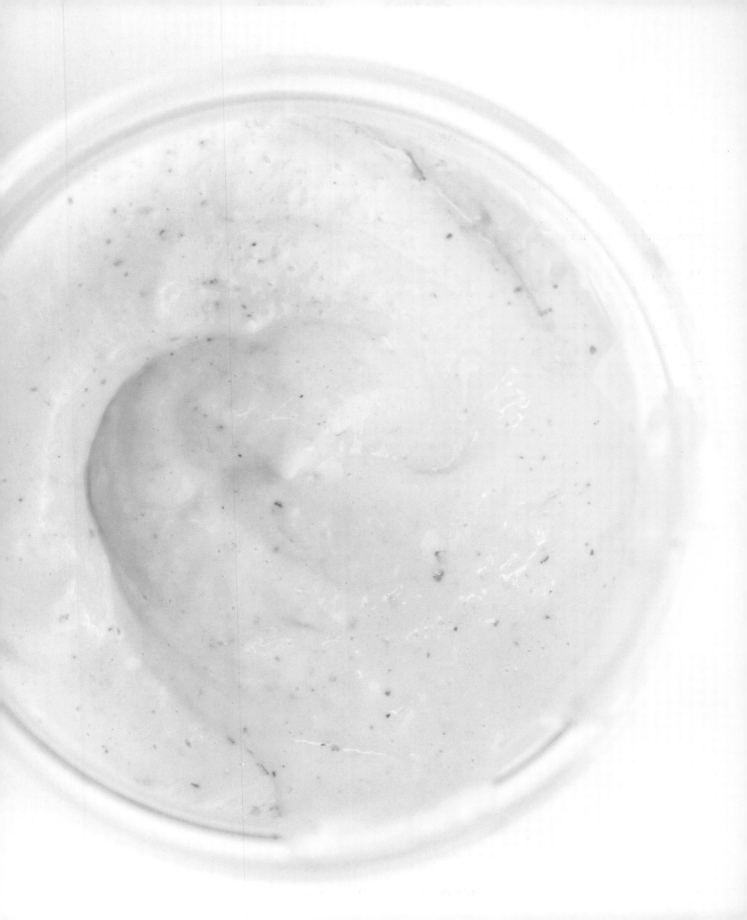

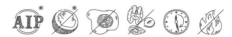

Balsamic Mustard Vinaigrette

Makes about 1 cup (2 tablespoons per serving) ○ Prep Time: 5 minutes

Forget the store-bought stuff! This vinaigrette is whisked together to give the ol' vinegar-and-oil dressing a little more body and jazzed up with some mustard for an extra kick. This versatile dressing is perfect for all your salad needs and doubles as a fantastic marinade!

2 tablespoons aged balsamic vinegar (see notes, page 90)

2 tablespoons coconut aminos

2 tablespoons spicy brown or Dijon mustard

½ teaspoon dried oregano leaves

½ teaspoon fine salt

½ teaspoon ground black pepper

¾ cup avocado oil or extra-virgin olive oil

○ In a medium-sized bowl, whisk together all of the ingredients except the oil. While whisking at a moderate pace, drizzle in the oil in a very thin and constant stream until fully incorporated. Store in the fridge for up to 3 weeks.

modifications: *To make this dressing AIP compliant, omit the mustard and black pepper and add another tablespoon of vinegar to compensate. To make it coconut-free, use ½ teaspoon yacón syrup or honey instead of the coconut aminos.*

variation: creamy balsamic mustard dressing. *If you like a creamy, extra-rich dressing, add 2 egg yolks to the vinegar and mustard mixture and continue the recipe as written.*

Per serving: Calories **244** · Fat **27.3g** · Total Carbs **1.0g** · Fiber **0.1g** · Protein **0g**

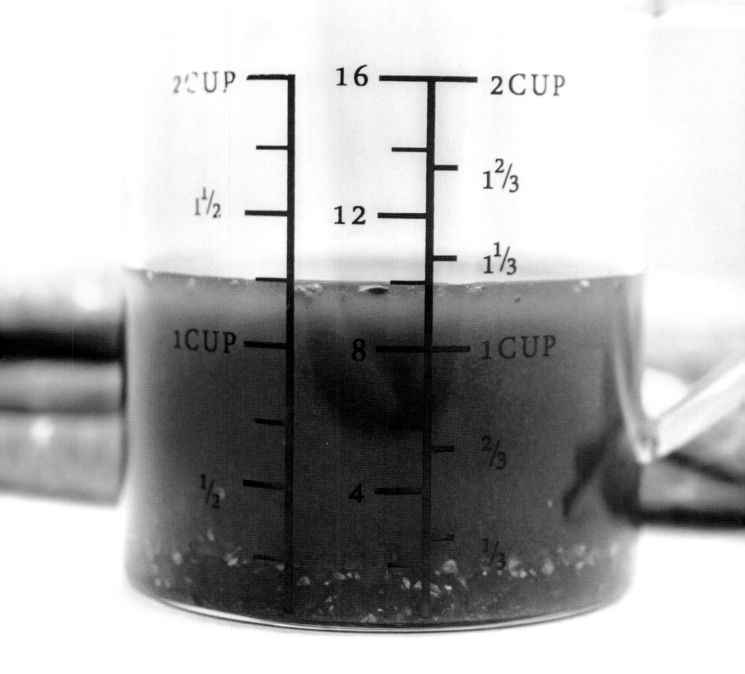

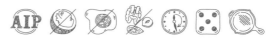

Green Onion Relish

Makes 2 cups (2 tablespoons per serving) ◦ Prep Time: 10 minutes ◦ Cook Time: 10 minutes

Prepare to become addicted to this amazing condiment. I first tasted it as a dinner guest at my friend Margaret's home in Miami Beach. She made it with leeks and ginger, and it was to die for. I forget where she said she learned the recipe, but I can tell you that I have been thinking about it ever since, and now I've made a version for you that's dreamy. I used green onions and garlic because I love garlic, but minced fresh ginger would work wonderfully as well.

6 green onions, roughly chopped

4 cloves garlic, peeled

2 teaspoons fine salt

⅔ cup extra-virgin olive oil

½ cup avocado oil

◦ Place the green onions and garlic in a food processor and pulse until finely minced.

◦ Open the food processor and mix in the salt. Set aside.

◦ In a large saucepan, heat the oils over medium-high heat until they reach deep-fry temperature (about 375°F)—when the end of a wooden spoon handle sizzles when inserted into the oil, it's ready.

◦ Remove the pot from the heat and place it on a stable heatproof surface. Add the green onion mixture to the hot oil and whisk to combine, then transfer the mixture to a heatproof glass jar. Let cool before sealing with a tight-fitting lid.

◦ Store in a cool, dry place for up to 5 days. The sauce won't go bad that fast, but it will lose its bite after 5 days.

Per serving: Calories **71** · Fat **7.9g** · Total Carbs **0.3g** · Fiber **0.1g** · Protein **0.1g**

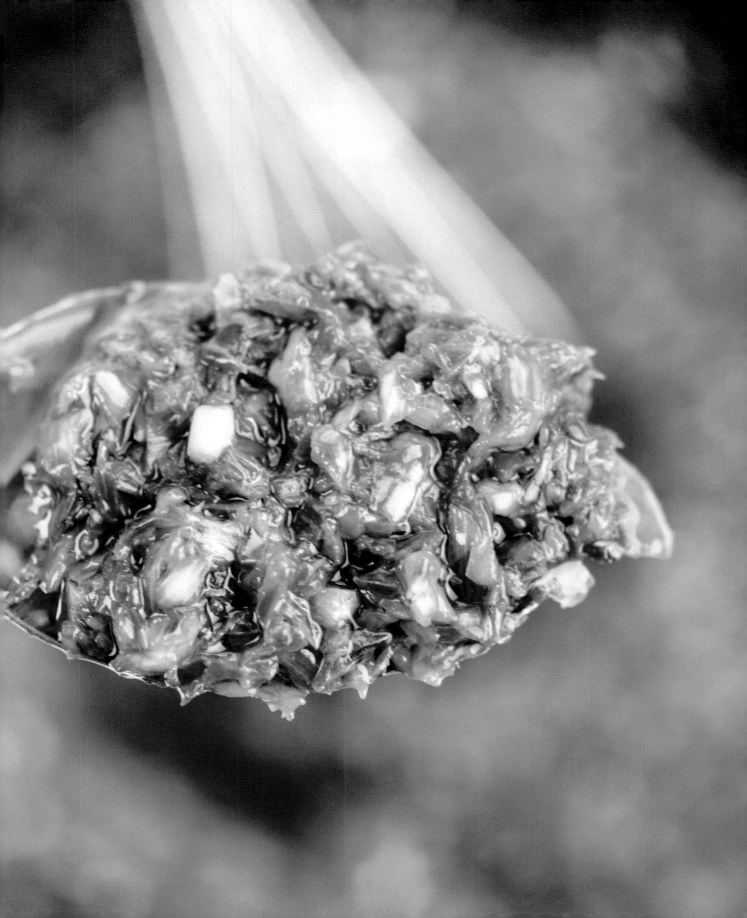

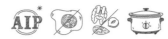

Slow Cooker Blueberry BBQ Sauce

Makes 3 cups (2 tablespoons per serving) ◦ Prep Time: 5 minutes ◦ Cook Time: 16 hours

This squeaky-clean, sweet-and-tangy sauce is made without nightshades or sugar. And it simmers all night, making it an easy hands-off recipe.

---

3 cups fresh or frozen blueberries

1½ cups apple cider vinegar

¼ cup coconut aminos

1 tablespoon fish sauce

2 cloves garlic, peeled

2 whole cloves

1 teaspoon cumin seeds

1 cinnamon stick

½ teaspoon stevia glycerite (see note)

◦ Combine all of the ingredients except the stevia in a slow cooker. Cover and cook on high for 3 to 4 hours, until the blueberries are broken down and the mixture is a dark blueish-purple soup of sorts.

◦ Open the lid and fish out the cinnamon stick and cloves with a spoon. Blend the sauce with an immersion blender until pureed. Add the stevia, cover with the lid, and cook on low for 12 hours.

◦ Stir well and strain into a quart-sized jar, removing the solids. Let cool for 30 minutes before sealing and putting in the fridge.

◦ Store in the fridge for up to 2 months or in the freezer for up to 6 months.

note: *Stevia glycerite is less sweet than regular stevia drops. If using regular stevia, reduce the amount to 10 drops. You may also use 1 tablespoon of raw honey instead of the stevia.*

modifications: *To make this sauce AIP compliant, omit the cumin seeds and stevia and add 1 teaspoon yacón syrup.*

Per serving: Calories **18** · Fat **0.1g** · Total Carbs **3.7g** · Fiber **0.5g** · Protein **0.2g**

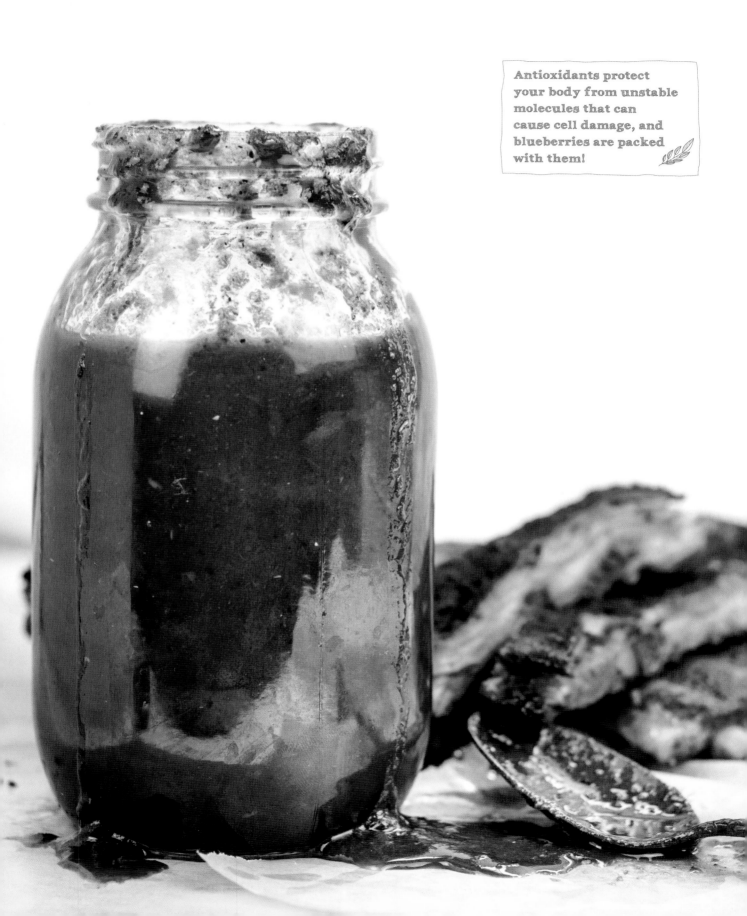

Antioxidants protect your body from unstable molecules that can cause cell damage, and blueberries are packed with them!

Homemade Kraut

Makes 2 quarts (1 cup per serving) ○ Prep Time: 30 minutes, plus 3 weeks to ferment

Fermented foods feed the good bacteria in your gut. While there are a lot of great probiotics on the market, they can be pricey. A couple of heads of cabbage and some salt will cost you less than $5, and that's all you need to make sauerkraut at home. I like using red cabbage for the added polyphenols—and because it's just so dang pretty.

2 small heads red cabbage (about 2 pounds total)

4 teaspoons fine salt, plus more for sprinkling (see notes)

notes: *When fermenting foods, do not use a salt that contains iodine, such as table salt. An unrefined salt like Redmond Real Salt will work well here.*

If the fermented cabbage smells foul or has black spots, the batch was contaminated and must be tossed. The best way to avoid contaminated kraut is to make sure the jars, lids, and tamper are sterile before you begin.

○ Sterilize two quart-sized or one 64-ounce jar(s) with lid(s), and a tamper: To sterilize your jars, lids, and tamper, submerge them in a large stockpot full of hot water and boil for at least 10 minutes. Use clean tongs to remove them from the boiling water and place them on clean paper towels until you're ready to use them. Make sure you have a cool, dark place to put the jars while they ferment (65°F to 72°F is ideal).

○ To shred the cabbage, cut the heads into quarters, core them, and run them through a food processor fitted with the thin slicer attachment—works like a charm. You can also shred it by hand with a sharp knife, very thinly slicing the cored quarters crosswise.

○ Divide the shredded cabbage into two batches. Put one batch in a large bowl and sprinkle it with 2 teaspoons of the salt. Massage the cabbage with the salt until it is tender and releasing fluid, about 5 minutes. Put the prepared cabbage in the jar and use the sterilized tamper or wooden spoon to press down as much as possible. Repeat with the remaining cabbage and salt.

○ Use the tamper to press down on the cabbage until it is just below the level of the fluid, then sprinkle a little extra salt on top. Close the lid(s) tightly and place the jar(s) in a cool, dark place for 3 weeks.

○ In 3 weeks, it's harvest day! Open the jars; you may need to give the lid a light tap on the counter to relieve the pressure. The kraut will smell like roasting broccoli—you know, the scent that cruciferous vegetables have; it's not pleasant, but it's not a putrid smell, either. If there are vile odors or visible mold, toss it.

○ Use a clean fork to toss the kraut and mix it up a bit, then taste it. You can now store the kraut in the fridge for up to a month. Always use a clean utensil to serve it.

Per serving: Calories **27** · Fat **0.2g** · Total Carbs **6g** · Fiber **4.1g** · Protein **1.3g**

The cheapest and best probiotic you will ever have.

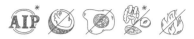

Mozz Blocks

Makes twelve 1-inch blocks (1 block per serving) ◦ Prep Time: 30 minutes, plus 1 hour to set

In my first book, there's a recipe for nut-free "cheese" made from cauliflower and nutritional yeast, and it's a killer yellow cheese recipe. For this book, I wanted to make a cauliflower- and coconut-free cheese that can replace creamy-dreamy mozzarella! While cashews and parsnips may seem like an unlikely pairing, they hit a home run here. This creamy, dairy-free cheese hits the spot: snack on it as is or melt it into noodles or on your favorite pizza crust (such as "Cheesy" Mushroom Meatzas, page 230).

1 medium parsnip (about 4 ounces)

½ cup filtered water

¾ cup raw cashews (about 4 ounces)

¼ cup unflavored grass-fed beef gelatin

1 tablespoon fish sauce

2 teaspoons white wine vinegar

1 teaspoon garlic powder

¼ teaspoon ground black pepper

¼ cup extra-virgin olive oil

¼ cup boiling filtered water

⅛ teaspoon fine salt (optional)

◦ Dice the parsnip and place it in a small saucepan with ½ cup of water. Cover with the lid and bring to a simmer over medium heat. Simmer for 5 minutes, or until the parsnip is tender. Remove from the heat and drain.

◦ Put the steamed parsnip, cashews, gelatin, fish sauce, vinegar, garlic powder, and pepper in a high-powered blender or food processor and blend until smooth. With the machine running, slowly drizzle in the olive oil until a thick cream forms. Then slowly pour in the boiling water until it is fully incorporated. Taste the mixture and add the salt, if needed.

◦ Pour the mixture into 12 wells of a silicone ice cube mold or a 9 by 5-inch loaf pan lined with parchment paper. Place in the fridge for about 1 hour to firm up.

◦ Remove the cheese from the mold or loaf pan; if you used a loaf pan, cut the cheese into twelve 1-inch blocks. Store in the fridge for up to a week.

modifications: *To make this "cheese" AIP compliant and nut-free, replace the cashews with 4 ounces peeled and steamed zucchini or cauliflower.*

Per serving: Calories **112** · Fat **8.7g** · Total Carbs **4.2g** · Fiber **0.8g** · Protein **4.8g**

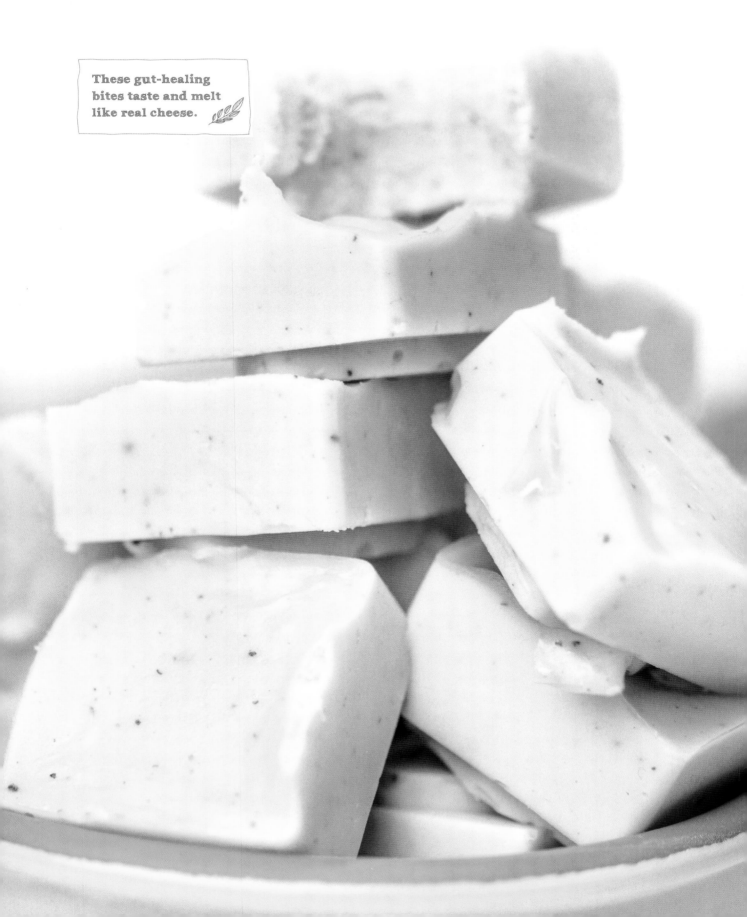

These gut-healing bites taste and melt like real cheese.

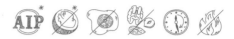

Green Basil Curry Sauce

Makes 2 cups (¼ cup per serving) ○ Prep Time: 20 minutes

I once worked on a food truck in San Diego. We were a staple at the Hillcrest Farmers Market, and there, in front of the truck, my friend Chef Gage would set up a stir-fry station with his big wok. He made the best bowls with a rainbow of sauces. The creamy basil curry was my favorite. This is a nightshade-free ode to that sauce. This bright and creamy condiment is perfect for stir-fries or to jazz up fried eggs. It pairs well with grilled meats and roasted vegetables alike; try it with Hail Mary Chicken (page 258) or Cumin-Dusted Mahi-Mahi (page 274).

1 packed cup fresh basil leaves

1 cup chopped celery

1 cup chopped green onions

3 cloves garlic, peeled

1 (2-inch) knob fresh ginger, peeled and minced

2 tablespoons Citrus Curry Powder (page 82)

1 teaspoon ground coriander

1 teaspoon ground sumac

1 teaspoon ground white pepper

Grated zest of 3 limes

Juice of 3 limes

⅔ cup canned unsweetened full-fat coconut milk

○ Put all of the ingredients in a blender or food processor and blend until smooth.

○ Store in a glass jar in the fridge for up to 5 days or in the freezer for up to a month.

> Basil is an excellent source of vitamins A and K. In this curry sauce, these fat-soluble vitamins are paired with the fats they need to be properly absorbed.

modifications: *To make this sauce AIP compliant, use the AIP version of the curry powder; omit the coriander, sumac, and white pepper; and add 1 teaspoon ground cinnamon and 1 teaspoon ginger powder. To make it coconut-free, use cashew milk or Salted Cashew Cream (page 76) instead of the coconut milk.*

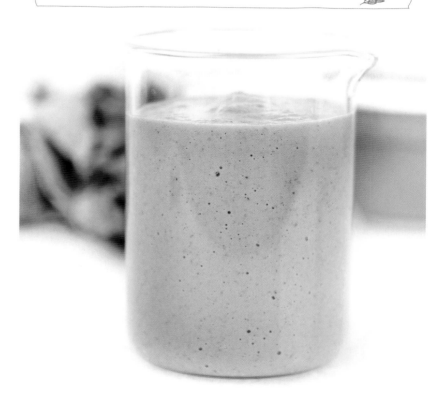

Per serving: Calories **78** · Fat **6.4g** · Total Carbs **4.2g** · Fiber **1.9g** · Protein **1.4g**

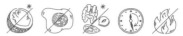

Stir-In Coffee Creamer

Makes 3 cups (2 tablespoons per serving) ○ Prep Time: 10 minutes

Giving up coffee creamer is hard for most people. It's one thing I see time and time again online: "What am I going to put in my coffee?" And let's be honest, most of the store-bought dairy-free options are not very good—they are thin, bland, lacking in flavor, and full of emulsifiers and other ingredients we don't want to start the day with. This recipe is tried, true, and loved by many. It's thick and creamy and stirs in like a dream. It's an absolute game changer!

¾ cup raw cashews

¾ cup unsweetened canned coconut cream

¾ cup filtered water

¼ cup collagen peptides

¼ cup MCT oil

1 teaspoon vanilla extract

1 teaspoon ground cinnamon

⅛ teaspoon fine salt

notes: *If you don't have MCT oil, increase the amount of coconut cream to 1 cup.*

Soaking nuts or seeds with a pinch of salt for 4 to 8 hours reduces their phytic acid content and makes them easier to digest. See page 62 for more information.

modifications: *To make this creamer coconut-free, omit the coconut cream, add ¾ cup dairy-free milk of choice, and use a palm oil–based MCT oil or ghee. To make it nut-free, use ¾ cup shelled hemp seeds (aka hemp hearts) or pumpkin seeds instead of the cashews.*

○ Put all of the ingredients in a high-powered blender and blend until smooth. If you're using a regular blender, blend for 2 minutes, then strain the mixture through a fine-mesh sieve.

○ Store in a glass jar in the fridge for up to a week. Stir into hot or cold coffee or tea!

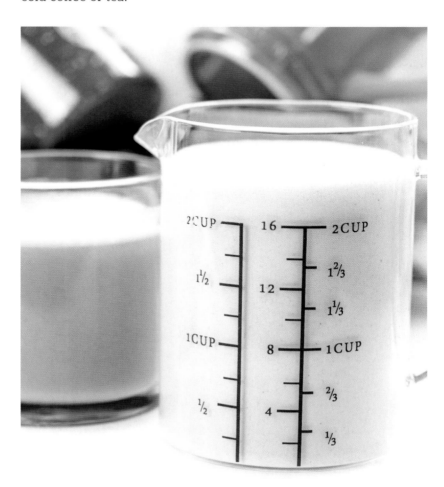

Per serving: Calories **76** · Fat **6.4g** · Total Carbs **1.5g** · Fiber **0.3g** · Protein **4g**

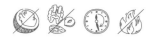

Cilantro Aioli

Makes 1½ cups (1 tablespoon per serving) ◦ Prep Time: 10 minutes

I hope my mom doesn't mind that I borrowed this recipe from her Miami restaurant, Green Gables Café. They used to serve an amazing pulled turkey sandwich with cilantro aioli, and I made that sauce hundreds of times while I was the chef there. Here, I've scaled down the recipe for a home-cooked version that you will be adding to every meal. Use it on meats, eggs, or salads or as a dip!

Leaves from 1 bunch fresh cilantro, roughly chopped (about 2 cups)

3 cloves garlic, peeled

1 tablespoon Dijon mustard

½ teaspoon fine salt

½ teaspoon grated lemon zest

Juice of 1 lemon

3 large egg yolks, room temperature

1¼ cups avocado oil

◦ Put the cilantro, garlic, mustard, salt, lemon zest, and lemon juice in a food processor and pulse until minced. Turn off the food processor.

◦ Add the egg yolks and turn on the food processor. Immediately begin to drizzle in the avocado oil in a needle-thin stream. Most food processors come with a tube that fits into the top and has a tiny hole at the bottom. It is meant for exactly this purpose: pour the oil through this attachment.

◦ Keep blending until all of the oil is incorporated and the aioli is thick and creamy. Turn off the food processor and use a spatula to transfer the aioli to a glass jar. Store in the fridge for up to 10 days.

notes: *You may use parsley or arugula in this recipe if you're one of those folks with an aversion to cilantro.*

You may also use extra-virgin olive oil instead of avocado oil. While I love cooking with olive oil, I feel the flavor is too strong for mayo, but that's a personal preference.

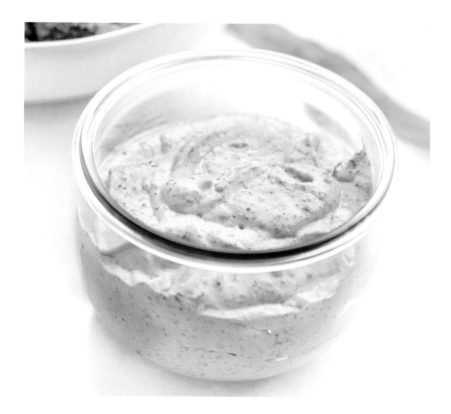

Per serving: Calories **109** · Fat **12g** · Total Carbs **0.4g** · Fiber **0.1g** · Protein **0.4g**

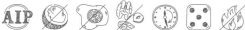

Frozen Herb Blocks

Makes twelve 1 by 1½-inch blocks (1 block per serving) ◦ Prep Time: 15 minutes

I use a lot of fresh herbs in my cooking, but not always enough to use an entire bunch—I often end up with extras that are beginning to wilt in the fridge. Waste not, want not is my motto. I run a minimal-waste kitchen. So what to do with the extras? This method shows you how to transform any combination of herbs into flavor bombs that won't expire. I use them to make my Perfect Roast Chicken (page 254) and Herbed Yellowfin Tuna Steaks (page 276). Let these herbaceous fat blocks melt in a skillet to spice up a stir-fry or use them to top a steak before serving.

4 cups fresh herb leaves of choice, any combination

1 cup extra-virgin olive oil

2 cloves garlic, peeled

◦ Put all of the ingredients in a blender or food processor and puree until smooth. Transfer to an ice cube tray or silicone mold and freeze.

◦ You can keep the blocks in the tray or unmold them and store in a reusable container in the freezer for up to 3 months.

note: *I use a lot of cilantro, dill, parsley, oregano, and rosemary, so my blocks usually contain a mix of these herbs, but truly any combination works. They all taste amazing!*

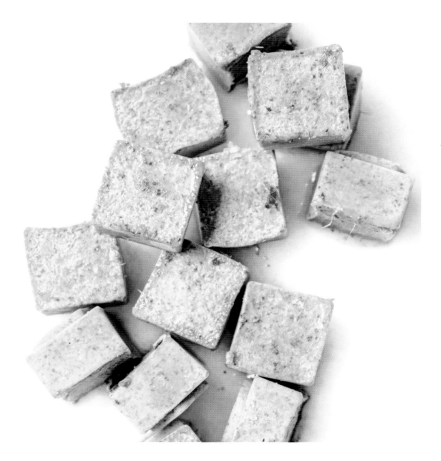

Per block: Calories **161** · Fat **18g** · Total Carbs **0.4g** · Fiber **0.2g** · Protein **0.1g**

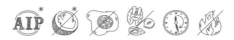

Blender Guac

Makes 2 cups (¼ cup per serving) ○ Prep Time: 10 minutes

All the deliciousness of guacamole, hold the messy kitchen. This dreamy, creamy guac is perfect for dollops or scoops. I like using unsweetened coconut milk yogurt for the probiotics and extra creaminess, but any unsweetened dairy-free yogurt or good ol' canned coconut cream will do. If you fare well with dairy, Greek yogurt will work too.

1 bunch fresh cilantro

4 ripe Hass avocados, peeled, halved, and pitted

½ cup extra-virgin olive oil

2 tablespoons apple cider vinegar

2 tablespoons unsweetened plain coconut milk yogurt

2 cloves garlic, peeled

1 teaspoon grated lemon zest

Juice of 2 lemons

1 teaspoon ground cumin

1 teaspoon fine salt

½ teaspoon ground black pepper

○ Trim the ends off the cilantro stems.

○ Put all of the ingredients in a blender and puree until smooth. Use a rubber spatula to transfer everything to an airtight container. Store in the fridge for up to 5 days.

modifications: *To make this guac AIP compliant, omit the black pepper and cumin and add ½ teaspoon onion powder and ½ teaspoon garlic powder.*

Per serving: Calories **249** · Fat **25g** · Total Carbs **7.3g** · Fiber **4.9g** · Protein **1.7g**

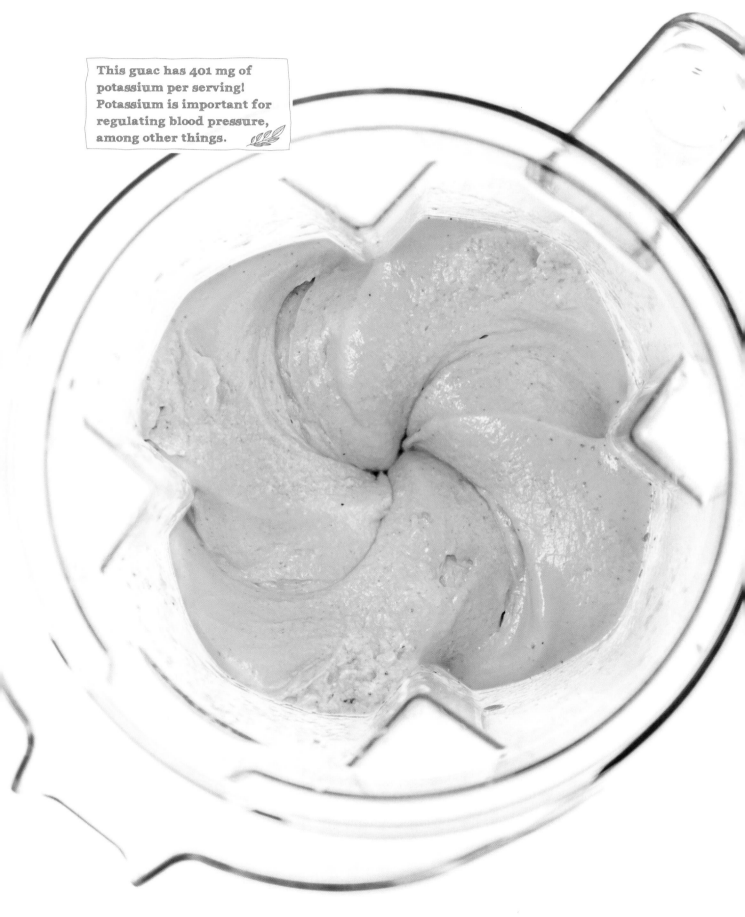

This guac has 401 mg of potassium per serving! Potassium is important for regulating blood pressure, among other things.

BREAKFAST

For me, crispy fried eggs are as good as it gets. In case you want to get a bit more creative, this chapter has more than a few ideas for the incredible edible egg! Egg whites are packed with protein, and the yolks contain lots of great fats. Eggs are also a good source of iodine. If you can't do eggs, I've included some delicious egg-free dishes for you too. From sweet to savory, there's a nourishing breakfast recipe here for everyone.

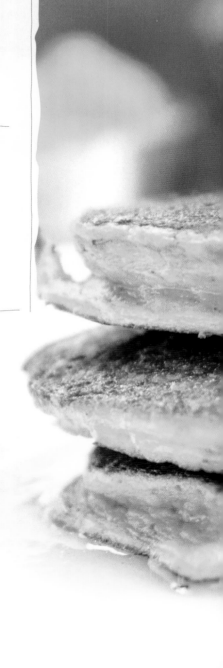

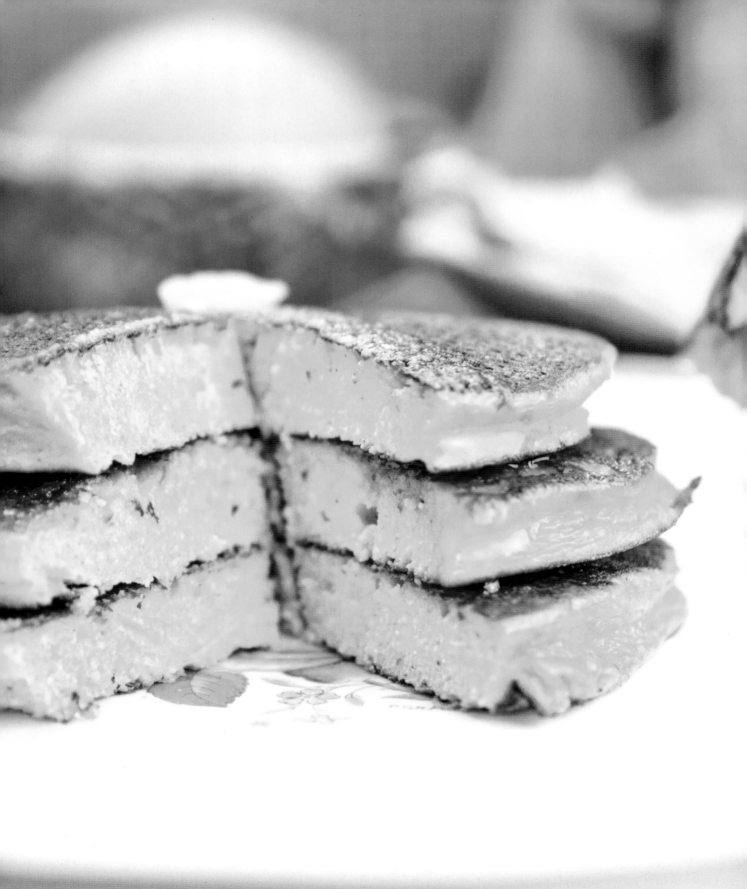

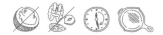

Eggs Bianca

Serves 2 ◦ Prep Time: 10 minutes ◦ Cook Time: 20 minutes

I love dishes like shakshuka or "eggs in purgatory," where the eggs simmer gently in a flavorful vegetable sauce. Here I forgo the usual tomato base for a creamy white sauce with Italian flavors. It's the perfect brunch recipe or quick dinner for two.

1 tablespoon extra-virgin olive oil

1 large zucchini, spiral sliced into noodles (about 3 cups noodles)

2 cloves garlic, minced

1 teaspoon fine salt, divided

2 cups Cauliflower Sour Cream (page 74)

4 large eggs

½ teaspoon ground black pepper

5 fresh basil leaves, chopped, for garnish

1 green onion, sliced, for garnish

◦ Heat a large skillet over medium heat. When it's hot, drizzle in the olive oil.

◦ Add the zucchini noodles, garlic, and ½ teaspoon of the salt to the skillet and sauté for 2 to 3 minutes, until the noodles are tender. Spread the sour cream over the noodles, then bring the contents of the skillet to a gentle simmer.

◦ Make 4 wells in the creamy zoodles and crack the eggs into the wells. Sprinkle with the remaining ½ teaspoon of salt and the pepper. Cover with a tight-fitting lid and simmer over low heat for 8 to 10 minutes, until the eggs are cooked through.

◦ Remove the skillet from the heat and garnish with the basil and green onion.

Per serving: Calories **351** · Fat **24.5g** · Total Carbs **16.2g** · Fiber **4.8g** · Protein **17.7g**

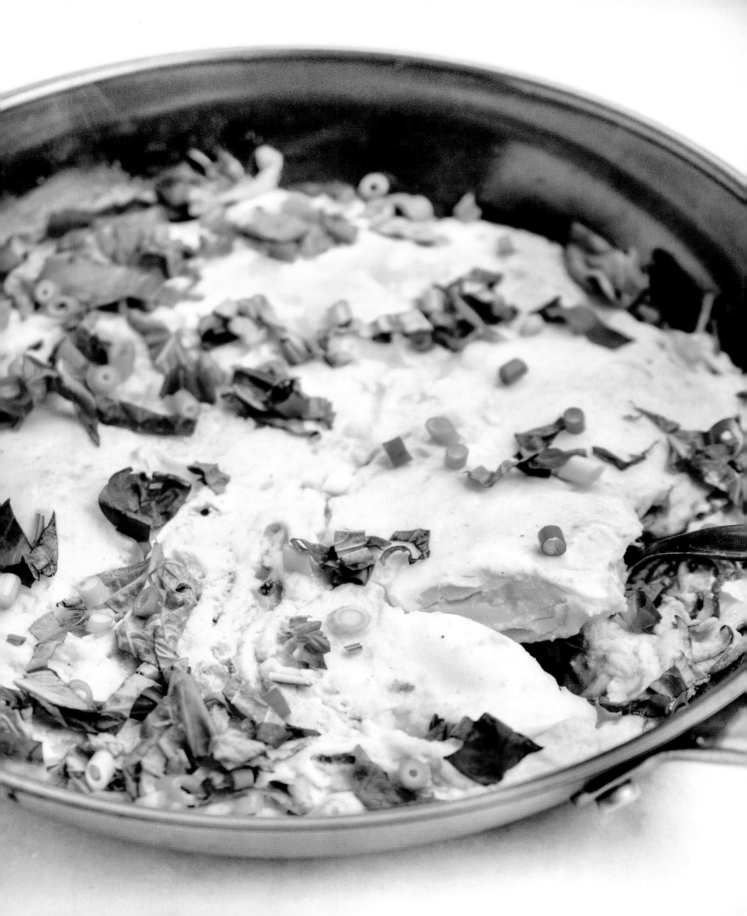

Broccoli Noodle Egg Skillet

Serves 2 ◦ Prep Time: 10 minutes ◦ Cook Time: 20 minutes

This egg-and-noodle creation might use some unlikely ingredients, but it just works. The noodles are tender and go so well with the savory sautéed onions and broccoli. The eggs add a creamy, saucy element, and the coconut butter drizzle adds a tad of richness. Yum!

2 tablespoons ghee or coconut oil

1½ cups broccoli florets

¼ cup minced white onions

1 (7-ounce) bag shirataki noodles

4 large eggs

½ teaspoon fine salt

1 green onion, sliced, for garnish

1 teaspoon everything bagel seasoning, for garnish

2 tablespoons coconut butter, melted, for garnish

modifications: *To make this dish coconut-free, use ghee and replace the coconut butter with tahini or avocado oil mayo.*

◦ Heat a 15-inch skillet over medium heat. When it's hot, melt the ghee in the skillet, then add the broccoli and onions. Sauté for 5 to 8 minutes, until the vegetables are tender and a little browned.

◦ While the veggies cook, empty the noodles into a colander and rinse them with fresh water. Shake off the excess water and add the noodles to the skillet. Sauté for 5 minutes, mixing the noodles with the veggies, then spread them evenly in the skillet.

◦ Make 4 wells in the noodle-and-veggie mixture, then crack the eggs into the wells and sprinkle everything with the salt.

◦ Use a spatula to spread the egg whites around in the noodles without breaking the yolks. Then let everything cook undisturbed until the egg whites are cooked through, about 8 minutes.

◦ Remove the skillet from the heat and sprinkle with the sliced green onion and everything bagel seasoning. Drizzle the coconut butter over the eggs and serve hot!

Per serving: Calories **423** · Fat **34.6g** · Total Carbs **14.4g** · Fiber **6.4g** · Protein **15.8g**

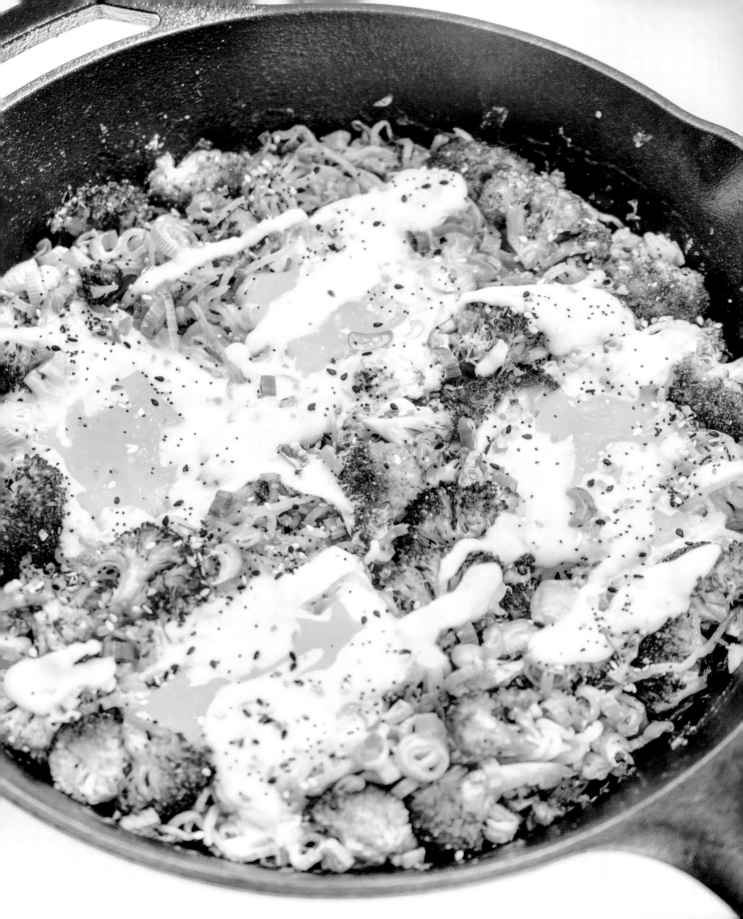

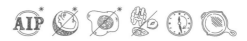

Sweet Onion Breakfast Bowls

Serves 4　◦　Prep Time: 10 minutes　◦　Cook Time: 20 minutes

This is my kind of Saturday morning meal. It's warm and filling and comes together really easily. The ground pork is just drowning in tender onions, and the spicy-sweet flavor will wake up your taste buds. The eggs are optional, but a good eight-minute egg is always welcome. Peppery arugula is my favorite plate filler if you need an easy side dish—it's so yummy on its own or wilted into a hot meal.

1 tablespoon lard, coconut oil, or ghee

2 large onions, finely diced (about 2 cups)

1 bay leaf

4 cups arugula

4 hard-boiled eggs, peeled and halved (see note)

2 pounds ground pork

1 teaspoon fine salt

1 teaspoon dried rosemary needles

1 teaspoon garlic powder

½ teaspoon turmeric powder

1 tablespoon coconut aminos

◦ Heat a large skillet over medium heat. When it's hot, melt the lard in the skillet, then add the onions and bay leaf. Cook, stirring occasionally, for 10 minutes, until the onions are tender and browned. Meanwhile, divide the arugula and hard-boiled eggs among 4 serving bowls.

◦ Stir the ground pork into the onions, breaking it up as you go, then add the dried seasonings. Keep stirring and breaking up the pork until it has fully browned, about 8 minutes.

◦ Stir in the coconut aminos and mix well. Divide the pork among the bowls with the arugula and eggs. Serve hot.

◦ Store leftovers in the fridge for up to 4 days. To reheat, sauté in a skillet over medium heat for 5 minutes.

note: *Keeping a dozen hard-boiled eggs in the fridge at all times is always a good idea! To make the perfect hard-boiled eggs, bring 3 cups of water to a boil in a 1½-quart saucepan. Use a spoon to gently lower the eggs into the boiling water. Boil for 8 minutes. Drain the water and fill the pot with cold tap water and ice. Chill the eggs in the ice bath for 2 minutes, then peel them.*

modifications: *To make this dish AIP compliant and egg-free, just leave out the eggs. To make it coconut-free, use aged balsamic vinegar instead of the coconut aminos.*

Per serving: Calories **60** · Fat **41.6g** · Total Carbs **7.6g** · Fiber **1.3g** · Protein **49.2g**

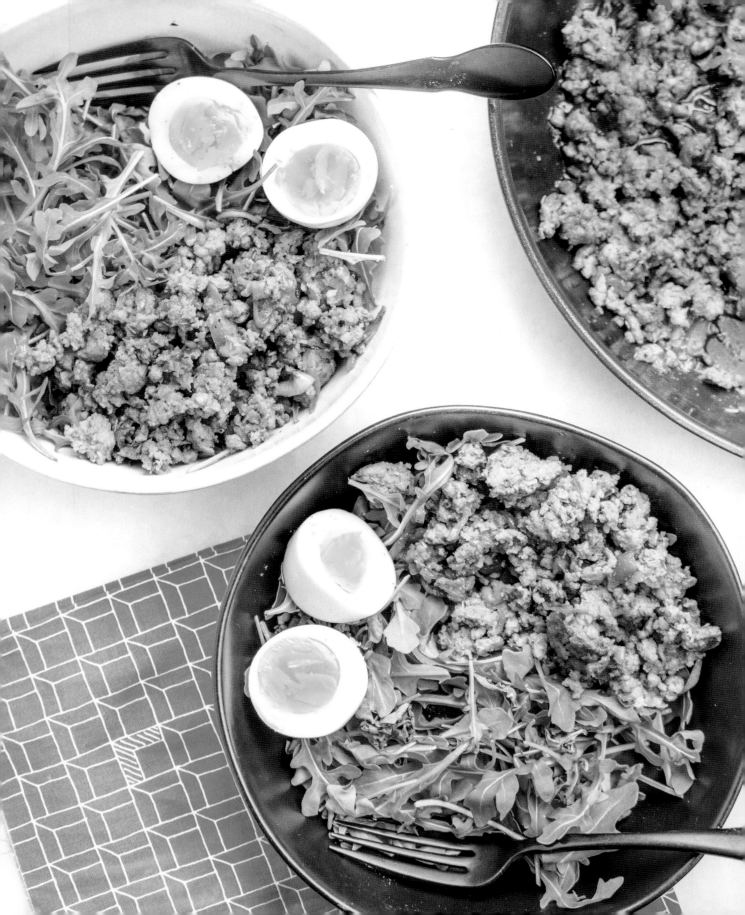

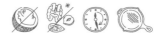

Pumpkin Pancakes

Make three 3-inch pancakes (1 serving) ○ Prep Time: 10 minutes ○ Cook Time: 5 minutes

These super easy, super fast pancakes need only three ingredients—pumpkin puree, cashew butter, and an egg—the rest are just for fun! This is a twist on the common banana, nut butter, and egg Paleo pancake recipe that uses pumpkin instead of banana so the pancakes have less of an impact on your blood sugar. The pumpkin still brings plenty of natural sweetness!

¼ cup 100% pumpkin puree

2 tablespoons unsweetened, unsalted cashew butter or sunflower seed butter

1 large egg

½ teaspoon ground cinnamon

¼ teaspoon ground cardamom (optional)

Pinch of fine salt

1 tablespoon ghee, for the pan, plus melted ghee for topping if desired

○ Heat a large skillet over medium heat. While it heats, whisk together the pumpkin, cashew butter, egg, cinnamon, cardamom, and salt in a medium-sized bowl until smooth.

○ Melt the ghee in the hot skillet. Use a rubber spatula to scrape the batter out of the bowl and make 3 pancakes in the skillet, each about 3 inches in diameter. Cook for 2 to 3 minutes, until they look dry around the edges and little bubbles have formed across the surface. Use a thin spatula to carefully flip them over and cook for another 3 minutes.

○ Remove from the skillet, stack, and top with melted ghee if desired. Dig in!

note: *If you want a sweet topping, add a drop or two of stevia glycerite to the melted ghee.*

Per serving (without ghee topping): Calories **409** · Fat **34.2g** · Total Carbs **14.1g** · Fiber **3.1g** · Protein **12.6g**

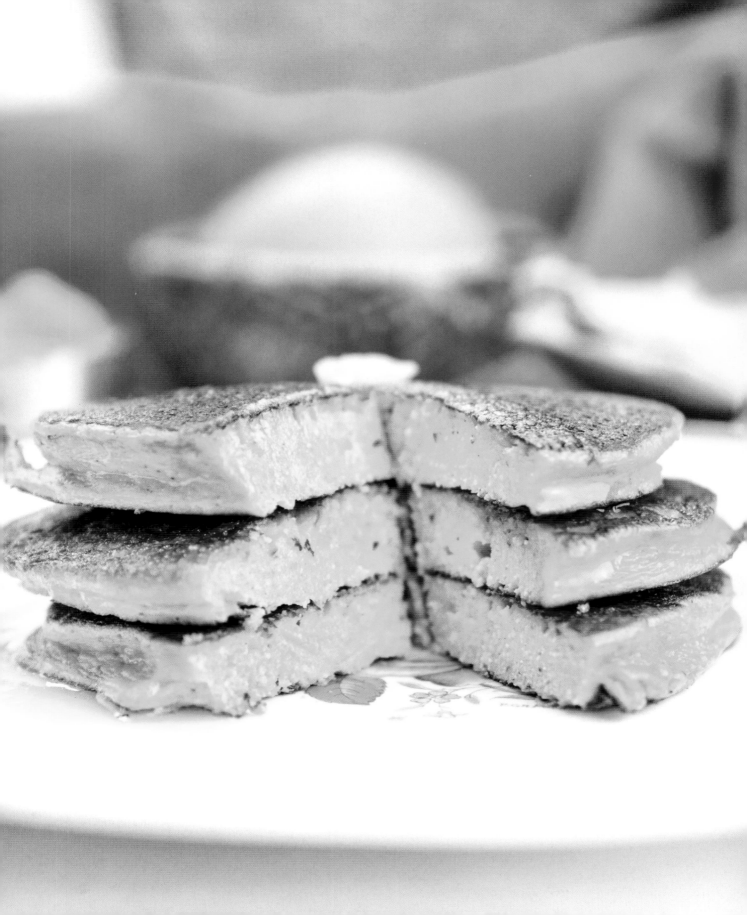

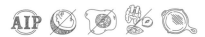

Radish + Pork Belly Hash Browns

Serves 2 ◦ Prep Time: 15 minutes ◦ Cook Time: 25 minutes

While sweet potatoes are an obvious choice for hash browns when you can't have regular potatoes, I find them too sweet for the flavor profile I'm looking for. However, radishes, when properly prepared, work very well—and you get the bonus of an anti-inflammatory and low-starch meal. It's the perfect way to start the day.

8 ounces pork belly, cut into ¼-inch pieces

1 teaspoon fine salt

1 teaspoon dried rosemary needles

1 teaspoon garlic powder

1 teaspoon onion powder

1 teaspoon lard or ghee

1 pound radishes, shredded

1 green onion, sliced on the bias, for garnish

- Put the pork belly in a 15-inch skillet and cook over medium heat, stirring occasionally, until it's well browned, 8 to 10 minutes. Add the dried seasonings and lard to the skillet and mix well. Continue to cook until the pork belly becomes crispy, about 5 minutes, stirring once or twice.

- Meanwhile, place the shredded radishes in a clean kitchen towel and squeeze to release as much water as possible. Then add the radishes to the skillet and mix them with the seasoned crispy pork belly.

- Spread the mixture evenly across the bottom of the pan, then flatten it well with a spatula. Cook undisturbed for 5 minutes, then use the spatula to turn the hash over in sections and flatten it to the bottom of the pan again. Cook undisturbed for another 5 minutes. Finally, scrape everything up and mix it all together. Garnish with the green onion and serve hot.

Per serving: Calories **654** · Fat **62.6g** · Total Carbs **10.1g** · Fiber **4.2g** · Protein **12.6g**

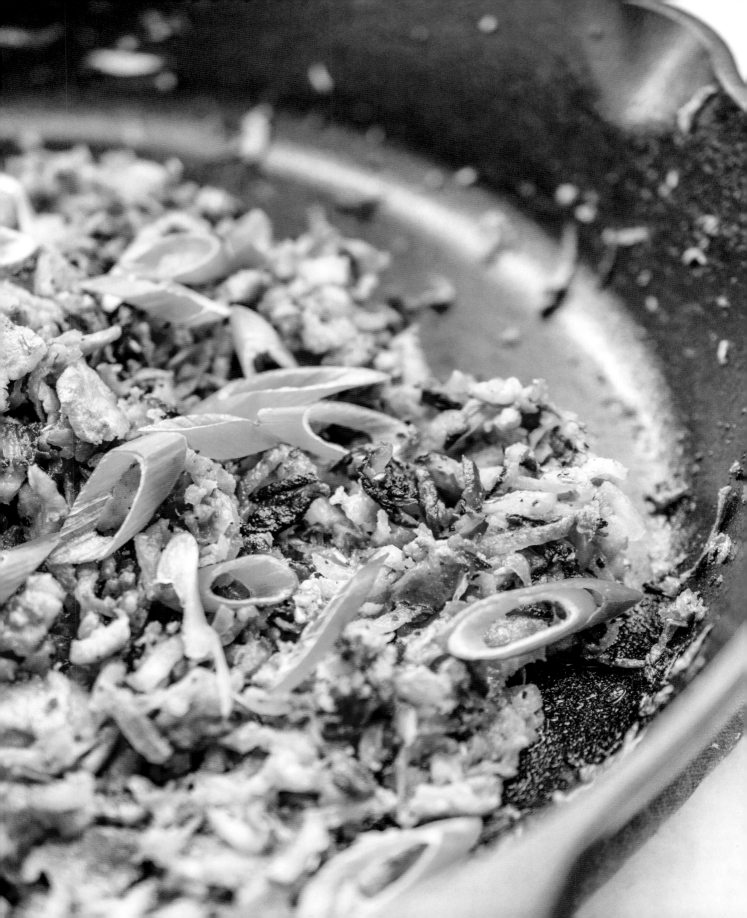

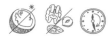

Protein Avocado Toast

Serves 1 ◦ Prep Time: 5 minutes ◦ Cook Time: 5 minutes

This hearty "mug bread" recipe crisps up in a skillet for a super slice of toast. The consistency of the bread is more like a biscuit—it's tender yet filling and has a lovely nutty flavor. It makes a perfect base for avocado toast, and with plenty of healthy fats, 13 grams of protein, and almost 11 grams of fiber, this avocado toast is anything but basic. Top the mashed avocado with kelp granules for added iodine; when paired with the selenium-rich tahini in the bread, it's a perfect team for thyroid support!

1½ tablespoons tahini

1 large egg

1 tablespoon plus 2 teaspoons coconut flour

¼ teaspoon fine salt, divided

1 tablespoon extra-virgin olive oil or ghee, for toasting

½ ripe Hass avocado, peeled

1 teaspoon kelp granules (optional)

◦ In a 4-inch square microwave-safe glass container, mix the tahini and egg until smooth. Stir in the coconut flour and ⅛ teaspoon of the salt until well combined. Microwave on high for 1 minute, or until the center is set and the edges have pulled away from the sides.

◦ Heat the olive oil in a skillet over medium heat. Use a spatula to remove the bread from the glass container. Toast the bread in the hot skillet for 2 minutes on each side.

◦ In the meantime, mash the avocado gently with a fork.

◦ Spread the mashed avocado on the toasted bread, then sprinkle with the remaining ⅛ teaspoon of salt and the kelp granules, if using. Slice the toast in half and enjoy.

notes: *If you don't do sesame seeds, you can use 2 tablespoons ghee in place of the tahini.*

To make the bread in the oven, bake it at 350°F for 20 minutes, or until the center is set and the edges have pulled away from the sides. You may use a small metal baking pan or a ramekin instead of a glass baking dish if you prefer.

I use a Pyrex sandwich-size food storage container for this single-serving bread.

modifications: *To make this dish coconut-free, use 3 tablespoons blanched almond flour in place of the coconut flour.*

Per serving: Calories **487** · Fat **42.3g** · Total Carbs **17.9g** · Fiber **10.9g** · Protein **13.2g**

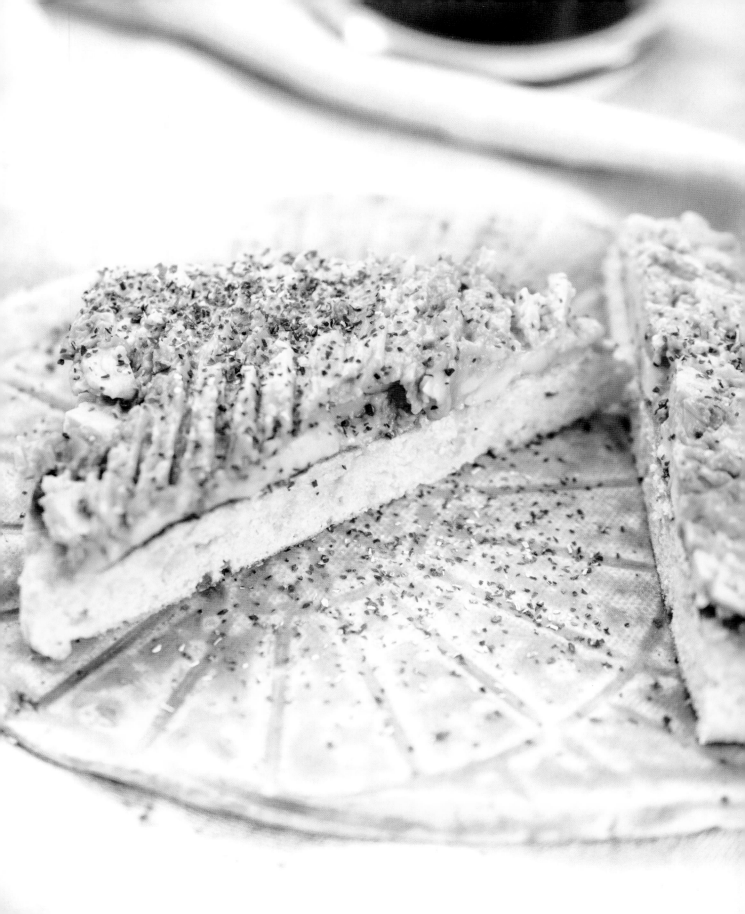

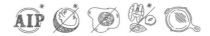

Protein Waffles

Makes 8 waffles (1 waffle per serving) ◦ Prep Time: 10 minutes ◦ Cook Time: 30 minutes

You can make waffles out of anything, and these savory broccoli-and-sausage concoctions are no exception. Yeah, sure, you could fry them up as patties, but where is the fun in that?

1 pound ground breakfast sausage

1 cup finely chopped broccoli florets

¼ cup almond meal, or 1 tablespoon coconut flour

2 cloves garlic, minced

2 teaspoons yacón syrup (optional; see note)

½ teaspoon fine salt

Special equipment:

Waffle iron

- Preheat a waffle iron according to the manufacturer's instructions.

- Put all of the ingredients in a large bowl and mix well. Shape the mixture into 8 evenly sized balls and gently flatten.

- Cook the patties one at a time in the waffle iron on high heat for about 4 minutes, until browned and crispy. Cooking times may vary. Make sure to close the iron well to flatten the patties.

- Serve hot! Store wrapped tightly in the fridge for up to 5 days. Reheat in a skillet over medium heat, toasting for 2 to 3 minutes per side.

note: *You may swap honey for the yacón syrup or omit the sweetener altogether.*

modifications: *To make these waffles AIP compliant, be sure to use an AIP-friendly sausage. I use ButcherBox ground breakfast sausage; it's made with pork and is nightshade-free. You can use your preferred brand, even if it's made with chicken or turkey.*

Per serving: Calories **218** · Fat **17.8g** · Total Carbs **4.2g** · Fiber **0.7g** · Protein **9.1g**

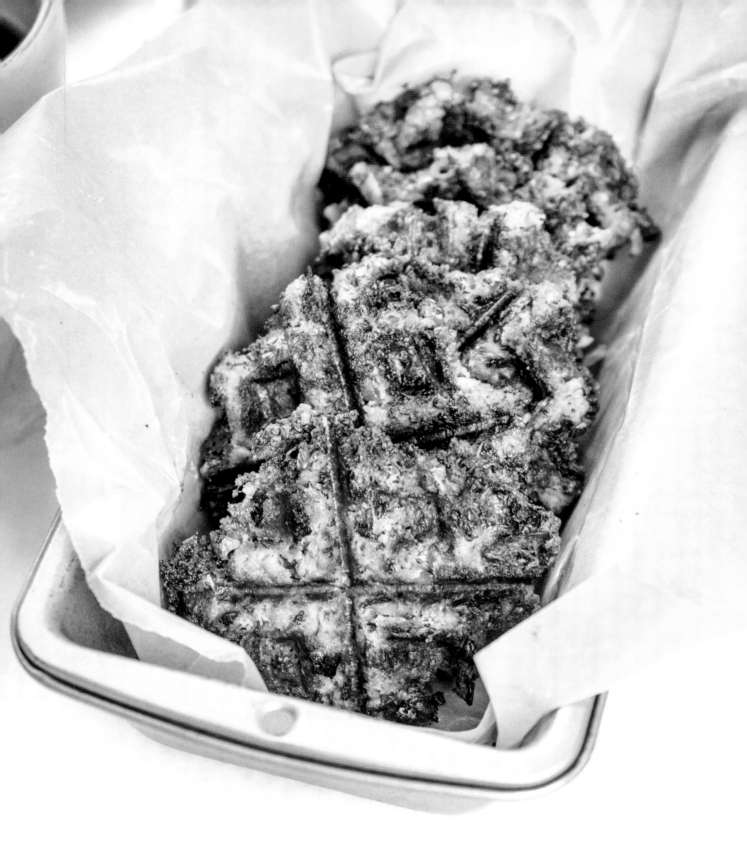

Sheet Pan Breakfast

Serves 2 ◦ Prep Time: 10 minutes ◦ Cook Time: 25 minutes

This recipe makes use of adorable delicata squash rings for a fun and delicious breakfast! The season for delicata squash is short, but it's glorious. This winter squash is small and has a mild sweet flavor. And unlike most winter squash, there's no need to peel the delicate and flavorful skin; it cooks beautifully and is easy to cut and eat. Delicata squash is another wonderful source of vitamin C.

1 delicata squash (about 1 pound)

6 slices bacon

5 large eggs

1 teaspoon fine salt

1 tablespoon chopped fresh parsley, for garnish

◦ Place an oven rack in the middle position. Preheat the oven to 400°F.

◦ Cut the squash crosswise into 9 slices, each about ½ inch thick. Use a spoon or knife to scoop out the seeds.

◦ Line up the squash rings on a sheet pan. Put a wire rack in the pan and line up the bacon on the rack, right over the squash. Put the pan in the oven on the middle rack and roast for 15 minutes.

◦ Remove the pan from the oven, then carefully lift off the rack with the bacon and set it in another sheet pan to catch the drips. Use a spatula to flip the squash rings over.

◦ Crack the eggs into five of the rings and sprinkle everything with the salt. Return the bacon rack to the sheet pan with the squash and eggs and put the sheet pan back in the oven.

◦ Roast for another 10 minutes, or until the bacon is crispy and the eggs are cooked through. Remove from the oven and use a spatula to scrape up and plate the eggs and squash. Garnish with the parsley and serve with the bacon on the side.

note: *Use only 4 eggs if you prefer to serve 2 whole eggs to each person, without having to split a fifth egg in half. I often throw the extra egg on there if I'm feeding someone who eats more or I'm feeding one adult and one child.*

Per serving: Calories **336** · Fat **21.7g** · Total Carbs **9.9g** · Fiber **2.1g** · Protein **24.9g**

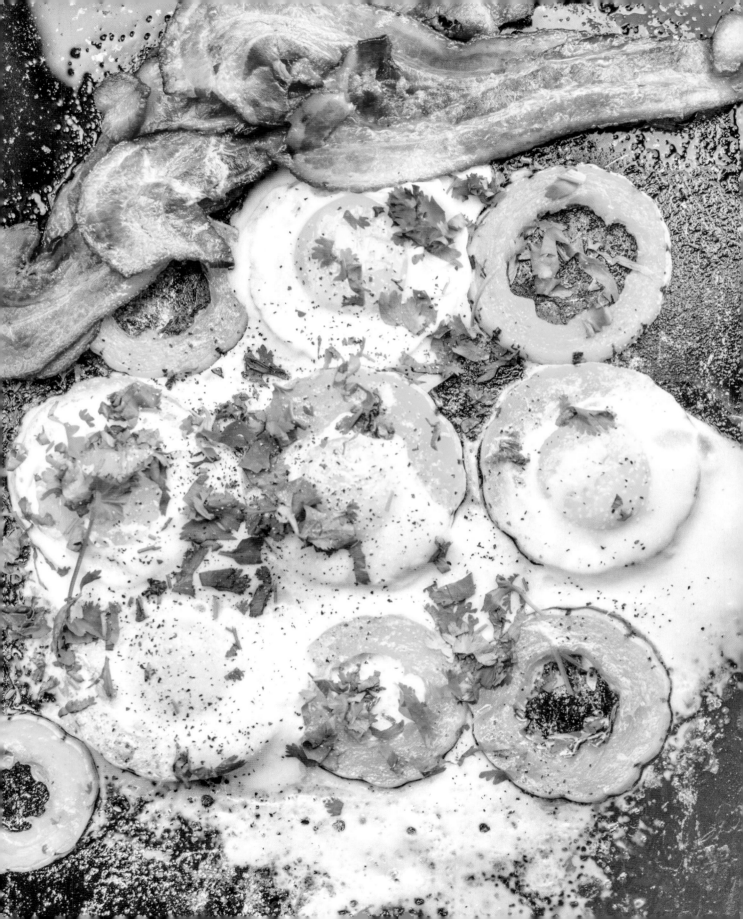

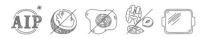

Breakfast Rice Bowls

Serves 2 ◦ Prep Time: 8 minutes ◦ Cook Time: 25 minutes

Enjoy a warm breakfast bowl in the morning without the insulin spike! Don't let the cinnamon throw you off—it is often used for sweet breakfast dishes, but cinnamon on savory roasted vegetables is delicious, and you can quote me on that. Plus, did you know that cinnamon helps with blood sugar regulation? With the addition of vitamin C–packed cauliflower and loads of healthy fats, this truly is a breakfast of champions!

2 (12-ounce) bags frozen riced cauliflower

1 teaspoon fine salt

1 teaspoon ground black pepper

1 teaspoon mustard seeds

½ teaspoon ginger powder

½ teaspoon ground cinnamon

6 slices bacon

1 green onion, sliced on the bias, for garnish

◦ Place an oven rack in the middle position. Preheat the oven to 400°F.

◦ Pour the riced cauliflower onto a sheet pan and season it with the salt, pepper, mustard seeds, ginger powder, and cinnamon. Toss to mix thoroughly, then spread the cauliflower evenly across the sheet pan, breaking apart any clumps.

◦ Lay the bacon flat on top of the cauliflower, spacing it evenly. Put the sheet pan in the oven on the middle rack and roast for 25 minutes, or until the bacon is crispy and bits of the rice are toasty and browned.

◦ Remove the pan from the oven and use tongs to transfer the bacon slices to a cutting board. Chop the crispy bacon into large pieces, then add it back to the cauliflower rice and mix everything together.

◦ Use a large spatula or spoon to scoop up the bacon and rice mixture and serve it in 2 bowls. Garnish with the sliced green onion.

◦ Store leftovers in the fridge for up to 5 days. To reheat, microwave on high for 1 minute or sauté in a skillet over medium heat for 10 minutes.

modifications: *To make this dish AIP compliant, omit the black pepper and mustard seeds and double the ginger and cinnamon.*

awesome additions: *If you can do eggs, put some Everything Sauce (page 72) on these bad boys, or add more protein to the dish by putting an egg on top.*

You can also beef up this meal by adding cooked ground beef.

Per serving: Calories **301** · Fat **21.2g** · Total Carbs **17.7g** · Fiber **7.2g** · Protein **13.9g**

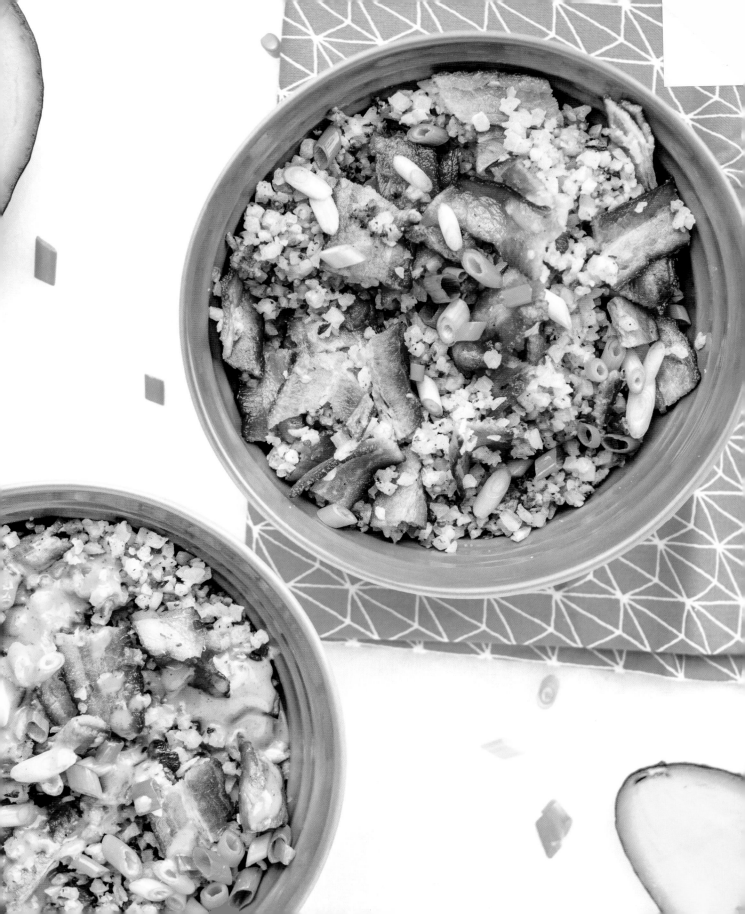

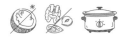

Slow Cooker Frittata

Serves 6 ◦ Prep Time: 15 minutes ◦ Cook Time: 2 or 4 hours

Take the pressure out of cooking a frittata with this easy slow cooker version. There's no watching the oven so the frittata won't burn. I love setting this to cook early on a weekend morning so that it's hot and ready to eat when we get back from walking our dog, Bruce, or riding our bikes—or, better yet, on a lazy weekend when we stay in our PJs until noon! You can add any veggies you want to this recipe, or even cooked sausage. Frittatas are so flexible.

1 tablespoon ghee or coconut oil, plus more for the slow cooker

1 cup chopped broccoli

1 cup diced onions

1 cup sliced mushrooms of choice (about 4 ounces)

1½ teaspoons fine salt, divided

12 large eggs

1 teaspoon dried oregano leaves

1 teaspoon garlic powder

1 teaspoon ground black pepper

1 teaspoon fish sauce

½ cup unsweetened dairy-free milk of choice

¼ cup extra-virgin olive oil

◦ Heat a large skillet over medium heat. When it's hot, melt the ghee in the skillet. Add the broccoli, onions, mushrooms, and ½ teaspoon of the salt. Sauté for 8 to 10 minutes, until tender.

◦ While the veggies cook, put the eggs, oregano, garlic powder, pepper, fish sauce, and remaining teaspoon of salt in a blender. Blend on medium speed until frothy. Lower the speed and slowly pour in the milk and then the olive oil.

◦ Lightly grease the inside of a slow cooker. Transfer the cooked vegetables to the pot and spread them out. Pour in the egg mixture.

◦ Cook on high for 1½ to 2 hours or on low for 3 to 4 hours, until the center is set and the edge of the frittata has pulled away from the side of the slow cooker.

◦ Remove the lid and gently run a rubber spatula around the edge and under the frittata to release it, in case it has stuck to the bottom of the slow cooker. Cut into 6 pieces and use a spatula to serve.

◦ Store leftovers in the fridge for up to 4 days. To reheat, bake in a preheated 300°F oven for 5 minutes.

note: *Instead of the dairy-free milk and olive oil, you may use ¾ cup Salted Cashew Cream (page 76), coconut cream, or heavy cream.*

Per serving: Calories **270** · Fat **20.7g** · Total Carbs **6.7g** · Fiber **1.3g** · Protein **14.2g**

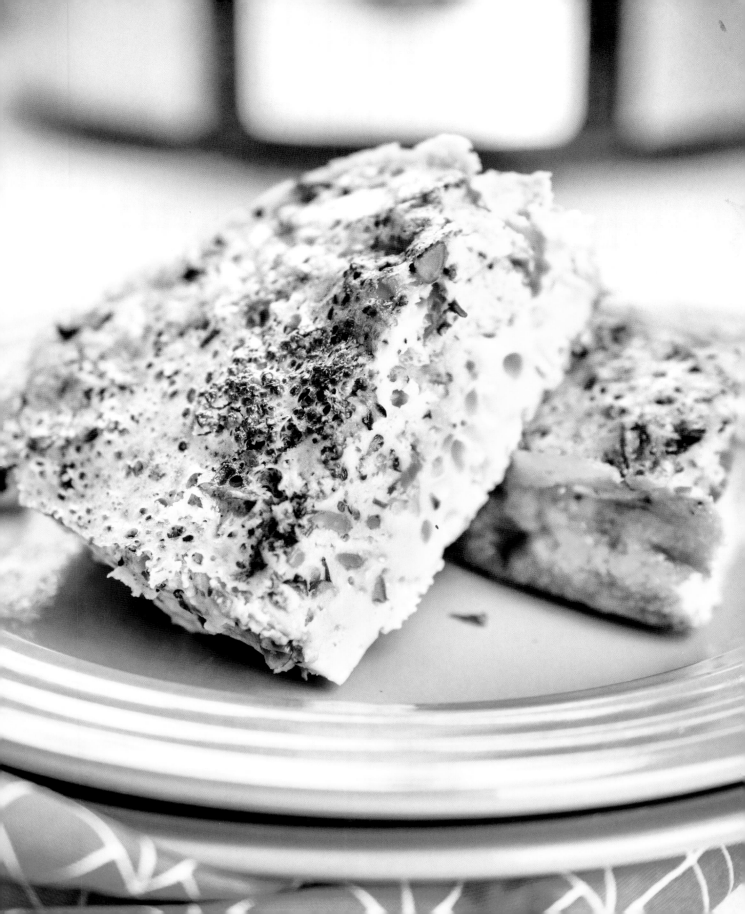

BEEF

Beef is my favorite protein. After seafood, grass-fed beef has some of the most favorable fat profiles to fight inflammation. Red meat is also high in B6, B12, iron, niacin, phosphorus, and zinc, with a really high absorption rate. Using extra-virgin olive oil and anti-inflammatory herbs and spices to cook beef helps protect your body from any oxidation that may occur when cooking the meat. In this book, we do all that!

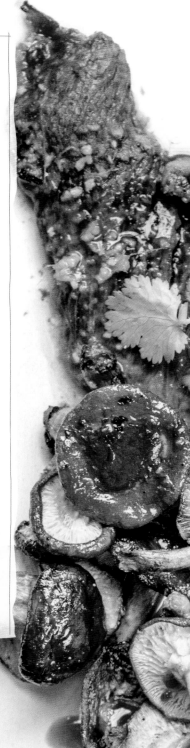

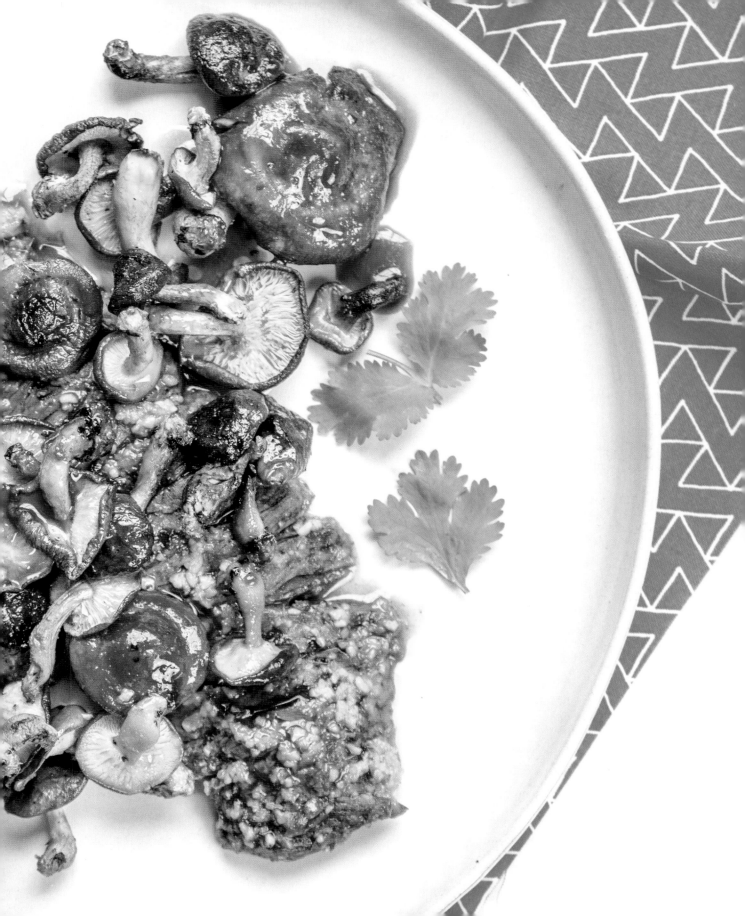

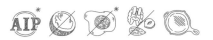

Burger Bar

Serves 6 ○ Prep Time: 15 minutes ○ Cook Time: 20 minutes

Who doesn't love a good build-a-burger bar? Fry up some perfectly seasoned grass-fed beef patties and serve them on a platter with all the fixings. These juicy burgers have a killer crust and an incredible flavor from the Cuban Sazón. (Don't worry; you probably already have the dried seasonings you'll need to make this blend in your pantry.) I've suggested some toppings for these delicious patties, but really, you can use anything you like.

2 pounds ground beef (85% lean)

1 tablespoon Cuban Sazón (page 83)

1 tablespoon pork panko, store-bought or homemade (page 80)

2 teaspoons fine salt

3 tablespoons extra-virgin olive oil or avocado oil, for the pan

12 large Bibb lettuce leaves, for serving

Suggested toppings:

1½ cups Pickled Radishes (page 84)

1 ripe Hass avocado, peeled, pitted, and sliced

1 cup broccoli sprouts

¼ cup plus 2 tablespoons Onion + Bacon Spread (page 88)

3 hard-boiled eggs (see note, page 118), sliced

○ Heat a 15-inch cast-iron skillet over medium heat. While it heats, mix the ground beef with the Cuban Sazón, pork panko, and salt in a large bowl until well combined. Shape the mixture into 6 evenly sized meatballs, about 2 inches in diameter. Gently flatten them into ½-inch-thick patties and make an indentation in the center of each patty with your finger.

○ Pour the oil into the hot skillet, then arrange 3 or 4 patties in the skillet, being careful not to overcrowd the pan. Cook the patties for 5 minutes on each side, or until a nice thick crust forms and the burgers feel firm. Repeat with the remaining patties.

○ Arrange the lettuce leaves and any toppings, such as pickled radishes, avocado slices, broccoli sprouts, Onion + Bacon Spread, and hard-boiled eggs, on a platter. Serve right away; have your guests build their burgers with the toppings they like.

○ Store the patties in the fridge for up to 5 days. To reheat, warm in a covered skillet over medium heat for 3 to 4 minutes per side.

modifications: *To make these burgers AIP compliant, use the AIP version of the Cuban Sazón. Do not serve with eggs.*

Per burger with toppings (except egg): Calories **410** · Fat **28.2g** · Total Carbs **5.4g** · Fiber **2.4g** · Protein **31.6g**

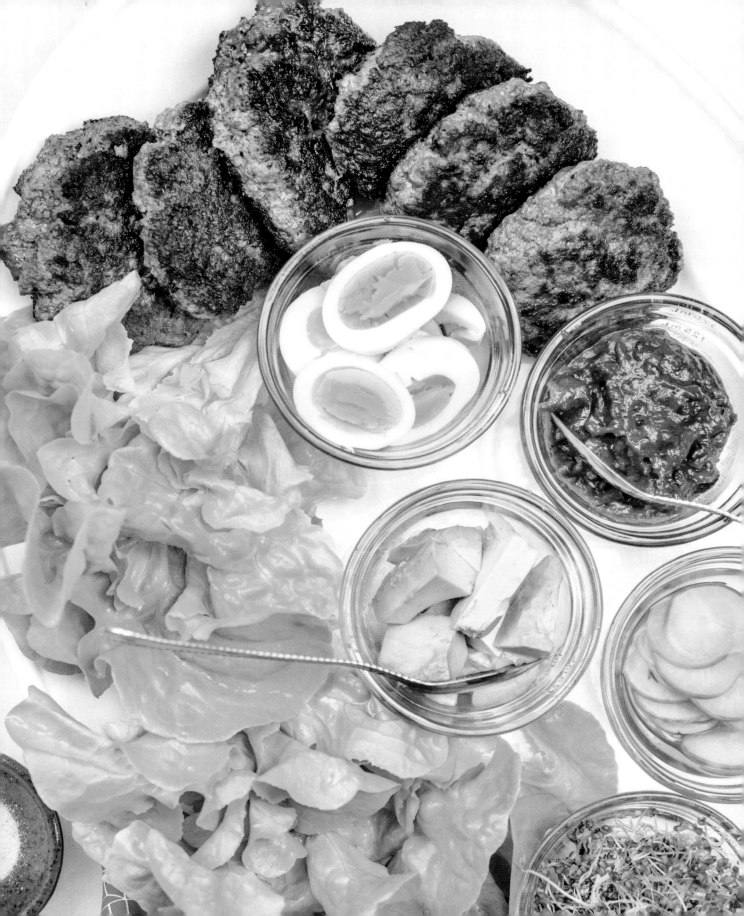

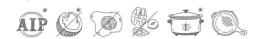

Sweet Osso Buco

Serves 3 ◦ Prep Time: 20 minutes ◦ Cook Time: 3 hours 20 minutes

This recipe reminds me of another time, a slower time, a time when sauces simmered all day and back doors were never locked. Perhaps it's because it uses an old-school Dutch oven, or maybe it's the rich flavors of the sauce, which build during its long cooking time. This one-pot dish goes from stovetop to oven for a warm, hearty meal that is perfect for Sunday supper or a holiday dinner, yet easy enough to make any day you've got the time.

---

3 beef shanks (about 3½ pounds)

3 teaspoons fine salt, divided

2 tablespoons extra-virgin olive oil

4 celery ribs, diced (about 2 cups)

3 medium carrots, diced (about 1½ cups)

1 large white onion, diced (about 1 cup)

4 cloves garlic, minced

2 bay leaves

¼ teaspoon ground nutmeg

1 teaspoon dried rubbed sage

½ teaspoon dried rosemary or thyme leaves

¼ cup coconut aminos

Juice of 1 orange

1 tablespoon apple cider vinegar

2 cups bone broth

modifications: *To make this dish AIP compliant, use ginger powder instead of the nutmeg. To make it coconut-free, replace the coconut aminos with low-sodium gluten-free tamari or aged balsamic vinegar.*

- Place an oven rack in the middle position. Preheat the oven to 300°F.

- Heat a 6-quart Dutch oven or heavy-bottomed pot on the stovetop over medium heat. While it heats, season the beef shanks with 2 teaspoons of the salt.

- Pour the olive oil into the pot, then arrange the shanks in the pot so they are not overlapping. Brown for 3 minutes per side, then remove the shanks from the pot and set aside.

- Put the celery, carrots, onion, garlic, and bay leaves in the pot and sauté for 7 minutes, or until the onion is tender and translucent. Add the remaining teaspoon of salt, the nutmeg, sage, and rosemary and mix well.

- Stir in the coconut aminos, orange juice, and vinegar and mix well, deglazing the bottom of the pot. Stir in the broth.

- When the mixture comes to a simmer, put the shanks back in the pot, nestling them among the saucy vegetable mixture so that only the top portions protrude above the surface of the liquid.

- Put the lid on the pot and transfer it to the middle rack of the oven. Cook for 3 hours, or until the shanks are nicely browned and tender.

- Remove the pot from the oven and fish out the bay leaves and shanks. Then use an immersion blender to puree the contents of the pot until you have a rich, creamy sauce.

- Put the shanks back in the pot and shred the meat with 2 forks, or serve the shanks whole with a ladleful of the sauce. Store leftovers in an airtight container in the fridge for up to 5 days. To reheat, warm in a skillet with a tight-fitting lid over medium heat for 10 to 15 minutes.

Slow Cooker Method: Complete the stovetop instructions using a large skillet, then transfer everything to a slow cooker and cook on low for 6 hours or on high for 3 hours.

Per serving: Calories **414** · Fat **22.5g** · Total Carbs **20.4g** · Fiber **4.4g** · Protein **31.7g**

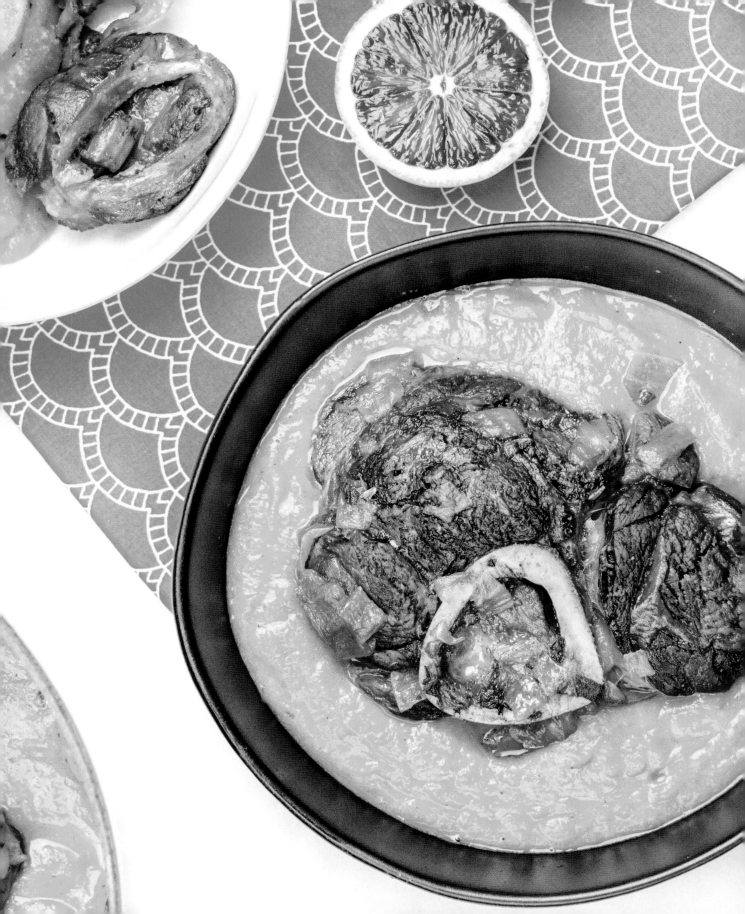

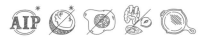

Pumpkin Bolognese

Serves 4 ◦ Prep Time: 15 minutes ◦ Cook Time: 25 minutes

Don't let the unconventional ingredients fool you—this meat sauce is delicious. Even my olive-hating husband loves this recipe! A blend of anti-inflammatory ingredients replaces tomatoes, and a blend of shredded cabbage and low-carb shirataki noodles subs for pasta.

For the noodles:

2 (7-ounce) bags angel hair shirataki noodles

2 tablespoons extra-virgin olive oil

2 cups shredded green cabbage

1 teaspoon fine salt

For the meat:

2 pounds ground beef (85% lean)

1 tablespoon Castaway Seed Blend (page 82)

2 teaspoons fine salt

1 teaspoon ground black pepper

For the sauce:

1 tablespoon extra-virgin olive oil or ghee

1 large onion, diced

4 cloves garlic, minced

1 bay leaf

1 cup 100% pumpkin puree

1 cup bone broth

½ cup green olives, pitted

2 teaspoons fish sauce

2 teaspoons Italian herb blend, plus more for garnish if desired

1 teaspoon aged balsamic vinegar (see notes, page 90) or coconut aminos

1 teaspoon fine salt

◦ Prepare the noodles: Heat a 15-inch skillet over medium heat. While it heats, drain the shirataki noodles in a colander and rinse them with fresh water.

◦ Pour the olive oil into the skillet and add the cabbage. Sauté for 2 to 3 minutes, until the cabbage begins to wilt. Add the shirataki noodles and salt and sauté, tossing frequently, until the cabbage and noodles are tender and well mixed, about 5 minutes. Transfer to a large bowl, cover, and set aside.

◦ Brown the meat: Return the skillet to the stovetop, still over medium heat. Crumble the ground beef into the skillet, then add the seed blend, salt, and pepper and stir to combine. Cook the beef, stirring to break it up, until well browned, about 8 minutes. Transfer the meat to a separate bowl and cover.

◦ Make the sauce: Return the skillet to the stovetop. Put the olive oil in the skillet along with the onion, garlic, and bay leaf. Sauté until tender, about 5 minutes. Add the pumpkin, broth, olives, fish sauce, Italian herb blend, vinegar, and salt. Stir well and simmer for 3 minutes.

◦ Transfer the contents of the skillet to a blender and puree until smooth. Pour the sauce back into the skillet and add the meat, then stir well, cover, and simmer on low until ready to serve.

◦ To serve, you can add the noodles to the meat sauce to warm them or warm the noodles separately, divide them among 4 shallow bowls, and ladle the meat sauce over them. Garnish each serving with a sprinkle of Italian herb blend, if desired.

◦ Store leftovers in an airtight container in the fridge for up to 4 days or freeze the sauce in a freezer-safe jar for up to 3 months. To reheat, simmer in a saucepan until warmed through.

note: *If you don't like pumpkin, sweet potato puree works well too!*

modifications: *To make this dish AIP compliant, replace the seed blend and black pepper used to season the meat with 2 teaspoons Italian herb blend.*

Per serving: Calories **481** · Fat **31.5g** · Total Carbs **15.1g** · Fiber **5.3g** · Protein **33.2g**

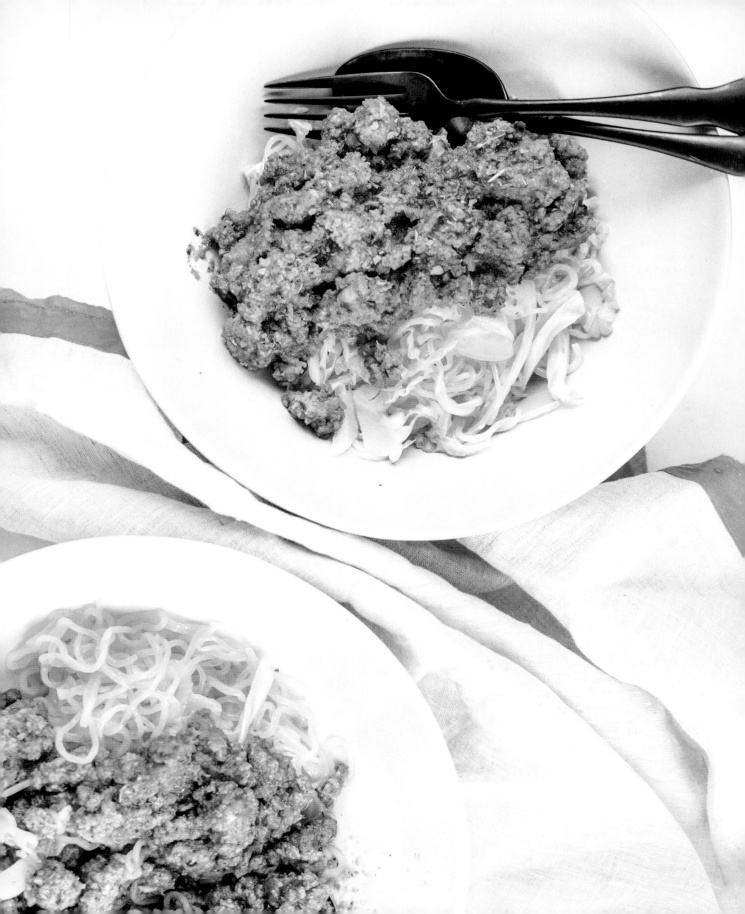

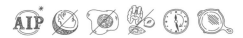

Perfect Ground Beef with Avocado

Serves 4 ◦ Prep Time: 10 minutes ◦ Cook Time: 20 minutes

Ground beef and avocado make a powerful pair. This bowl of hormone health goodness is loaded with important minerals like zinc, selenium, potassium, and magnesium, and hormones love minerals! High-quality ground beef contains bioavailable beta-carotene, anti-inflammatory omega-3 fatty acids, and most amino acids. I sneaked mushrooms in here too for their immune-boosting properties, and colorful sumac for its potent polyphenols. This perfectly seasoned yet simple meal is a staple in my home, and I'm sure it will be in yours as well!

2 tablespoons bacon fat, tallow, or ghee

½ cup shiitake mushrooms, minced (about 2 ounces)

4 cloves garlic, minced

2 green onions, sliced, white and green parts separated

2 pounds ground beef (85% lean)

2 teaspoons fine salt

2 teaspoons garlic powder

2 ripe Hass avocados, peeled, pitted, and diced, for serving

Juice of 2 limes, for serving

1 teaspoon ground sumac, for garnish

◦ Heat a 15-inch skillet over medium heat. Melt the bacon fat in the hot skillet, then add the mushrooms, garlic, and white parts of the green onions. Sauté for 3 minutes, or until the mushrooms are lightly browned and the onions start to become translucent.

◦ Crumble the ground beef into the skillet. Break it up with a wire whisk and mix it well with the veggies. Cook until the beef is browned, about 8 minutes. Add the salt and garlic powder and stir to combine. Continue cooking until the beef is dark brown and glossy and any fluid has cooked off, about 5 minutes more.

◦ Serve the beef in shallow bowls. Top with the diced avocados, lime juice, the green parts of the green onions, and the ground sumac.

◦ Store leftovers in the fridge for up to 5 days. To reheat, sauté in a skillet over medium heat for 5 minutes.

modifications: *To make this dish AIP compliant, omit the sumac.*

Per serving: Calories **558** · Fat **39.1g** · Total Carbs **10.7g** · Fiber **5.4g** · Protein **4.2g**

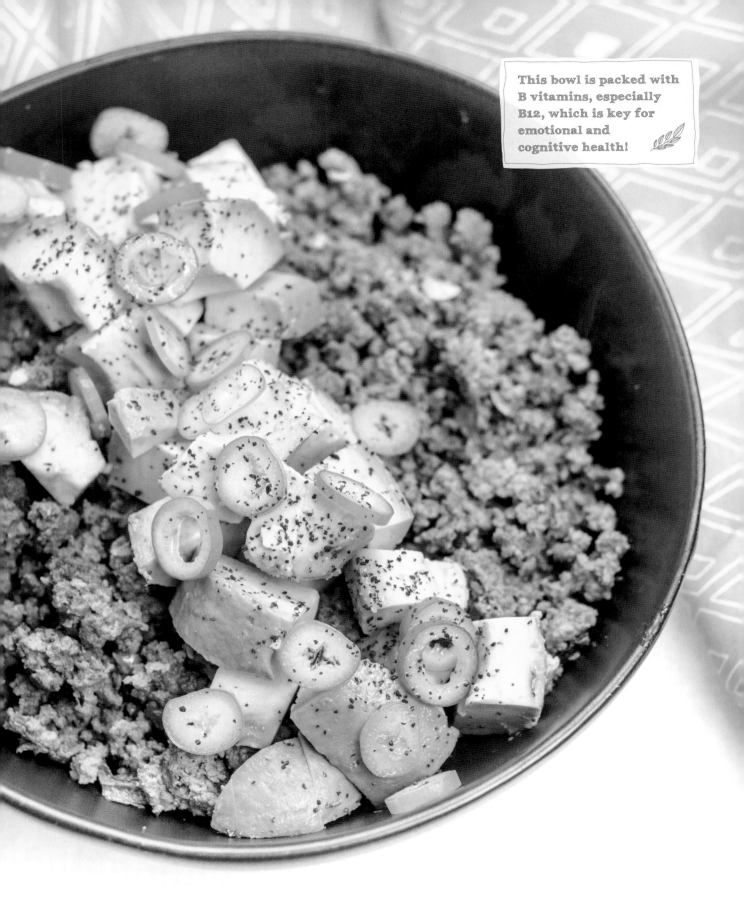

This bowl is packed with B vitamins, especially B12, which is key for emotional and cognitive health!

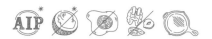

Superhero Bowls

Serves 4 ◦ Prep Time: 10 minutes ◦ Cook Time: 25 minutes

The liver isn't really a filter, so no, you're not eating trapped toxins when you eat liver. The liver actually transforms toxins, usually into something the body can process and eliminate. When you eat liver, you're supporting your own liver and helping it do its many important jobs even better. This recipe is a wonderful Asian-inspired stir-fry, but with a mega nutrient-density, superpower upgrade. The amazing stir-fry flavors really mask the organ meat, and I am happy to report that my husband and six-year-old have enjoyed this dish many times.

8 ounces beef liver, diced

1 pound ground beef (85% lean)

2 tablespoons Asian Garlic Compound Butter (page 78)

1 large onion, diced

2 teaspoons minced fresh rosemary

2 teaspoons fine salt

1 teaspoon ground cumin

1 (12-ounce) bag broccoli slaw (see notes)

2 teaspoons red wine vinegar

2 teaspoons toasted sesame oil

2 teaspoons spicy brown or Dijon mustard, for drizzling

1 teaspoon sesame seeds, for garnish

◦ Heat a 15-inch skillet over medium heat. While it heats, pulse the diced liver in a food processor or meat grinder until it's minced to the same texture as the ground beef. Transfer the liver to a large mixing bowl and add the ground beef. Mix the two meats together with your hands until well combined.

◦ Melt the compound butter in the hot skillet, then add the onion and sauté until translucent and tender, about 4 minutes. Add the beef and liver mixture along with the rosemary, salt, and cumin. Mix well and use a wire whisk to crumble the meat. Cook until the meat is browned, about 10 minutes.

◦ Mix in the broccoli slaw and cook, stirring occasionally, for 5 minutes, or until the slaw is tender. Mix in the vinegar and sesame oil, then remove the pan from the heat. Serve in bowls drizzled with the mustard and garnished with the sesame seeds.

◦ Store leftovers in the fridge for up to 5 days or in the freezer for up to 2 months. If you freeze it, thaw it in the fridge overnight. To reheat, sauté over high heat for 5 to 6 minutes.

notes: *If you don't have a batch of compound butter already made, you can use the same quantity of butter, lard, tallow, or coconut oil for this recipe—just add 1 teaspoon coconut aminos and 1 clove garlic, minced.*

You can find broccoli slaw at any grocery store or make it yourself at home. It's simply a mix of vegetables that are shredded or cut into matchsticks. I like to include broccoli stems, cauliflower stems, cabbage, and carrots. Coleslaw or any shredded cruciferous vegetable blend will work as a substitute in any recipe that calls for broccoli slaw.

modifications: *To make this dish AIP compliant, make the AIP version of the compound butter and omit the cumin, sesame oil, and mustard. Add 1 tablespoon prepared horseradish at the end for flavor. To make it coconut-free, use the coconut-free version of the compound butter. To make it dairy-free, use the dairy-free version of the compound butter.*

Per serving: Calories **409** · Fat **21.8g** · Total Carbs **12g** · Fiber **2.5g** · Protein **39.3g**

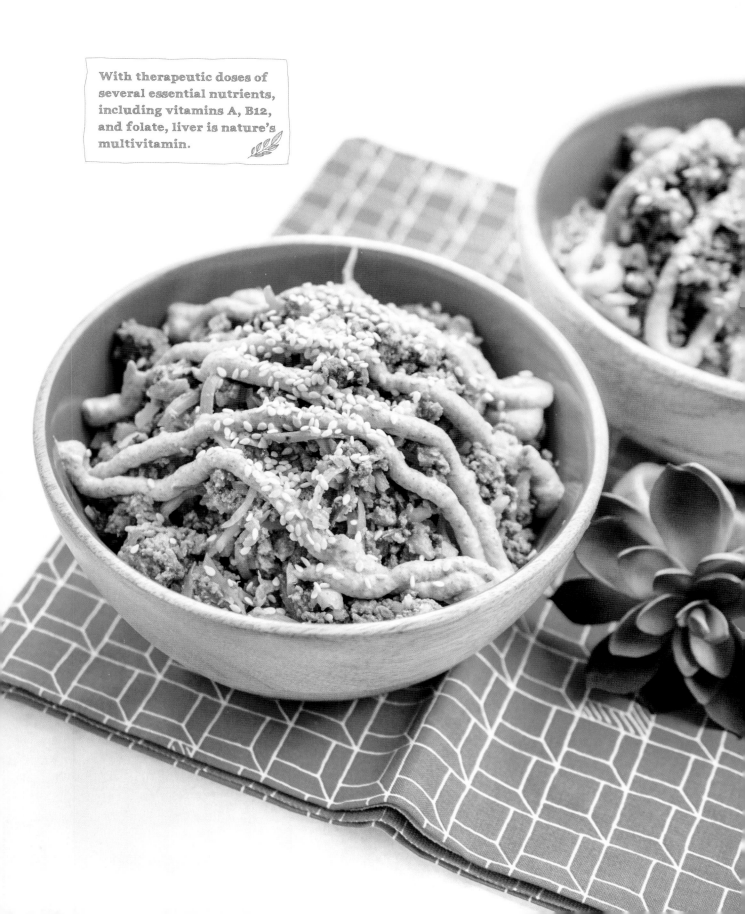

With therapeutic doses of several essential nutrients, including vitamins A, B12, and folate, liver is nature's multivitamin.

Marinated Steak + Buttery Cabbage

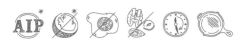

Serves 4 ⊙ Prep Time: 15 minutes ⊙ Cook Time: 15 minutes

Skip the labor of love that is shredding cabbage and pick up a bag of coleslaw mix instead! This super fine shredded veg mixture is perfect for stir-fries, and when cooked in copious amounts of ghee, as it is here, it's almost noodlelike. This one-pot meal of shredded cabbage topped with tender strips of flank steak is a surefire winner. If cruciferous vegetables give you bloat when they're raw, don't worry: cooking them makes them easier to digest.

1½ pounds flank steak

1 tablespoon extra-virgin olive oil

1 tablespoon spicy brown or Dijon mustard

1 teaspoon ginger powder

1 teaspoon ground cumin

3 teaspoons fine salt, divided

¼ cup ghee

6 cups coleslaw mix (about 1½ pounds)

1 tablespoon coconut aminos

¼ cup fresh parsley, minced

⊙ Cut the steak into very thin strips and toss it in a bowl with the olive oil, mustard, ginger, cumin, and 2 teaspoons of the salt. Set the steak aside to marinate while you cook the cabbage.

⊙ Heat a Dutch oven or large heavy-bottomed pot over medium heat. Melt the ghee in the pot, then add the coleslaw mix and sprinkle with the remaining teaspoon of salt. Cover with the lid and cook for 3 minutes, then remove the lid and sauté for another 3 minutes, until the cabbage is very tender. Transfer the cabbage to a bowl, then cover it and place it near the stove so it doesn't get cold.

⊙ Place half of the marinated steak strips in the pot one at a time so that each strip lies flat and they do not overlap. Brown the steak for 2 minutes per side, then remove from the pot. Repeat with the second half of the steak strips.

⊙ Return all of the steak to the pot and quickly stir in the coconut aminos and parsley, then remove the pot from the heat. Serve the steak over the cabbage.

⊙ Store leftovers in an airtight container in the fridge for up to 4 days. To reheat, sauté over medium heat for 5 minutes.

modifications: *To make this dish AIP compliant, marinate the steak in a mixture of 1 tablespoon olive oil, 1 tablespoon apple cider vinegar, 1 tablespoon garlic powder, and 1 teaspoon ginger powder. Use bacon fat or lard to cook the coleslaw mix. To make it coconut-free, use aged balsamic vinegar or low-sodium gluten-free tamari instead of the coconut aminos.*

Per serving: Calories **455.7** · Fat **32.8g** · Total Carbs **5.3g** · Fiber **1.9g** · Protein **33.6g**

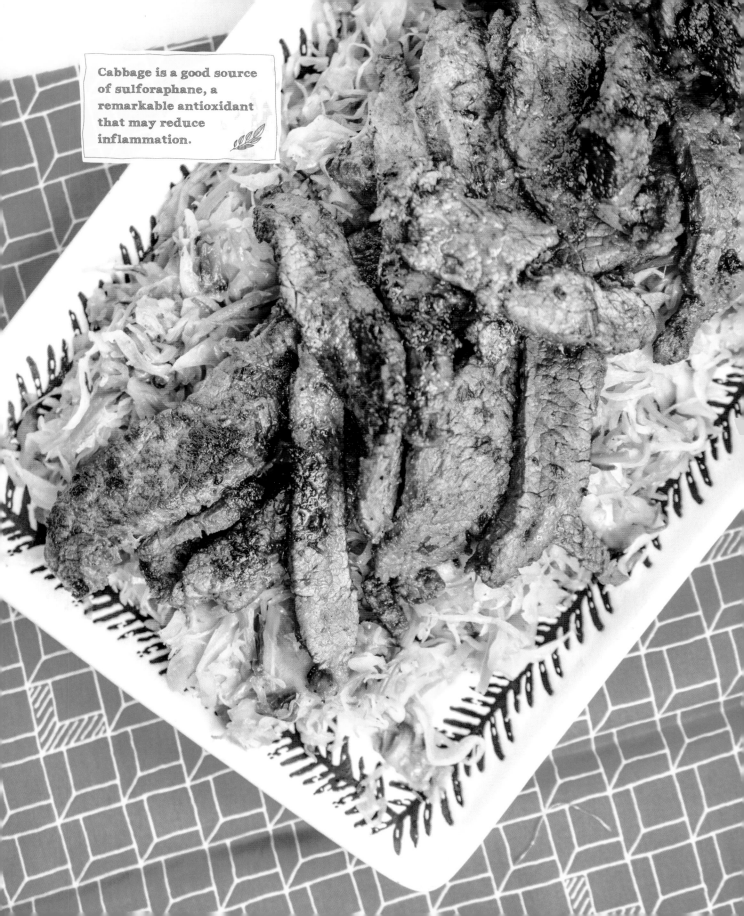

Cabbage is a good source of sulforaphane, a remarkable antioxidant that may reduce inflammation.

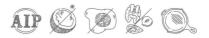

Lemon Herb Beef + Broccoli

Serves 4 ○ Prep Time: 15 minutes ○ Cook Time: 20 minutes

These perfectly browned morsels of beef are little bites of heaven. This is the kind of recipe I make for my mom when I go back home. It's a feel-good meal that delivers big flavor! Check out the note below for my allergen-free baking powder recipe; it's integral to the beef texture. The baking powder acts as a tenderizer while the other components create a coating that gives the beef the most wonderful color and mouthfeel! Finally, a pro tip: don't rush the browning process by trying to fit too many pieces of meat in the pan; an overcrowded pan is the enemy of great texture.

1½ pounds skirt steak, cut into ½-inch cubes

1 teaspoon baking powder (see note)

1 tablespoon coconut aminos

1 tablespoon fish sauce

2 sprigs fresh rosemary, plus more for garnish if desired

1 (1-inch) piece lemon rind

1 teaspoon fine salt, divided

3 tablespoons extra-virgin olive oil or avocado oil, divided

½ cup sliced onions

2 cloves garlic, minced

1 pound trimmed broccoli florets

Juice of 2 lemons

Lemon wedges, for serving (optional)

note: *To make corn-free baking powder, sift together equal parts baking soda, cream of tartar, and arrowroot starch. This method is no-fail! Store in an airtight jar in a cool, dry place for up to a month.*

modifications: *To make this dish coconut-free, replace the coconut aminos with low-sodium gluten-free tamari, liquid aminos, or aged balsamic vinegar.*

○ Heat a 15-inch skillet over medium heat. While it heats, toss the steak cubes with the baking powder in a large bowl until well coated, then add the coconut aminos, fish sauce, rosemary sprigs, lemon rind, and ¼ teaspoon of the salt. Mix well and let the steak marinate until the skillet gets hot.

○ When the skillet is hot, pour in 2 tablespoons of the oil. Put half of the beef in the skillet one piece at a time, making sure none of the pieces are touching. Cook undisturbed for 2 minutes, then use tongs to turn the pieces over. Cook for 2 minutes more, until the cubes have a nice, glossy dark crust on the sides that were browned.

○ Remove the cooked pieces from the skillet and brown the rest of the meat in the same way. Return all the meat to the skillet and add the rosemary, lemon rind, and any remaining marinade. Sauté for 2 minutes, then transfer the contents of the skillet to a bowl and set it aside. This last step should happen quickly so you don't overcook the beef.

○ Pour the remaining tablespoon of oil into the skillet, then add the onions and minced garlic. Sauté until tender, about 4 minutes. Add the broccoli and remaining ¾ teaspoon of salt and sauté until the broccoli is tender and bright green, about 6 minutes. Stir in the lemon juice, deglazing the skillet and mixing all the flavor into the broccoli.

○ Return the beef to the skillet, mix well, and serve right away! Garnish with a sprig of rosemary and serve with lemon wedges, if desired.

○ Store leftovers in the fridge for up to 5 days. To reheat, sauté over medium heat until warmed through.

Per serving: Calories **395** · Fat **20g** · Total Carbs **11g** · Fiber **3.1g** · Protein **46.1g**

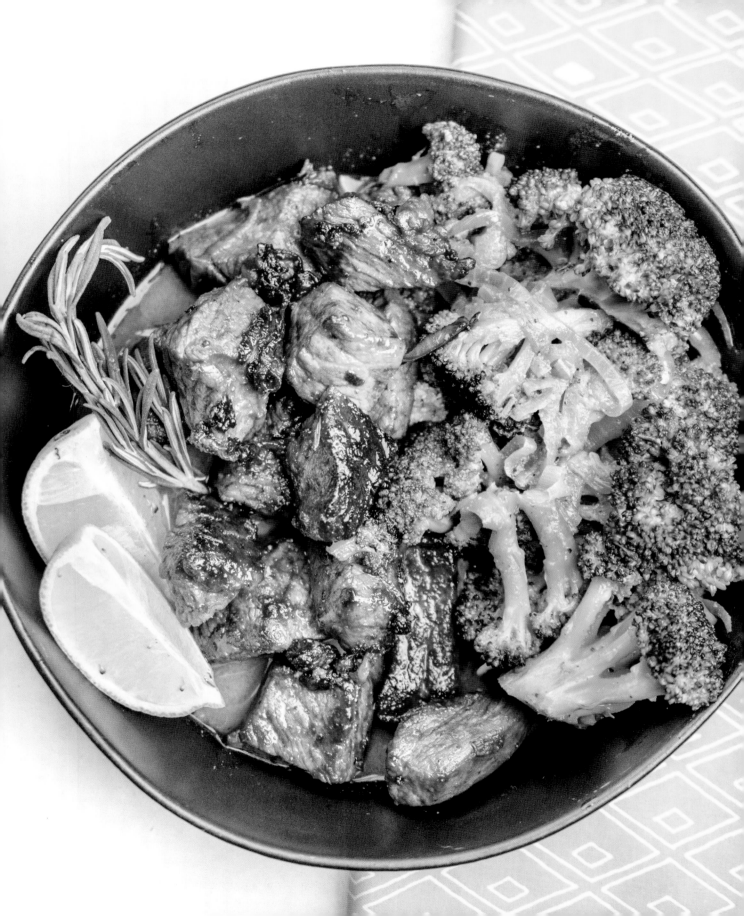

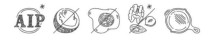

Steakhouse Stir-Fry

Serves 3 ◦ Prep Time: 20 minutes ◦ Cook Time: 25 minutes

If you feel like you can't cook a steak, this recipe is for you; you get the entire steakhouse experience in an easy stir-fry. It's funny how there is this pressure when cooking a steak, kind of like baking: you don't know if it turned out well until you're done. But stir-fry is the opposite—it's practically no-fail. In this dish, creamy horseradish, bacon, and Brussels sprouts are topped with a spiced sirloin that cooks up in no time.

4 slices bacon, diced

½ medium onion, diced (about ¼ cup)

1 (9-ounce) bag shredded Brussels sprouts (about 3 cups)

¼ cup Salted Cashew Cream (page 76)

1 tablespoon prepared horseradish

2 teaspoons fine salt, divided

¼ cup bone broth

1 teaspoon ground cumin

1 pound sirloin steak, cut into bite-sized pieces

2 tablespoons extra-virgin olive oil

1 tablespoon apple cider vinegar

◦ Heat a 15-inch skillet over medium heat. Put the bacon in the skillet and cook until browned and crispy, about 5 minutes. Add the onion and shredded Brussels sprouts to the pan and stir well. Cook, stirring occasionally, until the Brussels sprouts begin to brown, about 8 minutes.

◦ Stir in the cashew cream, horseradish, and 1 teaspoon of the salt. Mix until well combined and thick, then stir in the broth. Keep stirring until everything is tender and creamy, about 3 minutes. Transfer the veggies to a serving plate and cover with aluminum foil to keep warm.

◦ Sprinkle the remaining teaspoon of salt and the cumin over the beef. Drizzle the olive oil into the skillet, then add the sirloin, making sure the pieces are not crowded or overlapping—work in batches if needed to avoid overcrowding the pan. Allow to brown undisturbed for 3 minutes, then sauté for another 2 minutes, until browned all over.

◦ Stir in the vinegar and deglaze the skillet, scraping up the browned bits on the bottom. Serve the steak over the creamy Brussels sprouts.

◦ Store leftovers in an airtight container in the fridge for up to a week. To reheat, quickly sauté in a skillet over medium heat until warm.

notes: *If you can't find good-quality prepared horseradish, a good-quality wasabi powder will work too.*

If you've got Castaway Seed Blend (page 82) on hand, use that instead of the cumin for a flavor boost!

modifications: *To make this dish AIP compliant, use Cauliflower Sour Cream (page 74) instead of the cashew cream and replace the cumin with turmeric powder. To make it nut-free, use Cauliflower Sour Cream. If you can do dairy, heavy cream will work too.*

Per serving: Calories **524** · Fat **29.2g** · Total Carbs **12.8g** · Fiber **4.2g** · Protein **55.2g**

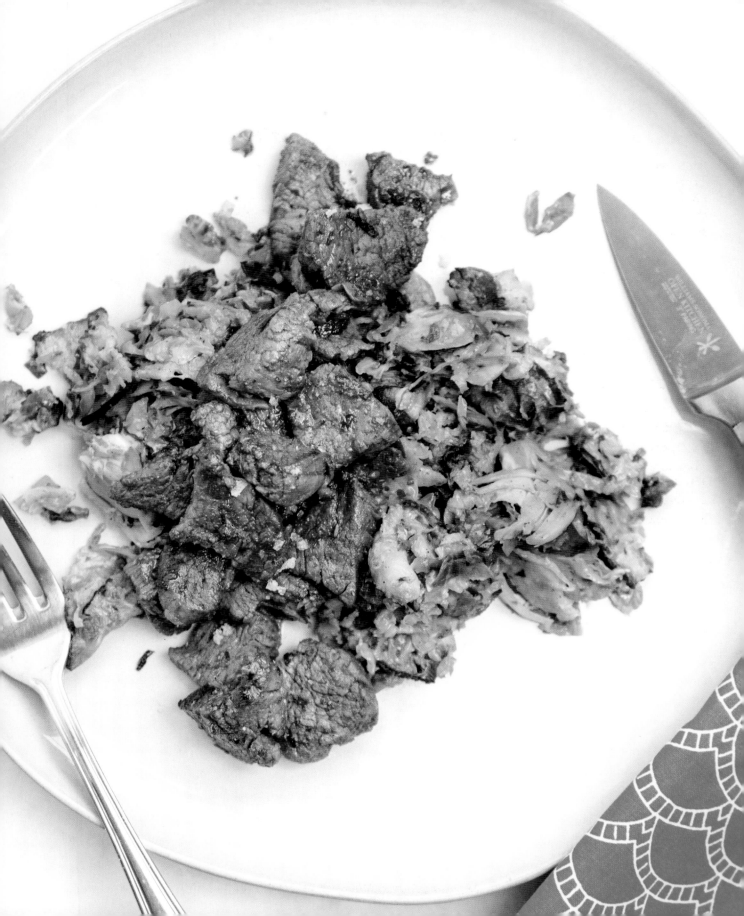

Balsamic Braised
Meatballs + Kale

Serves 4 ◦ Prep Time: 15 minutes ◦ Cook Time: 30 minutes

Braising is a delicious method for cooking meatballs; you get them nice and browned on the outside, and they finish cooking in a slow simmer, which lets them soak up flavor. The texture is quite special. I love this elegant dish with its umami mushrooms, robust leafy greens, and just enough sauce to tie it all together.

1 pound ground beef (85% lean)

1 pound ground pork

1 tablespoon whole psyllium husks or flaxseed meal

3 teaspoons fine salt, divided

2 teaspoons Castaway Seed Blend (page 82) or Cuban Sazón (page 83)

3 tablespoons lard, coconut oil, or ghee, divided

8 ounces sliced cremini mushrooms (about 2 cups)

1 small onion, sliced (about ½ cup)

2 cloves garlic, minced

Leaves from 2 sprigs fresh thyme, minced

¼ cup coconut cream

3 tablespoons aged balsamic vinegar (see notes, page 90), divided

2 cups chopped dinosaur kale, coarse stems removed

½ cup bone broth

◦ In a large bowl, mix together the ground beef, ground pork, psyllium husks, 2 teaspoons of the salt, and the seed blend. Shape the mixture into 16 large meatballs, about 3 inches in diameter.

◦ Heat a 15-inch skillet over medium heat. Melt 1 tablespoon of the lard in the skillet and arrange the meatballs in the pan so they are not touching each other. Brown the meatballs for 4 minutes on each side, 12 minutes total, turning them over with tongs. Transfer the meatballs to a plate, cover, and set aside.

◦ Melt the remaining 2 tablespoons of lard in the skillet, then add the mushrooms, onion, garlic, thyme, and remaining teaspoon of salt. Sauté until the mushrooms are lightly browned and tender, about 6 minutes. Mix in the coconut cream and 1 tablespoon of the vinegar. Turn the heat down to low.

◦ Return the meatballs to the pan and nestle them in the mushroom mixture. Arrange the kale leaves around the meatballs and cover the skillet. Cook for 5 to 7 minutes, then remove the lid and pour in the remaining 2 tablespoons of vinegar and the broth. Cover again and cook until the kale leaves have wilted, about 5 minutes more.

◦ Remove the lid and stir the veggies all together, turning the meatballs around in the sauce. Serve the meatballs with the greens, mushrooms, and sauce.

◦ Store leftovers in the fridge for up to 4 days. Reheat in a skillet covered with a lid over low heat for 10 minutes.

modifications: *To make this dish AIP compliant, use coconut flour instead of the psyllium husks or flaxseed meal and use a dried-herb-only seasoning, like Italian herb blend or herbes de Provence, for the meatballs. To make it coconut-free, use lard or ghee as the cooking fat and replace the coconut cream with Salted Cashew Cream (page 76), Cauliflower Sour Cream (page 74), or heavy cream if you can tolerate it.*

Per serving: Calories **602** · Fat **42.3g** · Total Carbs **9g** · Fiber **2.5g** · Protein **45.3g**

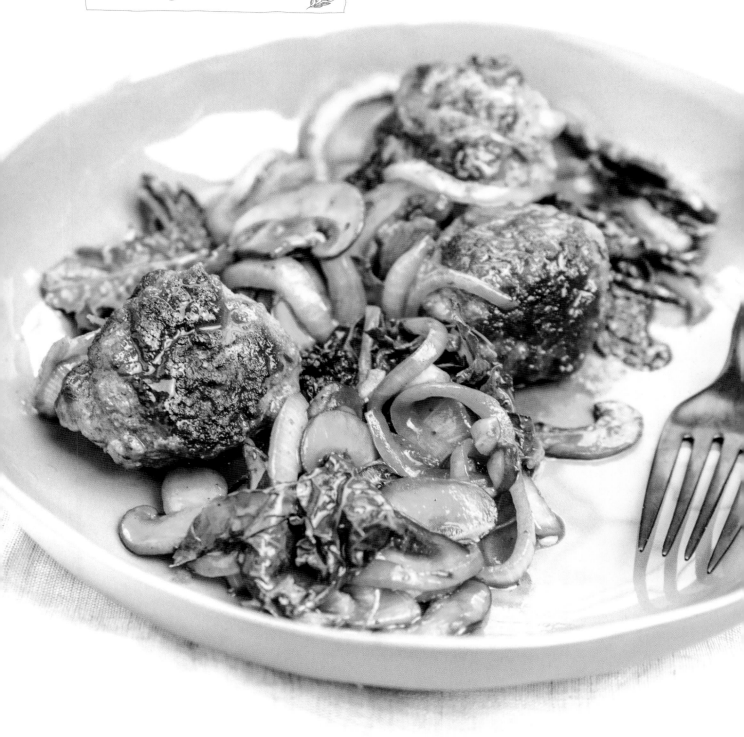

Leafy greens are a good source of calcium and manganese. Braising greens is a great way to make them easier to digest.

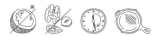

Hamburger Salad

Serves 6 ◦ Prep Time: 15 minutes ◦ Cook Time: 10 minutes

Think cobb salad meets Big Mac—with this dish, you get all the flavors of a burger in a delicious, warm salad. This salad is a version of my nightshade- and dairy-free Hamburger Soup recipe, which you can find on my website, TheCastawayKitchen.com. It is a reader favorite, but most people doubt it until they make it! Both the soup and this salad just work.

6 cups chopped romaine lettuce

½ cup Pickled Radishes (page 84)

1 Hass avocado, peeled, pitted, and diced

1 white or red onion, thinly sliced

¼ cup Horseradish Mayo (page 94)

3 hard-boiled eggs (see note, page 118)

1 tablespoon extra-virgin olive oil or ghee

2 pounds ground beef (85% lean)

1 tablespoon coconut aminos

1 tablespoon Dijon mustard

1 teaspoon everything bagel seasoning

¼ teaspoon fine salt

• Set up the main salad components without tossing everything together: Arrange the lettuce, pickled radishes, diced avocado, and onion slices in a large bowl. Place the mayo on one side. Peel and quarter the eggs and put them in as well. Set the bowl aside while you cook the beef.

• Heat a large skillet over medium heat. When it's hot, pour in the olive oil. Add the ground beef in 1-inch chunks. Cook undisturbed until the chunks brown on one side, about 2 minutes, then stir in the coconut aminos, mustard, everything bagel seasoning, and salt. Mix well, crumbling the beef with a wire whisk, and cook until all the meat is browned through, about 8 minutes more.

• Use a slotted spoon to transfer the beef from the skillet to the salad bowl. Mix everything together well with tongs, taste, and add more salt if needed. Serve right away!

• If you plan to save some for later, I recommend not mixing the ingredients. Store the beef and salad in separate airtight containers, with the mayo on the side, in the fridge for up to 3 days. Reheat the beef and combine the ingredients when ready to serve.

modifications: *To make this salad coconut-free, use low-sodium gluten-free tamari or liquid aminos instead of the coconut aminos.*

Per serving: Calories **466** · Fat **32.8g** · Total Carbs **6.1g** · Fiber **3g** · Protein **34.1g**

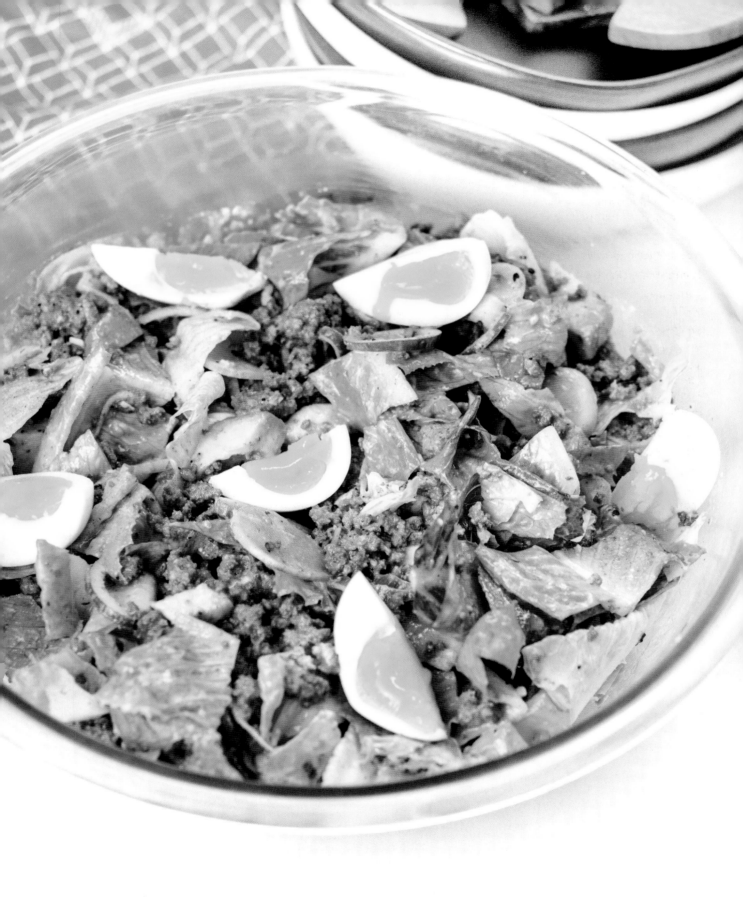

Beef + Broccoli Skillet Casserole

Serves 4 ◦ Prep Time: 5 minutes ◦ Cook Time: 40 minutes

Beef and broccoli are such a dynamic duo, one that appears in this book time and time again. You get all the amazing antioxidant, anti-inflammatory, detox-supporting goodness of broccoli with nutrient-dense, highly digestible, protein-packed beef. They come together beautifully in this dish, which has comfort food written all over it. Crispy, savory, creamy goodness that is kid approved!

1 tablespoon bacon fat or lard

2 pounds ground beef (85% lean)

2½ teaspoons fine salt, divided

2 teaspoons dried parsley

2 teaspoons garlic powder

2 teaspoons onion powder

2 large eggs, whisked

2 tablespoons unsweetened dairy-free milk of choice

1 tablespoon apple cider vinegar

1 pound fresh broccoli florets

2 tablespoons nutritional yeast

2 tablespoons unsweetened, unsalted cashew butter or sunflower seed butter

1 tablespoon extra-virgin olive oil or melted ghee

◦ Place an oven rack in the middle position. Preheat the oven to 400°F.

◦ Heat a 15-inch cast-iron skillet or other oven-safe skillet over medium heat. When it's hot, melt the bacon fat in the skillet, then crumble the ground beef into it. Cook, crumbling the meat with a whisk or spatula, until lightly browned, about 5 minutes. Stir in 2 teaspoons of the salt, the parsley, garlic powder, and onion powder. Continue to cook until the meat is completely browned, about 5 minutes more.

◦ Combine the eggs, milk, and vinegar in a small bowl and pour the mixture evenly over the beef. Remove the skillet from the heat.

◦ In a large bowl, quickly toss the broccoli with the remaining ½ teaspoon of salt, the nutritional yeast, cashew butter, and olive oil until well coated. Spread the florets over the ground beef in an even layer.

◦ Transfer the skillet to the middle rack of the oven and bake until the broccoli florets are browned and toasty and the egg mixture is cooked through, about 30 minutes.

◦ Remove the skillet from the oven and use a large spoon or spatula to serve the casserole hot! Store leftovers in the fridge for up to 4 days. To reheat, bake in a preheated 350°F oven for 10 minutes.

modifications: *To make this dish egg-free, omit the eggs and double the milk. Mix together the milk and vinegar as described above, but add 1 tablespoon grain-free flour to create a slurry. To make it AIP compliant, follow the instructions for the egg-free version, but use coconut flour or arrowroot starch for the slurry and use coconut butter instead of nut or seed butter on the broccoli.*

Per serving: Calories **568** · Fat **36g** · Total Carbs **11.1g** · Fiber **3.6g** · Protein **49.9g**

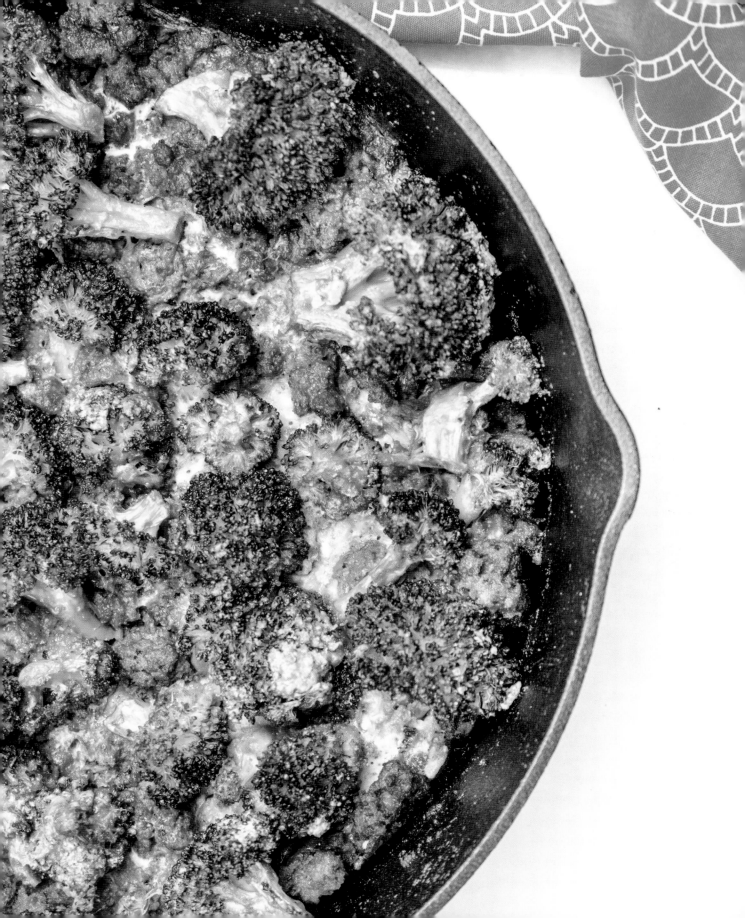

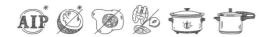

Rich Slow-Cooked Stew

Serves 5 ○ Prep Time: 15 minutes ○ Cook Time: 1 hour 20 minutes or 4½ hours, depending on method

This flavorful stew combines tender root vegetables, which are easy to digest, with fall-apart beef, anti-inflammatory spices, and the ultimate healing food, bone broth. It is perfect for sick days and winter nights. Move over, chicken noodle soup—there's a new classic in town. This dish can be made on the stovetop, in a slow cooker, or in a pressure cooker for convenience.

2 tablespoons tallow, lard, or ghee, divided

2 pounds beef stew meat

2½ teaspoons fine salt, divided

½ teaspoon baking powder (see note, page 148)

2 teaspoons garlic powder

2 teaspoons ground black pepper

1 teaspoon dried oregano leaves

1 teaspoon dried parsley

1 teaspoon ground cumin

½ teaspoon turmeric powder

3 medium celery ribs, diced

3 small carrots, diced

1 small onion, diced

1 small rutabaga, diced

3 cloves garlic, minced

1 bay leaf

2 tablespoons coconut aminos

2 tablespoons red wine vinegar

4 cups bone broth

• In a medium-sized heavy-bottomed pot or Dutch oven, melt 1 tablespoon of the tallow over medium heat. While it melts, toss the beef with 2 teaspoons of the salt and the baking powder in a large bowl. Add the beef to the pot and cook, stirring often, for 5 minutes, or until browned. Mix in the dried seasonings, then remove the beef from the pot and set aside.

• Melt the remaining tablespoon of tallow in the pot, then add all of the diced vegetables, the garlic, and bay leaf. Cook, stirring occasionally, for 10 minutes, or until the vegetables are tender and aromatic. Stir in the remaining ½ teaspoon of salt, the coconut aminos, and vinegar and deglaze the pot, using a wooden spoon to scrape up all the flavorful bits stuck on the bottom.

• Return the beef to the pot and mix it with the vegetables. Pour in the broth, stir well, and bring to a simmer, still over medium heat.

• **To make the stew on the stovetop,** cover the pot with a tight-fitting lid and simmer over low heat for 4 hours, or until the meat is very tender.

• **To make the stew in a slow cooker,** transfer the stew to a slow cooker, cover, and cook on high for 4 hours, or until the meat is very tender.

• **To make the stew in an electric pressure cooker,** transfer the stew to a pressure cooker, seal the lid, and cook on high pressure for 50 minutes. Release the pressure manually and open the lid.

• Keep warm until ready to serve. Store leftovers in the fridge for up to 6 days. To reheat, bring to a simmer in a saucepan.

note: *If you can't find a rutabaga, a turnip will do.*

modifications: *To make this dish AIP compliant, omit the black pepper and cumin and add 1 teaspoon ginger powder and 1 teaspoon onion powder. To make it coconut-free, use low-sodium gluten-free tamari instead of the coconut aminos.*

Per serving: Calories **682** · Fat **49.8g** · Total Carbs **10.1g** · Fiber **2.4g** · Protein **45.9g**

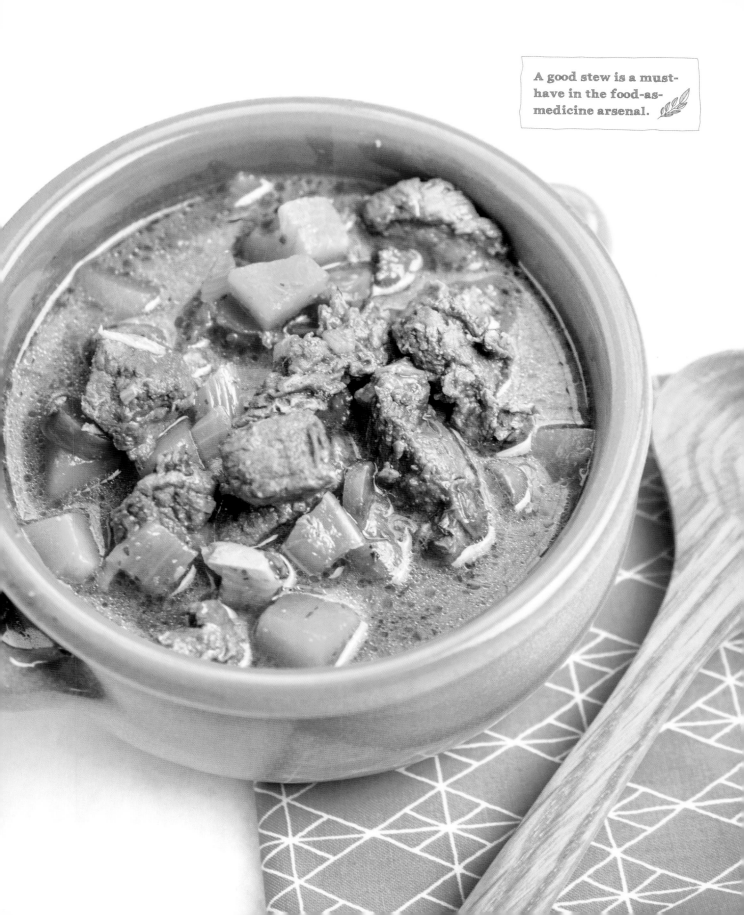

A good stew is a must-have in the food-as-medicine arsenal.

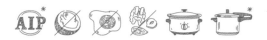

Meatballs + Mushroom Gravy

Serves 4 ○ Prep Time: 20 minutes ○ Cook Time: 4 hours 10 minutes

Think Swedish meatballs, but easier and much better for you. Folks can't believe this rich gravy is essentially mushroom puree! This slow cooker recipe has a wonderful texture and a comforting flavor. Serve it hot over cauliflower rice or with Warm Garlic Herb Radish Salad (page 298), or enjoy it as finger food! Pressure cooker instructions are also included.

For the meatballs:

2 pounds ground beef (85% lean)

2 tablespoons whole psyllium husks or flaxseed meal

2 teaspoons Castaway Seed Blend (page 82)

2 teaspoons fine salt

1 teaspoon garlic powder

½ teaspoon ground white pepper

¼ teaspoon ground nutmeg

For the mushroom gravy:

2 tablespoons ghee or lard

1 medium onion, diced

1¼ cups sliced cremini mushrooms (about 5 ounces)

Leaves from 2 sprigs fresh thyme, minced

1 teaspoon fine salt

Juice of 1 lemon

1 cup bone broth

2 tablespoons unsweetened dairy-free milk of choice

1 tablespoon extra-virgin olive oil, divided

¼ cup minced fresh chives, for garnish

modifications: To make this dish AIP compliant, replace the psyllium husks with 1 tablespoon unflavored grass-fed beef gelatin and 1 tablespoon coconut flour. Replace the seed blend with 1 teaspoon each onion powder and ginger powder, or use your favorite unsalted seasoning blend. Omit the white pepper.

○ Make the meatballs: In a large bowl, combine the ground beef, psyllium husks, seed blend, salt, garlic powder, white pepper, and nutmeg. Mix well and shape into 16 meatballs, about 2 inches in diameter. Set aside.

○ Make the mushroom gravy: Heat a large skillet over medium heat. When it's hot, melt the ghee in the skillet. Add the onion, mushrooms, thyme, and salt and sauté for 8 to 10 minutes, until the onion is very tender and aromatic. Stir in the lemon juice and deglaze the skillet.

○ Transfer the onion and mushroom mixture to a blender, then add the broth and milk and blend until smooth and creamy.

○ Cook the meatballs in the gravy: Drizzle 1½ teaspoons of the olive oil into a slow cooker, then pour in the gravy. Arrange the meatballs in the gravy so that they are mostly submerged. Drizzle the remaining 1½ teaspoons of oil over everything.

○ Cover and cook on low for 4 hours, or until the meatballs are cooked through and tender. Remove the lid and use a spoon to stir gently, turning the meatballs over in the sauce to coat them. Garnish with the chives before serving.

○ Store leftovers in the fridge for up to 5 days. Reheat in a skillet covered with a tight-fitting lid over low heat for 10 minutes.

Pressure Cooker Method: Make the meatballs as directed. Cook the mushrooms per the instructions in a pressure cooker using the sauté mode. After you deglaze the cooker with the lemon juice, add the broth and milk and use an immersion blender to puree everything into a smooth gravy. Add the meatballs and all of the olive oil. Seal the lid and cook on high pressure for 5 minutes. Let the pressure release naturally for 10 minutes, then release it manually. Open the lid, gently stir, and serve, garnished with the chives.

Per serving: Calories **481** · Fat **29.2g** · Total Carbs **8.9g** · Fiber **2.8g** · Protein **44.6g**

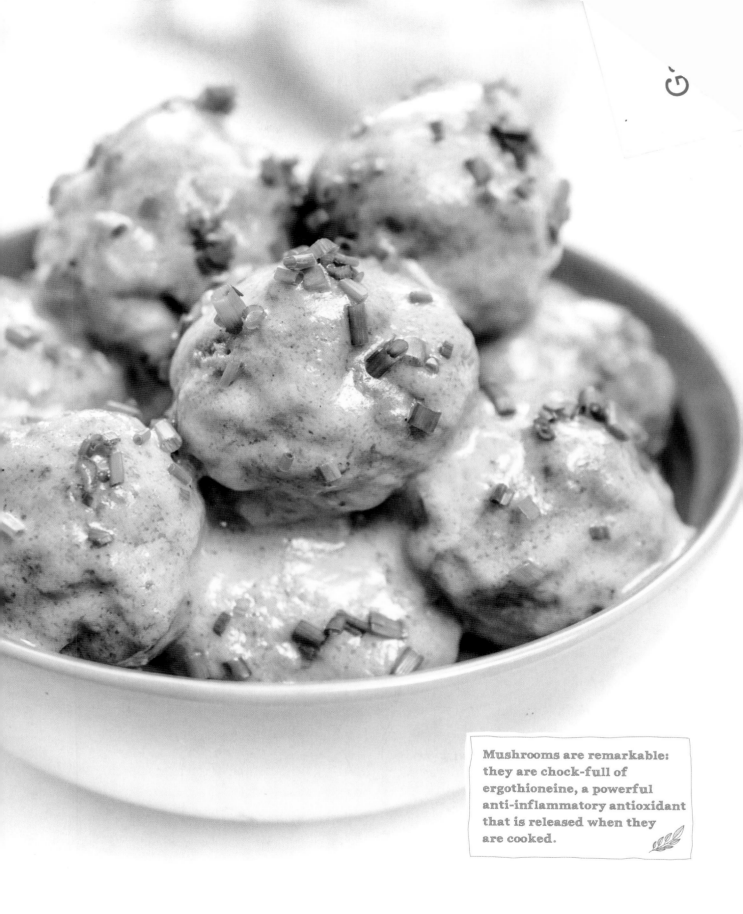

Mushrooms are remarkable: they are chock-full of ergothioneine, a powerful anti-inflammatory antioxidant that is released when they are cooked.

arlic Steak + Mushrooms

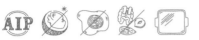

Serves 2 ◦ Prep Time: 12 minutes ◦ Cook Time: 22 minutes

One day, my mom called me in excitement: she had coated some mushrooms in fat, thrown them in the oven, and roasted them with some meat for a hurried weeknight meal. She hadn't anticipated anything special, but when she took the first bite, she just had to pick up the phone and tell me how amazing it was. A few experiments with this happy accident later, and we're officially hooked. Roasted meat and mushrooms, people! Tell your friends!

2 tablespoons extra-virgin olive oil

1 tablespoon minced fresh ginger

1 tablespoon minced garlic

1 teaspoon fish sauce

12 ounces skirt steak, hanger steak, or flap meat, cut crosswise into 2 pieces

4 cups whole shiitake or cremini mushrooms (about 6 ounces)

2 tablespoons ghee or lard, melted

1½ teaspoons fine salt

1 tablespoon coconut aminos, for drizzling

Leaves from 2 sprigs fresh cilantro, for garnish

notes: *The leftovers are great over salad or cauliflower rice. You can also add Gut-Healing Teriyaki Sauce (page 70) to create a stir-fry and serve it over Cauliflower "Fried" Rice (page 316).*

modifications: *To make this dish coconut-free, omit the coconut aminos or replace it with low-sodium gluten-free tamari.*

- Place an oven rack in the middle position. Preheat the oven to 400°F.

- In a small bowl, mix together the olive oil, ginger, garlic, and fish sauce and set aside.

- Lay the steak on a cutting board and pound it with a meat mallet or heavy-bottomed pot to tenderize it. Transfer the steaks to a sheet pan, pour the garlic-ginger mixture all over the steaks, and rub the mixture into the meat, coating evenly. Then lay the steaks flat, side by side but not overlapping, on one side of the sheet pan, leaving three-quarters of the pan free for the mushrooms.

- Clean the mushrooms by wiping the caps and steps with a damp cloth. If necessary, trim any of the stems that have stubborn dirt on them. If you're using cremini mushrooms, cut them into quarters.

- Put the mushrooms on the sheet pan next to the steaks. Pour the ghee over the mushrooms and use your hands to massage the ghee evenly into all of the mushrooms.

- Sprinkle the salt evenly over the steak and mushrooms. The higher you sprinkle from, the more evenly the salt will coat the food.

- Place the sheet pan in the oven on the middle rack and roast for 22 minutes. Remove from the oven. Place each steak on a plate and serve the mushrooms over the steaks. Carefully tilt the sheet pan to pour the sauce over the mushrooms. Drizzle the coconut aminos over everything and garnish with the cilantro.

- Store leftovers in the fridge for up to 4 days. To reheat, thinly slice the steak, place 1 teaspoon of olive oil in a skillet over medium heat, and gently sauté the steak with the mushrooms for 8 minutes.

Per serving: Calories **574** · Fat **42.2g** · Total Carbs **8.8g** · Fiber **2.1g** · Protein **39g**

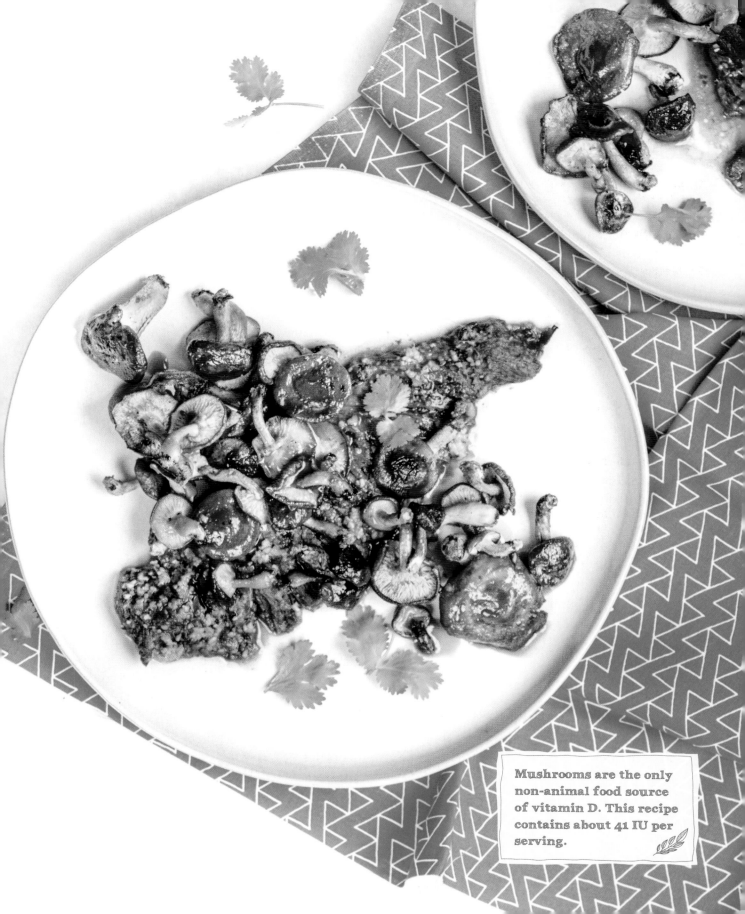

Mushrooms are the only non-animal food source of vitamin D. This recipe contains about 41 IU per serving.

Sesame Meatballs + Broccoli with Teriyaki Sauce

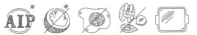

Serves 4 ◦ Prep Time: 15 minutes ◦ Cook Time: 30 minutes

Beef and broccoli is my favorite protein-and-veggie combination; not only do they taste amazing together, but the combo is a nutritionist's dream come true. In this dish, vitamins B6 (in the sesame seeds), B12 (in the beef), and folate (in the broccoli) work together to reduce the risk of heart disease by reducing levels of homocysteine. Get your takeout fakeout on while doing your body good!

4 cups broccoli florets

1 tablespoon extra-virgin olive oil

1½ teaspoons fine salt, divided

1 pound ground beef (85% lean)

1 medium Hass avocado, peeled, pitted, and mashed

1 tablespoon sesame seeds

2 teaspoons garlic powder

2 teaspoons ginger powder

1 teaspoon dried cilantro leaves

1 teaspoon Dijon mustard

2 tablespoons toasted sesame oil

¼ cup Gut-Healing Teriyaki Sauce (page 70), plus more if desired, for serving

◦ Place an oven rack in the middle position. Preheat the oven to 400°F.

◦ Put the broccoli florets on a sheet pan, then drizzle them with the olive oil and sprinkle with ½ teaspoon of the salt. Toss, massaging the oil into the florets, then spread them evenly over the sheet pan.

◦ Make the meatballs: In a large bowl, combine the ground beef, avocado, sesame seeds, garlic powder, ginger, cilantro, mustard, and remaining teaspoon of salt until thoroughly mixed. Shape the mixture into 12 meatballs, about 2 inches in diameter. Place the meatballs on the sheet pan among the broccoli florets. Drizzle the sesame oil over everything on the pan.

◦ Place the sheet pan in the oven on the middle rack and roast for 30 minutes. Remove the pan from the oven. The meatballs will be juicy and browned, and the broccoli nice and crispy!

◦ Drizzle a tablespoon of teriyaki sauce on each plate, or more to your liking. Enjoy! Store leftovers in an airtight container in the fridge for up to 4 days. To reheat, sauté in a skillet over medium heat until warmed through.

note: *You can use an equal amount of any fatty ground meat for this recipe, like dark meat turkey or pork.*

modifications: *To make this dish AIP compliant, omit the sesame seeds and mustard and replace the sesame oil with coconut oil. To make it coconut-free, use the coconut-free version of the teriyaki sauce.*

Per serving with Sauce: Calories **435** · Fat **32.4g** · Total Carbs **8.5g** · Fiber **3.3g** · Protein **27.1g**

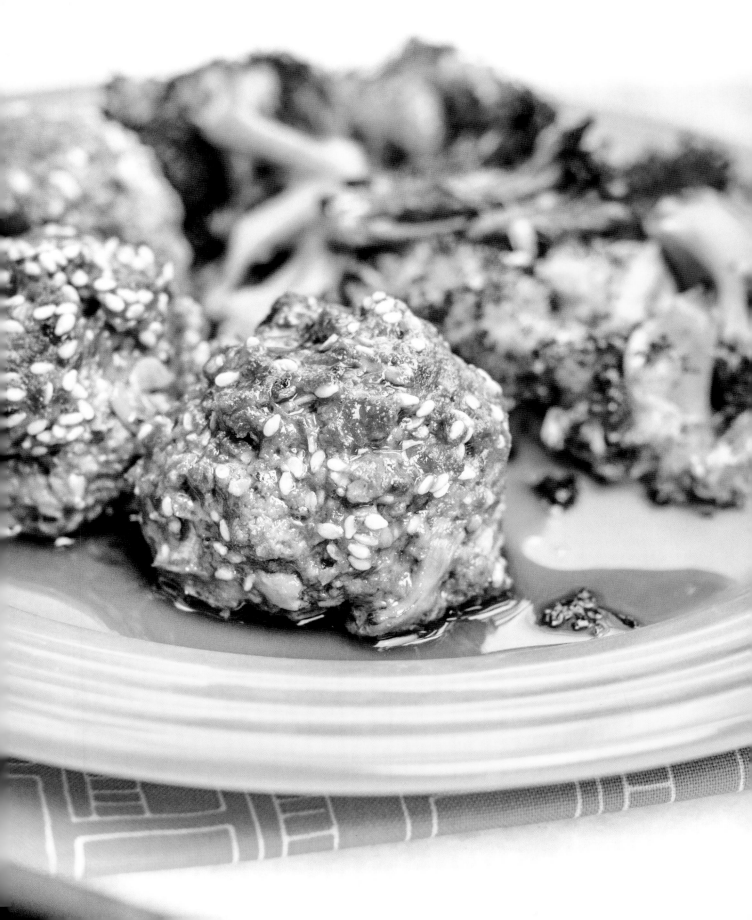

Ginger Cilantro Steak +
Tangy Cauliflower

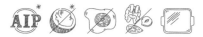

Serves 4 ◦ Prep Time: 10 minutes ◦ Cook Time: 30 minutes

Two flavor bomb recipes meet up in the oven for a dinner that comes together in forty minutes and tastes like a party in your mouth. You need two sheet pans for this recipe, so if you have only one, this recipe is a valid reason to pick up a second.

For the marinade:

1½ teaspoons fine salt

1 tablespoon minced fresh ginger

1 tablespoon minced garlic

2 tablespoons minced fresh cilantro

1½ teaspoons turmeric powder

¼ cup extra-virgin olive oil

1½ pounds skirt steak, hanger steak, or flat iron steak

For the cauliflower:

1 medium head cauliflower, cored and cut into florets

½ large onion, diced

½ teaspoon fine salt

1 teaspoon whole mustard seeds, or ½ teaspoon ground mustard seeds

½ teaspoon ground white pepper

¼ teaspoon Chinese five-spice powder

2 tablespoons coconut aminos

2 tablespoons extra-virgin olive oil

Juice of 2 lemons

Sprig of fresh cilantro, for garnish (optional)

◦ Place one oven rack in the middle position and another underneath the broiler. Preheat the oven to 400°F.

◦ In a bowl, combine all of the ingredients for the marinade and mix well. Put the steak in the bowl and massage the marinade into it, then set aside.

◦ Spread the cauliflower florets and onion on a sheet pan. Sprinkle with the salt and spices and toss to combine. Drizzle the coconut aminos, olive oil, and lemon juice over the vegetables and toss, mixing everything together and evenly coating the cauliflower. Spread the florets out on the pan and arrange them stem up.

◦ Put the sheet pan in the oven on the middle rack and roast for 30 minutes.

◦ When the cauliflower has roasted for 17 minutes, put the steak on another sheet pan and pour the extra marinade over it. Place the steak in the oven just below the broiler and roast for 7 minutes, then set the oven to the broil setting. Broil for 3 minutes, until the steak has a nice brown color. The cauliflower should be tender and the steak cooked to medium.

◦ Remove everything from the oven at the same time. Transfer the steak to a cutting board and let it rest for 5 minutes while you plate the cauliflower. Use a spatula to scrape up the crispy florets and onion pieces. Serve with the steak and garnish with a sprig of cilantro, if desired.

◦ Store leftovers in the fridge for up to 5 days. To reheat, sauté in a skillet over medium heat for 8 minutes.

modifications: *To make this dish coconut-free, replace the coconut aminos with 1 tablespoon molasses mixed with 1 tablespoon low-sodium gluten-free tamari.*

To enjoy this steak with an AIP-compliant side, I suggest Burnt Cabbage (page 232).

Steak, per 6-ounce serving: Calories **411** · Fat **28.7g** · Total Carbs **1.5g** · Fiber **0.2g** · Protein **33.1g**

Cauliflower, per serving: Calories **119** · Fat **7.6g** · Total Carbs **12.6g** · Fiber **3.7g** · Protein **3.3g**

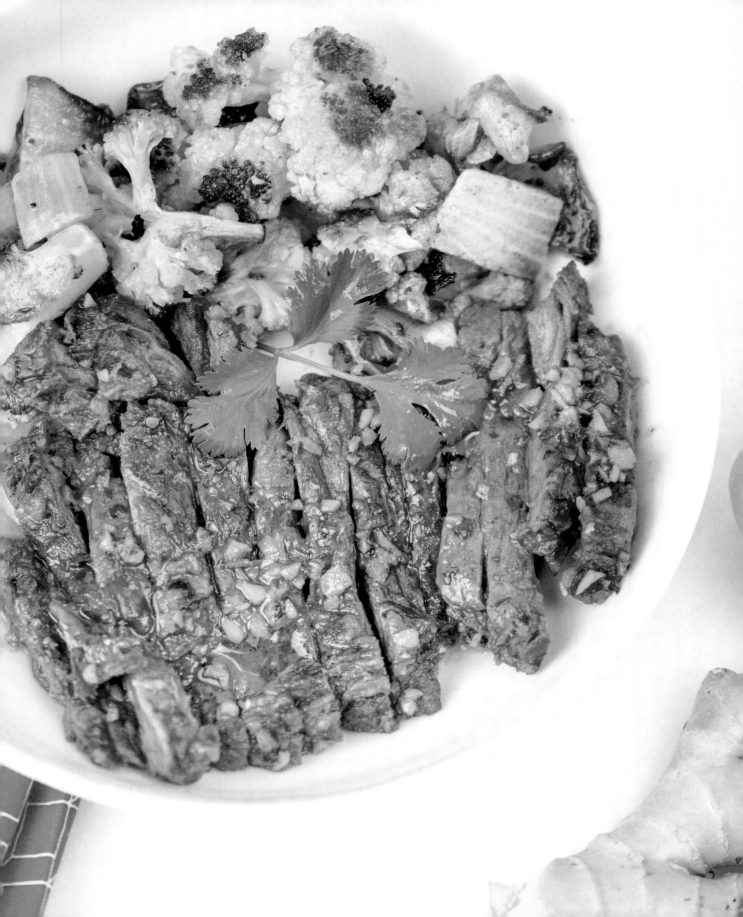

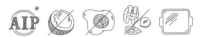

Carne Asada Meatballs

Serves 5 ◦ Prep Time: 15 minutes, plus 1 hour for marinade to infuse ◦ Cook Time: 25 minutes

This dish has been called "the best thing I have ever eaten" and "flavor bomb" by many a reader. It is one of the most popular recipes on my blog, *The Castaway Kitchen,* and a sheet pan recipe to boot! You are going to love this fun and easy take on carne asada, which pairs perfectly with Spicy Yellow Rice (page 320).

For the marinade:

½ large onion, finely diced

¼ cup minced fresh cilantro, plus more for garnish

2 cloves garlic, minced

2 tablespoons apple cider vinegar

2 tablespoons extra-virgin olive oil or avocado oil

Juice of 1 lemon

Juice of 1 lime

2 teaspoons fine salt

1 teaspoon ground black pepper

1 teaspoon dried oregano leaves

1 teaspoon ground cumin

For the meatballs:

2 pounds ground beef (85% lean)

2 tablespoons unflavored grass-fed beef gelatin

2 tablespoons whole psyllium husks or flaxseed meal

1 tablespoon melted bacon fat or ghee

5 lemon or lime wedges, for serving

◦ Mix together all of the marinade ingredients in a small bowl and set it in the fridge overnight or for at least for 1 hour.

◦ When you're ready to cook the meatballs, place an oven rack in the middle position and preheat the oven to 400°F.

◦ Pour the marinade into a large bowl. Add the ground beef, gelatin, and psyllium husks and mix well. Shape the mixture into 18 to 20 meatballs, about 2 inches in diameter. Place them on a sheet pan, 2 inches apart, and brush them with the bacon fat.

◦ Put the sheet pan in the oven on the middle rack and bake for 25 minutes, or until they are cooked through. Serve hot with lemon wedges and garnished with cilantro. Store leftovers in an airtight container in the fridge for up to 4 days. Reheat in a skillet covered with a tight-fitting lid over medium heat for 5 minutes.

modifications: To make this dish AIP compliant, omit the black pepper and cumin from the marinade and add 2 teaspoons garlic powder. Replace the psyllium husks or flaxseed meal in the meatballs with coconut flour.

Per serving: Calories **406** · Fat **26.1g** · Total Carbs **6.2g** · Fiber **2.2g** · Protein **35.3g**

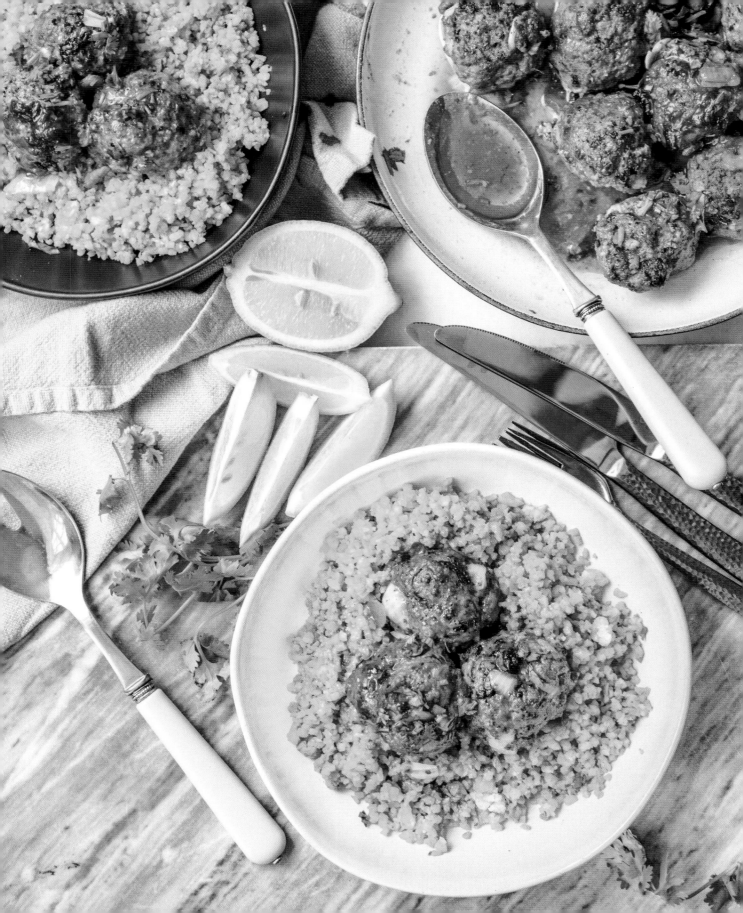

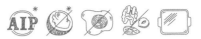

Kitchen Sink Casserole

Serves 8 ○ Prep Time: 15 minutes ○ Cook Time: 50 minutes

Everyone needs a good clean-out-the-fridge recipe, and this one really does the job! It calls for 3 pounds of ground beef and 6 cups of various diced veggies. Can you tell I developed this recipe when my CSA produce was about to go bad? Because that is totally what happened. You can use any combination of produce—not just what I happened to have on hand—to make this creamy-with-just-the-right-amount-of-crispy casserole.

---

7 celery ribs, finely diced

6 collard green leaves, finely chopped

2 broccoli stalks, finely diced

2 medium carrots, finely diced

1 medium parsnip, finely diced

1 medium red onion, finely diced

2 tablespoons extra-virgin olive oil, divided

1 tablespoon plus 1 teaspoon fine salt, divided

3 pounds ground beef (85% lean), pork, or turkey

1 tablespoon Castaway Seed Blend (page 82)

1 batch Cauliflower Sour Cream (page 74)

modifications: *To make this casserole AIP compliant, replace the seed blend with the AIP-compliant seasoning of your choice and use the AIP version of the Cauliflower Sour Cream. To make it coconut-free, use the coconut-free version of the sour cream.*

awesome additions: *This hearty casserole is a meal on its own, but it also pairs well with Charred Kale Soup (page 300).*

○ Preheat the oven to 400°F.

○ Roast the vegetables: In an 8 by 12-inch casserole dish, toss all of the vegetables with 1 tablespoon of the olive oil and 1 teaspoon of the salt. Put the casserole dish in the oven and roast the vegetables for 10 minutes while you brown the beef.

○ Heat a large skillet over medium heat. When it's hot, drizzle in the remaining tablespoon of oil. Crumble the ground beef into the skillet and season the meat with the remaining tablespoon of salt and the seed blend. Cook the beef, breaking it up with a wire whisk and stirring, until crumbled and browned, about 10 minutes. Continue cooking until any liquid that has pooled in the skillet simmers off, then remove the pan from the heat.

○ Use a spatula to turn over the vegetables in the casserole dish, then spread them back out. They should be softened but still vibrant in color.

○ Smear 1 cup of the sour cream over the veggies. Add the beef and spread it into an even layer. Finally, add the remaining sour cream and spread it evenly over the beef.

○ Put the casserole dish back in the oven and bake for 40 minutes, or until the sides are browned and the top looks firm and has begun to crack.

○ Remove the casserole from the oven and cut it into 8 large squares. Use a spatula to serve.

○ Store leftovers in the fridge for up to 5 days. To reheat, cover with aluminum foil and put in a preheated 350°F oven for 30 minutes. (Note: Never put a chilled casserole dish straight from the refrigerator into a preheated oven. Either allow the dish of food to come to room temperature first, or put the dish in a cold oven and then turn on the oven.)

Per serving: Calories **526** · Fat **39.3g** · Total Carbs **11.2g** · Fiber **3.6g** · Protein **31.3g**

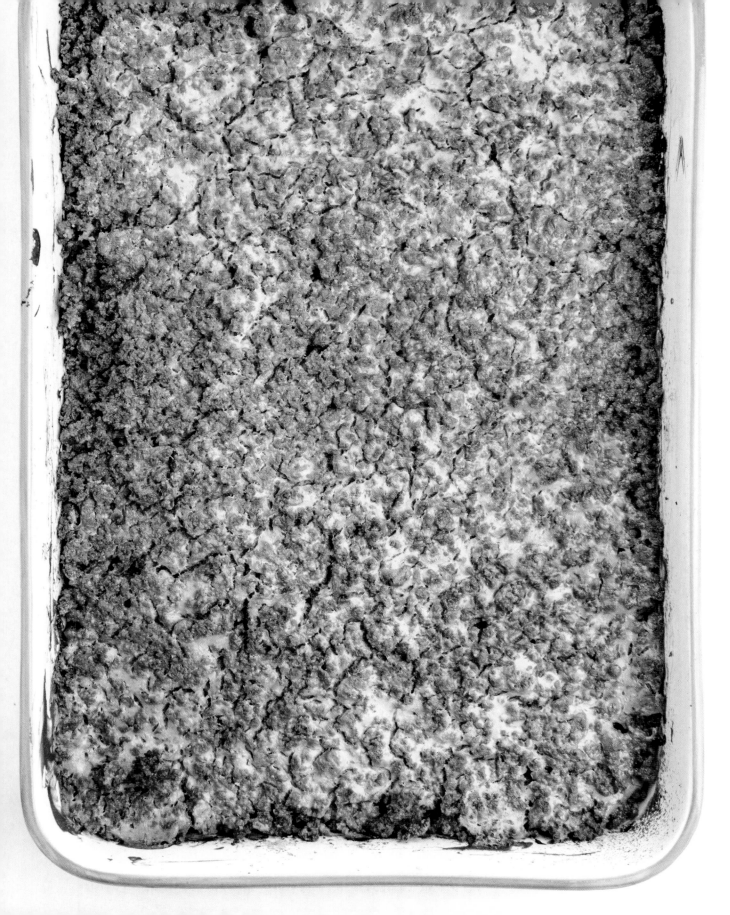

Mustard Beef + Broccoli Rice Sheet Pan Stir-Fry

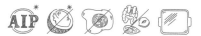

Serves 4 ◦ Prep Time: 20 minutes ◦ Cook Time: 20 minutes

Did you know that mustard and broccoli are a match made in heaven? Adding ground mustard seeds to cooked broccoli increases the bioavailability of broccoli's sulforaphane, an antioxidant that does a lot of cool stuff: it fights cancer, regulates blood sugar, and protects cells. Eating raw broccoli is a great way to get these benefits, but this easy sheet pan meal is way tastier!

1 pound sirloin strips

¼ teaspoon baking soda

6 cups fresh riced broccoli (see note)

1 cup sliced shiitake mushrooms (about 4 ounces)

4 cloves garlic, minced

1 teaspoon fine salt

1 teaspoon garlic powder

1 teaspoon ground mustard seeds

1 teaspoon onion powder

½ teaspoon ginger powder

1½ tablespoons coconut aminos

2 tablespoons extra-virgin olive oil

1 teaspoon fish sauce

1 tablespoon toasted sesame oil, for drizzling

1 tablespoon sesame seeds, for garnish

◦ Place an oven rack in the middle position. Preheat the oven to 400°F.

◦ Toss the beef and baking soda in a large bowl and let sit for 5 minutes.

◦ Add the remaining ingredients, except the sesame oil and sesame seeds, and toss to combine. Let everything marinate while the oven comes to temperature.

◦ Spread the beef and rice mixture over a sheet pan in a thin, even layer. If the layer is thicker than about 1 inch or the meat is crowded, divide the mixture between 2 sheet pans.

◦ Put the sheet pan in the oven on the middle rack and roast for 18 to 20 minutes, until the beef is just cooked through and the broccoli rice has toasty bits.

◦ Use a spatula to scrape up the stir-fry and serve in bowls. Drizzle with the sesame oil and garnish with the sesame seeds.

◦ Store leftovers in the fridge for up to 5 days. To reheat, sauté in a skillet over medium heat for 8 minutes.

note: *If you can't find riced broccoli at the store, make your own. Save the raw stems when you roast broccoli florets and just run them through a food processor. Store in the fridge for when you're in need of riced veggies!*

modifications: *To make this dish AIP compliant, use wasabi powder instead of the mustard powder (wasabi powder also has myrosinase, the important cofactor for sulforaphane bioavailability). Also omit the sesame oil and seeds. To make it coconut-free, use low-sodium gluten-free tamari instead of the coconut aminos.*

Per serving: Calories **359** · Fat **20g** · Total Carbs **14.6g** · Fiber **3.3g** · Protein **31.1g**

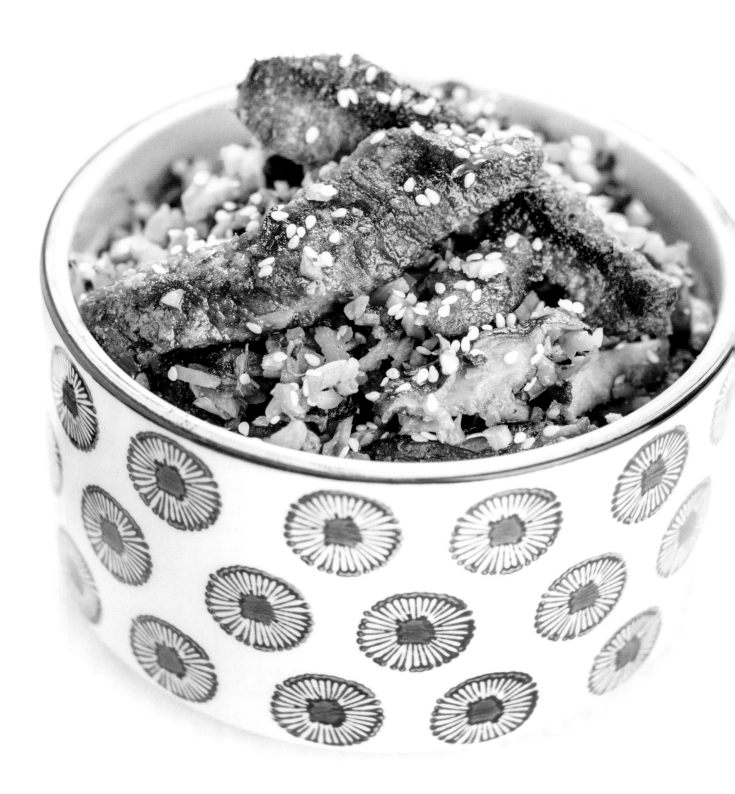

Mushroom Herb Meatballs with Cauliflower Steaks

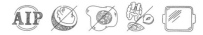

Serves 4 ○ Prep Time: 20 minutes ○ Cook Time: 35 minutes

My mushroom-hating husband had this to say, and I quote, "These are really good meatballs." Getting liver, olives, and mushrooms into his diet is one of my favorite pastimes, and I'm very sneaky about it.

For the cauliflower steaks:

1½ heads cauliflower (about 2½ pounds)

2 tablespoons extra-virgin olive oil

1 teaspoon fine salt

For the meatballs:

2 pounds ground beef (85% lean)

2 teaspoons fine salt

1 teaspoon onion powder

1 cup sliced cremini mushrooms (about 4 ounces)

3 cloves garlic, peeled

Needles from 2 sprigs fresh rosemary

2 tablespoons extra-virgin olive oil

For serving:

¼ cup Green Onion Relish (page 98), for serving

○ Place one oven rack in the middle position and another in the bottom position. Preheat the oven to 400°F.

○ Prepare the cauliflower steaks: Trim the cauliflower stems to create a flat surface. Place the whole head of cauliflower core end down on a cutting board. Cut the head in half and slice each half into 3 steaks, about ½ inch thick, starting from the cut side. Cut the half head of cauliflower into 2 steaks, about ½ inch thick. Lay the cauliflower steaks flat on a sheet pan. Drizzle the olive oil over them and sprinkle them with the salt. Put the pan in the oven on the middle rack and roast for 35 minutes.

○ Prepare the meatballs: Combine the ground beef, salt, and onion powder in a large bowl. In a food processor, pulse the mushrooms, garlic, rosemary, and olive oil until finely minced. Add the mushroom mixture to the meat and mix well, then shape the mixture into 12 meatballs, 2 inches in diameter. Arrange the meatballs on a second sheet pan. Place the second pan on the bottom rack of the oven and roast for 25 minutes.

○ Ideally, everything will be ready to come out of the oven at the same time. When done, the cauliflower steaks should be tender and golden brown and the meatballs cooked through and lightly browned. If necessary, pull out one pan and leave the other in the oven to cook until done.

○ Serve 2 cauliflower steaks with 3 meatballs and 1 tablespoon of the relish. Store leftovers in the fridge for up to 5 days. To reheat, sauté in a skillet over medium heat for 5 to 8 minutes.

note: *If you don't have Green Onion Relish on hand, any sauce will do here! The flavors of the meatballs and cauliflower are so good and flexible that they will go well with just about any condiment.*

Per serving: Calories **647** · Fat **46g** · Total Carbs **13.9g** · Fiber **5g** · Protein **45.9g**

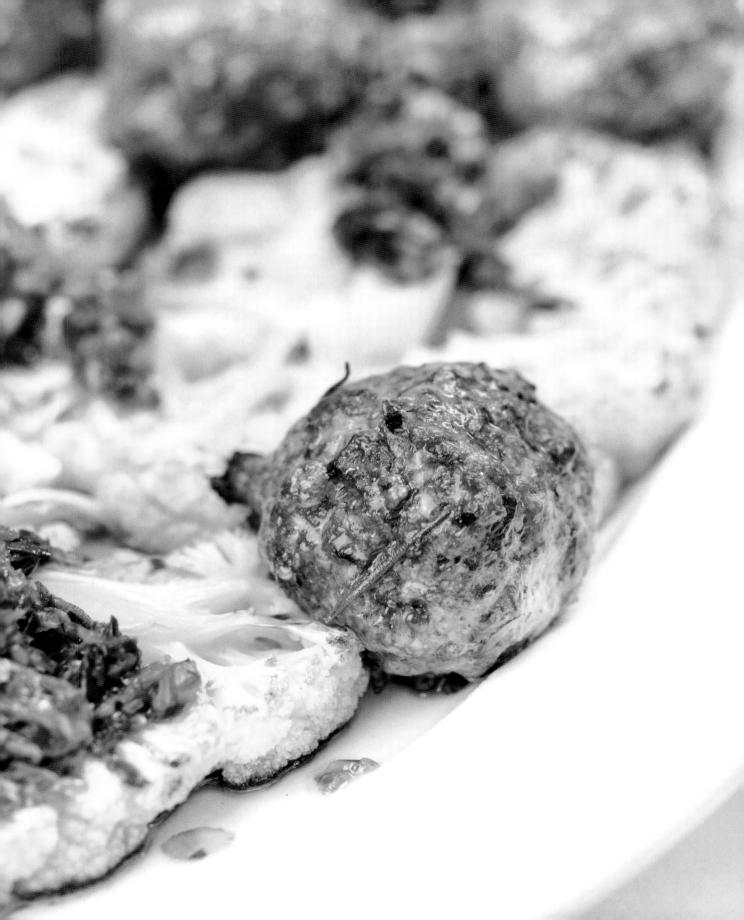

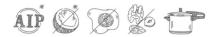

Creamy Beef + Bacon Soup

Serves 3 ◦ Prep Time: 10 minutes ◦ Cook Time: 25 minutes

This creamy soup is chock-full of hormone-healthy saturated fats, fiber, and wonderfully savory flavors. Something about bacon and ground beef in a creamy base gives me the warm fuzzies!

4 slices bacon, diced

1 pound ground beef (85% lean)

Leaves from 2 sprigs fresh thyme, minced

2 teaspoons coconut aminos

1 teaspoon fish sauce

1 teaspoon extra-virgin olive oil

½ large onion, diced

2 cloves garlic, minced

1 large head cauliflower, chopped (about 4 cups)

3 cups bone broth

2 tablespoons Dijon mustard

2 teaspoons fine salt

1 teaspoon ground black pepper

2 cups fresh baby spinach

◦ Put a pressure cooker in sauté mode. When it's hot, put the diced bacon in the pot and cook, stirring often, until crispy, about 8 minutes. Crumble the ground beef into the pot and cook, breaking it up with a wire whisk, until browned and crumbly, about 5 minutes. Stir in the thyme, coconut aminos, and fish sauce, then remove the beef and bacon from the cooker and set aside.

◦ Drizzle the olive oil into the pressure cooker. Add the onion and garlic and sauté for 5 minutes. Cancel the sauté function and add the cauliflower and broth. Seal the lid and cook on high pressure for 3 minutes. Release the pressure manually and open the lid.

◦ Add the mustard, salt, and pepper and use an immersion blender to puree the cauliflower and broth into a smooth, creamy soup.

◦ Stir in the reserved beef and bacon mixture and the spinach until well combined. Cook using the sauté mode until the spinach has wilted. Serve hot.

◦ Store leftovers in the fridge for up to 5 days. To reheat, bring to a simmer in a saucepan over medium heat.

notes: *If you don't like cauliflower or just want to make this soup a little starchier, you can use 3 cups peeled and diced Japanese sweet potato instead.*

modifications: *To make this soup AIP compliant, replace the mustard with 1 teaspoon apple cider vinegar and replace the black pepper with ½ teaspoon prepared horseradish or wasabi. To make it coconut-free, replace the coconut aminos with low-sodium gluten-free tamari or aged balsamic vinegar.*

Per serving: Calories **541** · Fat **34.6g** · Total Carbs **13.7g** · Fiber **4.3g** · Protein **44.2g**

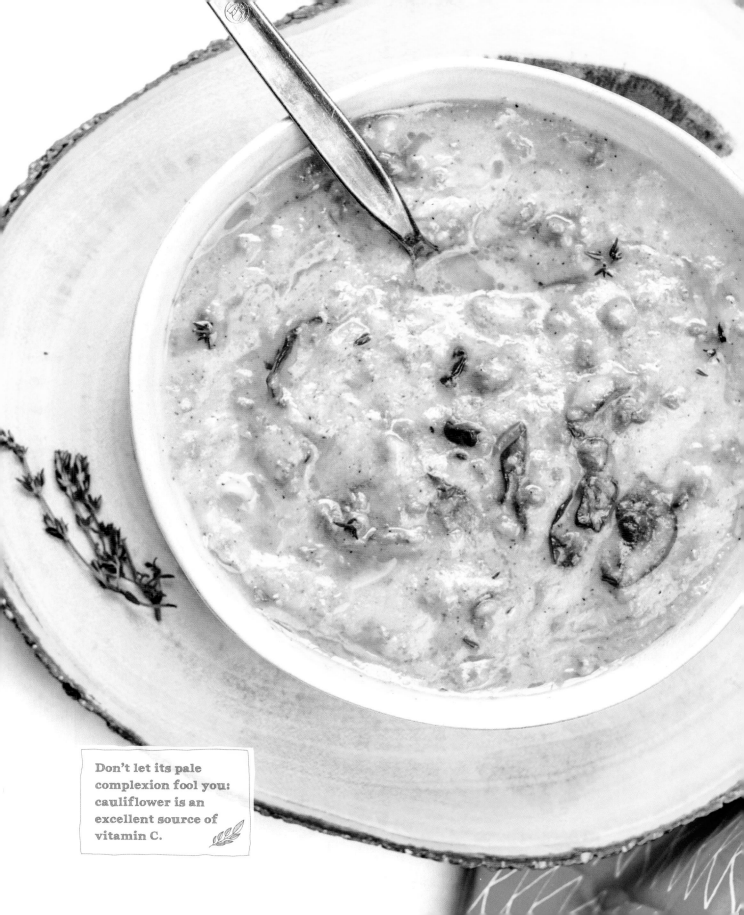

Don't let its pale complexion fool you: cauliflower is an excellent source of vitamin C.

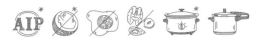

Beef Curry Bowls

Serves 4 ◦ Prep Time: 10 minutes ◦ Cook Time: 1 hour

East meets West in this pot roast–curry mash-up. Chuck roast is a tough but affordable cut of meat that is perfect for the magic of pressure cooking (though slow cooker instructions are also included). Here, perfectly cooked beef is served with all the fixings and a generous serving of Green Basil Curry Sauce, a nutrient powerhouse!

2½ pounds chuck roast

1 tablespoon fine salt

1 tablespoon extra-virgin olive oil

1 small onion, sliced

1 tablespoon coconut aminos

2 cups filtered water

4 cups fresh or frozen riced cauliflower (about 2 pounds)

For serving:

1 cup Green Basil Curry Sauce (page 106)

1 ripe Hass avocado, peeled, pitted, and sliced

3 tablespoons sprouted pumpkin seeds (see notes)

½ cup fresh cilantro leaves

◦ Season the chuck roast liberally with the salt, rubbing it into the meat. Place it in a pressure cooker and drizzle it with the olive oil. Add the onion and coconut aminos, then pour the water over everything. Seal the lid and cook on high pressure for 50 minutes. When it's done, release the pressure manually.

◦ Open the lid and use a slotted spoon to transfer the beef to a bowl. Set aside.

◦ Put the pressure cooker in sauté or reduce mode and bring the liquid in the pot to a simmer. Mix in the riced cauliflower and cook for 10 minutes, stirring occasionally, until the cauliflower is tender and warmed through. In the meantime, shred the beef with 2 forks.

◦ To serve, put a base layer of half cauliflower rice and half shredded beef in each of 4 bowls. Spoon ¼ cup of the curry sauce over the beef and load up the bowls with the avocado slices, pumpkin seeds, and cilantro.

Slow Cooker Method: Follow the instructions above, but add the riced cauliflower to the slow cooker with the beef, onion, coconut aminos, and water. Cook on high for 5 hours, then shred the beef and mix it with the cauliflower before dishing it into bowls and topping with the rest of the ingredients.

notes: *Change up the flavor profile of this dish by serving it with any delicious sauce from the Meal Makers chapter in place of the curry sauce. Green Onion Relish (page 98) or Gut-Healing Teriyaki Sauce (page 70) would be great here!*

Sprouted pumpkin seeds have been soaked and then dehydrated to make them easier to digest and prepare without oxidation. Go Raw is my preferred brand.

modifications: *To make this dish AIP compliant, make the AIP version of the curry sauce and omit the pumpkin seeds. To make it coconut-free, replace the coconut aminos with low-sodium gluten-free tamari and use the coconut-free version of the curry sauce.*

Per serving: Calories **843** · Fat **62.9g** · Total Carbs **14.6g** · Fiber **6.5g** · Protein **56.2g**

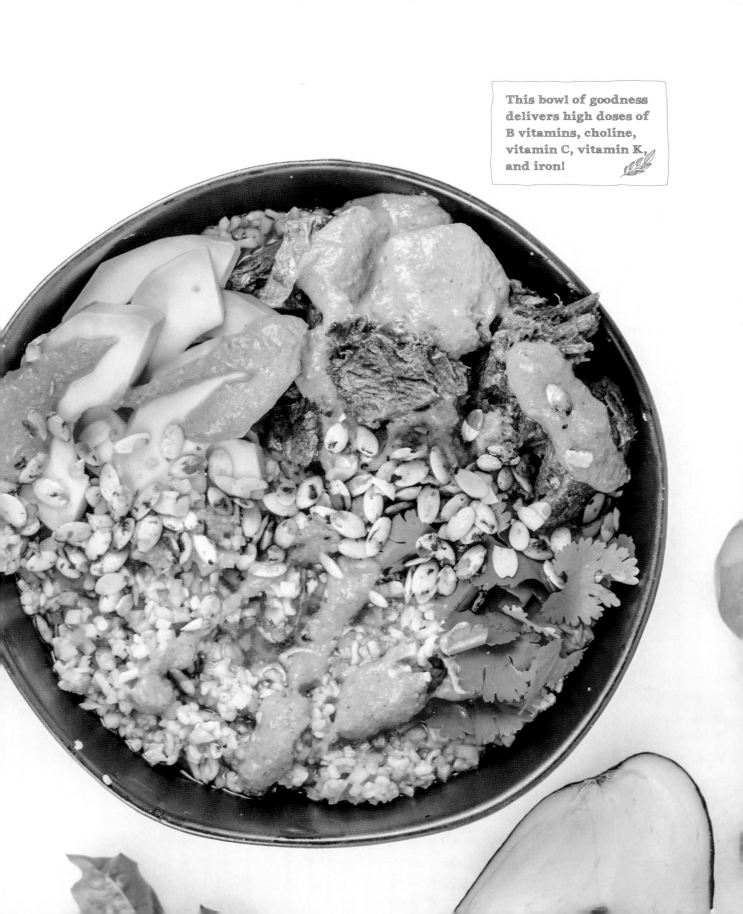

This bowl of goodness delivers high doses of B vitamins, choline, vitamin C, vitamin K, and iron!

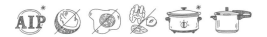

Savory Short Ribs

Serves 5 ◦ Prep Time: 15 minutes ◦ Cook Time: 1 hour 10 minutes

Fall-off-the-bone, melty meat in a super flavorful vegetable base! This one-pot pressure cooker recipe (though I've also included slow cooker instructions) recruits okra for added vitamin C and gut-healing goodness. Okra's mucilage is a type of soluble fiber that not only works as a thickening agent but also aids in eliminating toxins from the body.

15 (2-inch) English-cut beef short ribs (about 3 pounds)

1 tablespoon fine salt

1 tablespoon Cuban Sazón (page 83)

Leaves from 2 sprigs fresh sage, minced

1 teaspoon turmeric powder

2 teaspoons extra-virgin olive oil

2 cups sliced okra, fresh or frozen

1 cup diced white onions

1 cup sliced shiitake mushrooms (about 4 ounces)

⅔ cup sliced carrots

2 cloves garlic, minced

2 cups bone broth

2 tablespoons aged balsamic vinegar (see notes, page 90)

◦ Put a pressure cooker in sauté mode. While it heats, place the short ribs in a bowl and toss with the salt, Cuban Sazón, minced sage, and turmeric until well coated.

◦ Drizzle the olive oil into the cooker, then brown the short ribs in 3 batches, 5 ribs at a time, for 2 minutes per side, until nicely browned. Return all of the ribs to the bowl in which they were seasoned and set aside.

◦ Put all of the vegetables in the pressure cooker and sauté until tender, about 8 minutes, then stir in the broth and vinegar. Return the short ribs to the cooker and mix well. Cancel the sauté function.

◦ Seal the lid and cook on high pressure for 50 minutes. When it's done, release the pressure manually. Serve 3 short ribs per person with a ladleful of saucy vegetables.

Slow Cooker Method: Using a medium-sized pot on the stovetop, follow the recipe as written up to the last step. Then transfer everything to a slow cooker and cook on high for 4 hours.

modifications: *To make this dish AIP compliant, be sure to follow the modifications in the Cuban Sazón recipe.*

Per serving: Calories **716** · Fat **58.8g** · Total Carbs **10.7g** · Fiber **3g** · Protein **35.1g**

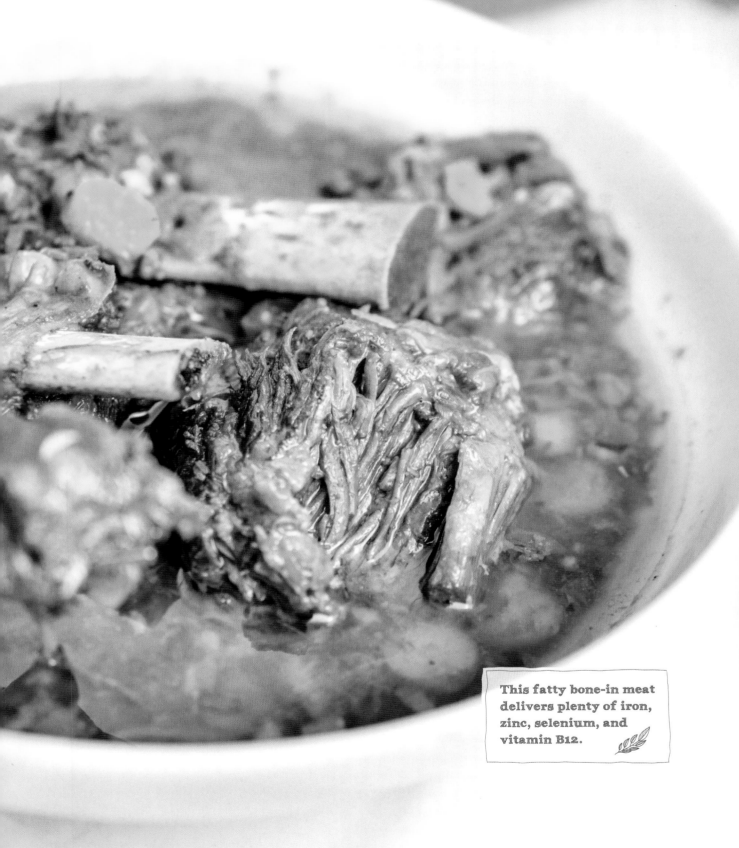

This fatty bone-in meat delivers plenty of iron, zinc, selenium, and vitamin B12.

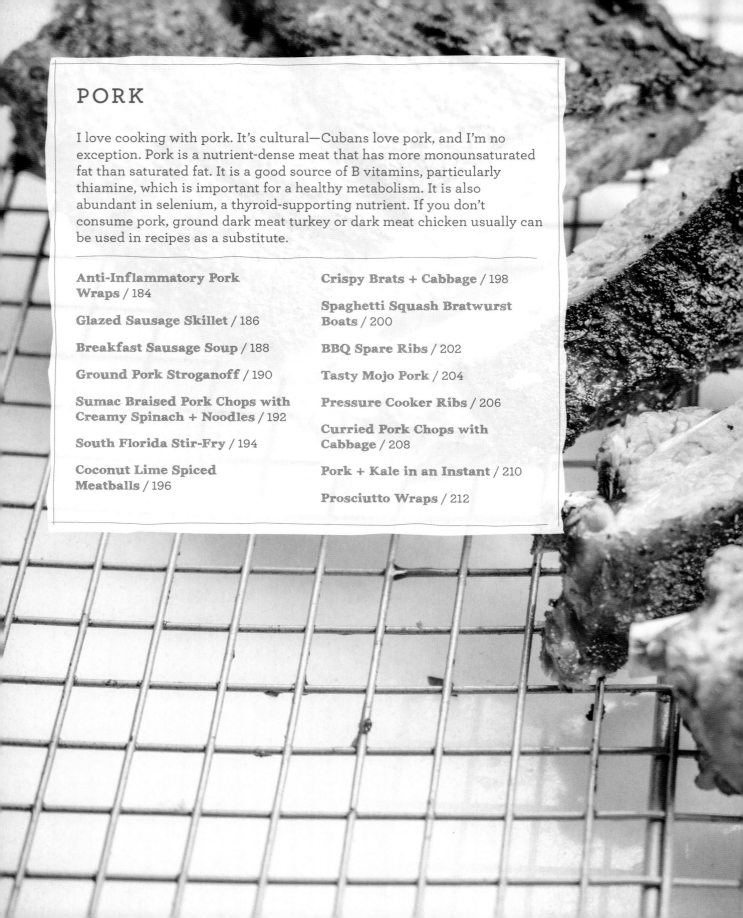

PORK

I love cooking with pork. It's cultural—Cubans love pork, and I'm no exception. Pork is a nutrient-dense meat that has more monounsaturated fat than saturated fat. It is a good source of B vitamins, particularly thiamine, which is important for a healthy metabolism. It is also abundant in selenium, a thyroid-supporting nutrient. If you don't consume pork, ground dark meat turkey or dark meat chicken usually can be used in recipes as a substitute.

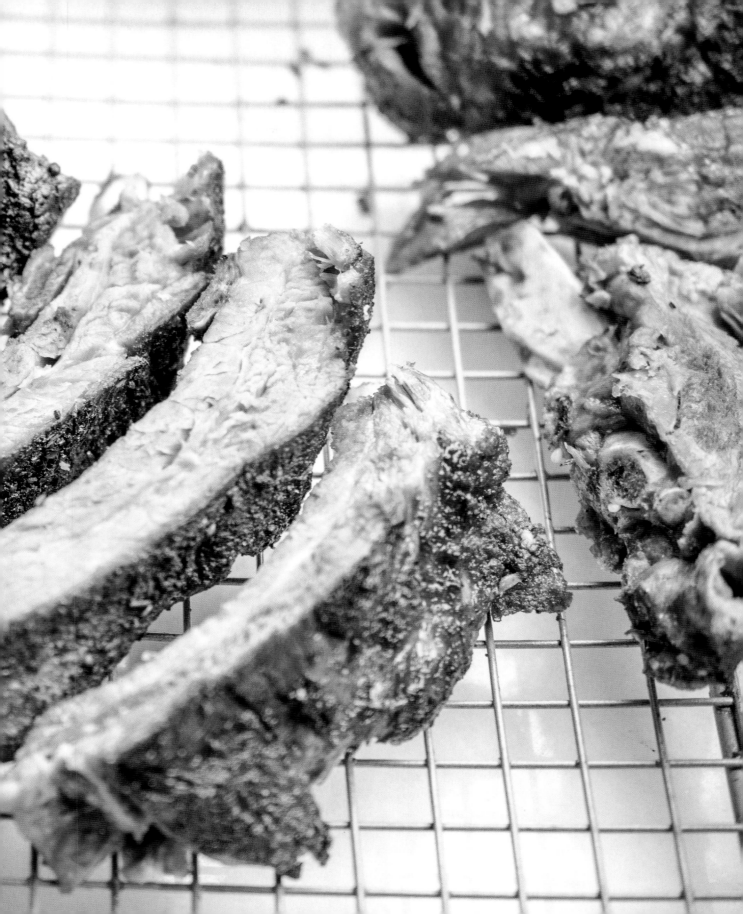

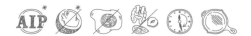

Anti-Inflammatory Pork Wraps

Serves 3 ◦ Prep Time: 10 minutes ◦ Cook Time: 20 minutes

With warm spices, a creamy texture, and toasty sesame flavors, this dish is reminiscent of curry. It's a lovely bouquet of Eastern flavors in a minced meat dish that is perfect scooped up in lettuce wraps!

2 tablespoons Asian Garlic Compound Butter (page 78)

1 small carrot, diced (about ½ cup)

1 small onion, diced (about ½ cup)

1 pound ground pork

1 teaspoon fine salt

1½ teaspoons garlic powder

1 teaspoon ginger powder

1 teaspoon ground mustard seeds

1 teaspoon turmeric powder

½ teaspoon ground black pepper

1 tablespoon toasted sesame oil

1 tablespoon unsweetened, unsalted sunflower seed butter

Juice of 1 lemon

For serving:

¼ cup cilantro leaves

1 tablespoon sesame seeds

1 head Boston lettuce, leaves separated

◦ Heat a large skillet over medium heat. Melt the compound butter in the skillet, then add the carrot and onion. Sauté for 6 minutes, or until tender.

◦ Crumble the ground pork into the skillet and cook, breaking up the meat as it cooks, until it begins to brown, about 5 minutes. Stir in the salt and spices and continue to cook until the pork is cooked through, about 10 minutes.

◦ Stir in the sesame oil, sunflower seed butter, and lemon juice until the mixture is creamy. Remove from the heat and spoon into bowls. Garnish with the cilantro leaves and sesame seeds and serve with lettuce leaves for wrapping and a spoon for scooping.

◦ Store leftover pork mixture in the fridge for up to 4 days. To reheat, bring to a light simmer in a skillet over low heat.

modifications: *To make this dish dairy-free, use the dairy-free version of the compound butter. To make it AIP compliant, use the dairy-free version of the compound butter and omit the mustard seeds, black pepper, sesame oil, and sesame seeds. Use coconut butter or coconut cream instead of the sunflower seed butter. Need it coconut-free? Use the coconut-free version of the compound butter. Alternatively, in place of the compound butter, you can use 2 tablespoons of any cooking fat you like and add 1 clove garlic, minced, and 1 teaspoon coconut aminos or low-sodium gluten-free tamari.*

Per serving: Calories **560** · Fat **43.1g** · Total Carbs **11.8g** · Fiber **3.6g** · Protein **33.3g**

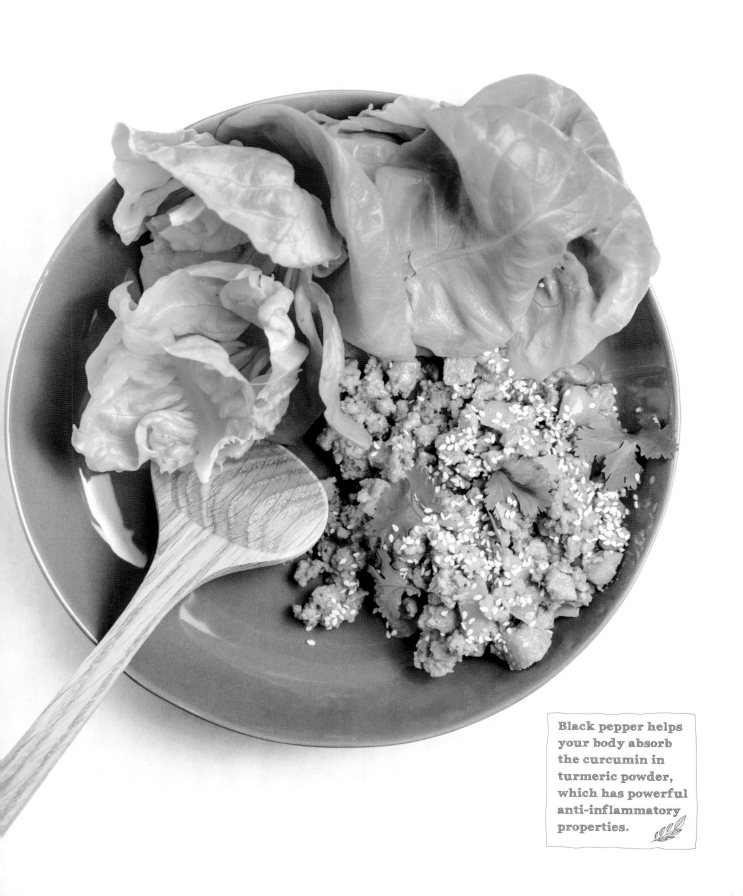

Black pepper helps your body absorb the curcumin in turmeric powder, which has powerful anti-inflammatory properties.

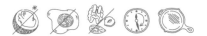

Glazed Sausage Skillet

Serves 4 ◦ Prep Time: 5 minutes ◦ Cook Time: 15 minutes

A quintessential skillet meal—this one is all about the quality of the bratwurst you use. I pretty much eat only Niman Ranch brats, which are nightshade-free and top-notch. I've found them at Whole Foods in every state I've lived in (Florida, California, Hawaii, and Virginia). You can also find quality bratwurst and sausages online at US Wellness Meats. A simple sauté brings this dish to life, and Gut-Healing Teriyaki Sauce pulls it all together.

5 fully cooked bratwursts (about 15 ounces), sliced

2 tablespoons ghee or lard

1 (1-pound) bag shredded Brussels sprouts

1 teaspoon garlic powder

1 teaspoon mustard seeds

½ teaspoon fine salt

¼ cup Gut-Healing Teriyaki Sauce (page 70)

◦ Heat a 15-inch skillet over medium heat. Place the sliced bratwursts in the pan and cook, stirring occasionally, until crispy, about 5 minutes.

◦ Stir in the ghee until melted, then add the Brussels sprouts, spices, and salt. Stir well, then press the mixture into the bottom of the skillet. Cover with the lid and cook for 5 minutes, or until the sprouts soften.

◦ Remove the lid and use a spatula to scrape up and turn over the mixture. Sauté for 5 minutes, or until the sprouts have some toasty bits. Stir in the teriyaki sauce and serve hot!

◦ Store leftovers in the fridge for up to 4 days. To reheat, sauté in a skillet over medium heat.

note: *If you don't eat pork, you can use beef bratwurst or chicken sausage.*

modifications: *To make this dish coconut-free, use the coconut-free version of the teriyaki sauce.*

Per serving: Calories **422** · Fat **30.5g** · Total Carbs **14.4g** · Fiber **4.4g** · Protein **23.7g**

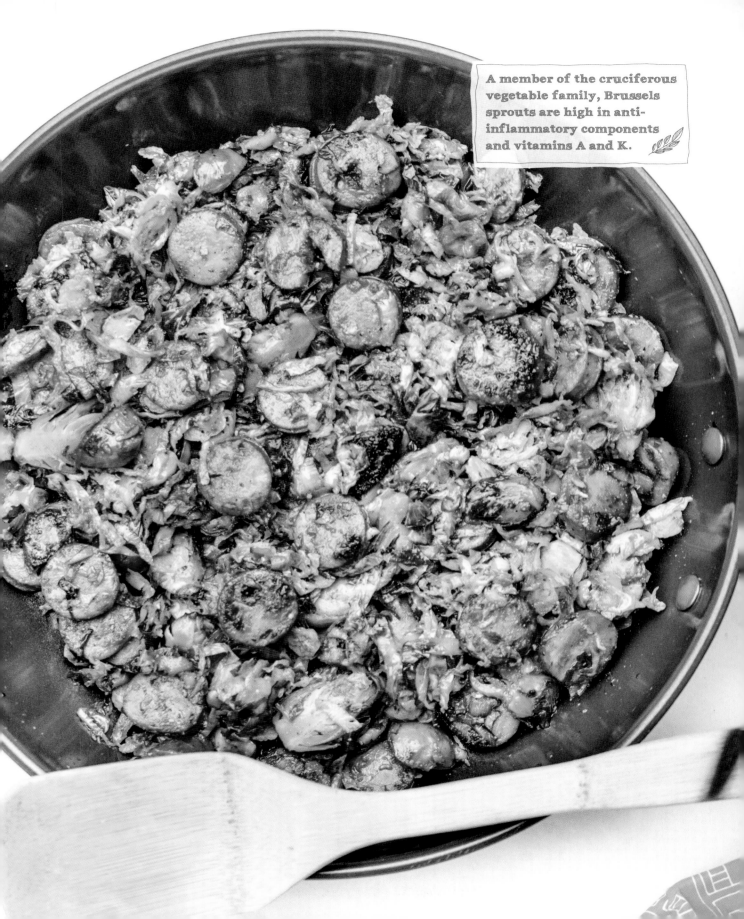

A member of the cruciferous vegetable family, Brussels sprouts are high in anti-inflammatory components and vitamins A and K.

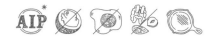

Breakfast Sausage Soup

Serves 6 ◦ Prep Time: 10 minutes ◦ Cook Time: 30 minutes

Breakfast sausage isn't just for breakfast! This soup uses breakfast sausage for the protein. I source nightshade-free breakfast sausage from ButcherBox, where I get most of my protein. However, any kind of ground protein, paired with your favorite seasoning blend, would work in this colorful, delicious soup. The best recipe is a flexible recipe.

2 tablespoons ghee or extra-virgin olive oil, divided

2 pounds ground breakfast sausage

3 cups shredded red cabbage

1 cup diced celery

1 cup diced white onions

1 teaspoon fine salt

½ teaspoon garlic powder

½ teaspoon ground black pepper

2 tablespoons apple cider vinegar

3 cups baby spinach

6 cups bone broth

◦ Heat a Dutch oven or large heavy-bottomed pot over medium heat. Once it's hot, put 1 tablespoon of the ghee in the pot, then add the sausage. Break up the meat with a wire whisk or spatula until crumbly. Cook, stirring occasionally, for 8 minutes, or until browned. Remove the sausage from the pot and set aside.

◦ Put the remaining tablespoon of ghee in the pot, then add the cabbage, celery, onions, salt, garlic powder, and pepper. Cook, stirring occasionally, until the vegetables are tender and aromatic, about 10 minutes. Stir in the vinegar and deglaze the pot, scraping the browned bits off the bottom.

◦ Add the spinach and cook, stirring occasionally, until wilted, about 2 minutes. Mix in the cooked sausage and pour in the broth. Bring to a boil, then turn the heat down to low and simmer for 5 minutes. Stir well and serve hot.

modifications: *To make this dish AIP compliant, use an AIP-friendly breakfast sausage or use any ground protein, such as beef, pork, or turkey, with 2 teaspoons of an AIP-friendly salted seasoning.*

awesome additions: *If you need more carbs, add a 10-ounce bag of frozen butternut squash cubes to the soup when you add the bone broth.*

Per serving: Calories **432** · Fat **28.5g** · Total Carbs **7g** · Fiber **1.9g** · Protein **35.5g**

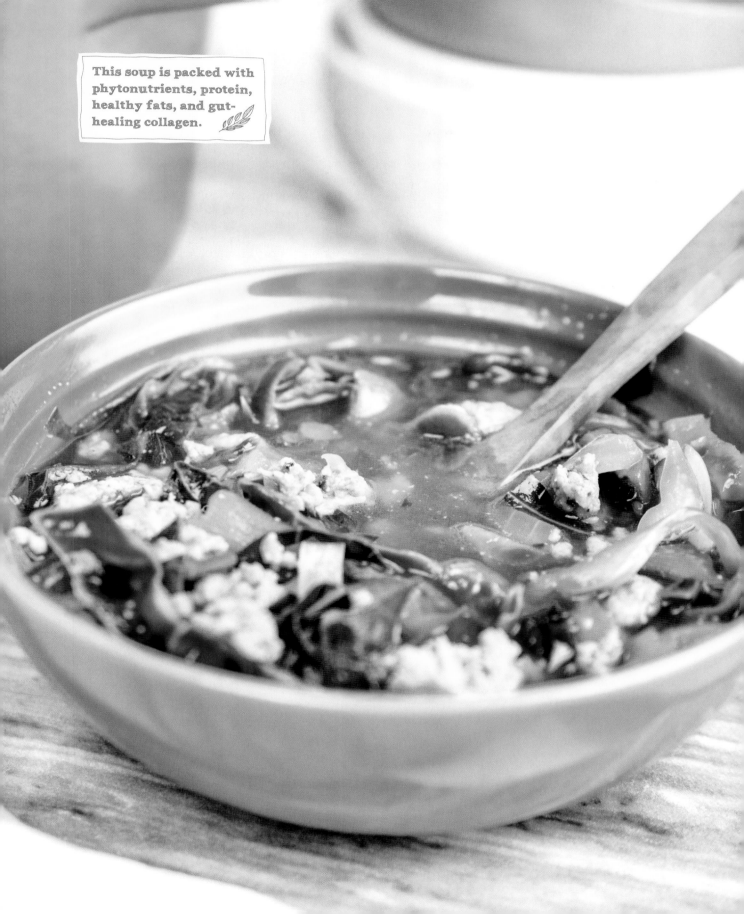

This soup is packed with phytonutrients, protein, healthy fats, and gut-healing collagen.

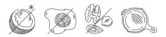

Ground Pork Stroganoff

Serves 4 ◦ Prep Time: 10 minutes ◦ Cook Time: 25 minutes

Traditional Russian beef stroganoff is made with pieces of beef in a creamy mushroom sauce served over pasta. We're deviating quite a bit by using ground pork and cauliflower cream, but I promise the flavor is spot-on. I think Babushka would approve! After all, grandmas are the original real-food healers, and this dish is as good for you as it is delicious.

2 tablespoons ghee or extra-virgin olive oil

2 pounds ground pork

2 tablespoons spicy brown mustard

2 teaspoons fine salt

2 teaspoons garlic powder

1 large white onion, diced

1 pound sliced cremini mushrooms (about 4 cups)

1 cup bone broth

1 cup Cauliflower Sour Cream (page 74) (see note)

1 large zucchini, spiral sliced into noodles (about 4 cups)

2 tablespoons chopped fresh parsley, for garnish

Ground black pepper, for garnish (optional)

◦ Heat a 15-inch skillet over medium heat. Once it's hot, melt the ghee in the skillet, then crumble in the ground pork. Stir in the mustard, salt, and garlic powder. Cook, stirring occasionally with a wooden spoon, until the pork is fully browned, 8 to 10 minutes.

◦ Move the browned pork to one side of the skillet, then add the onion and mushrooms to the other side. Sauté the onion and mushrooms for 5 minutes, then mix everything together until well combined.

◦ Pour in the broth, stir, and bring to a simmer, then whisk in the sour cream and continue to cook until the mixture is creamy and thick, 2 to 4 minutes.

◦ Serve with zucchini noodles and garnish with parsley and a dusting of black pepper if desired.

note: *You may use Salted Cashew Cream (page 76) instead of the Cauliflower Sour Cream, but add a splash of lemon juice for tang. If you handle dairy well, regular sour cream will work well too.*

modifications: *To make this dish coconut-free, use the coconut-free version of the sour cream.*

Per serving: Calories **616** · Fat **43.1g** · Total Carbs **10.6g** · Fiber **3.2g** · Protein **49.5g**

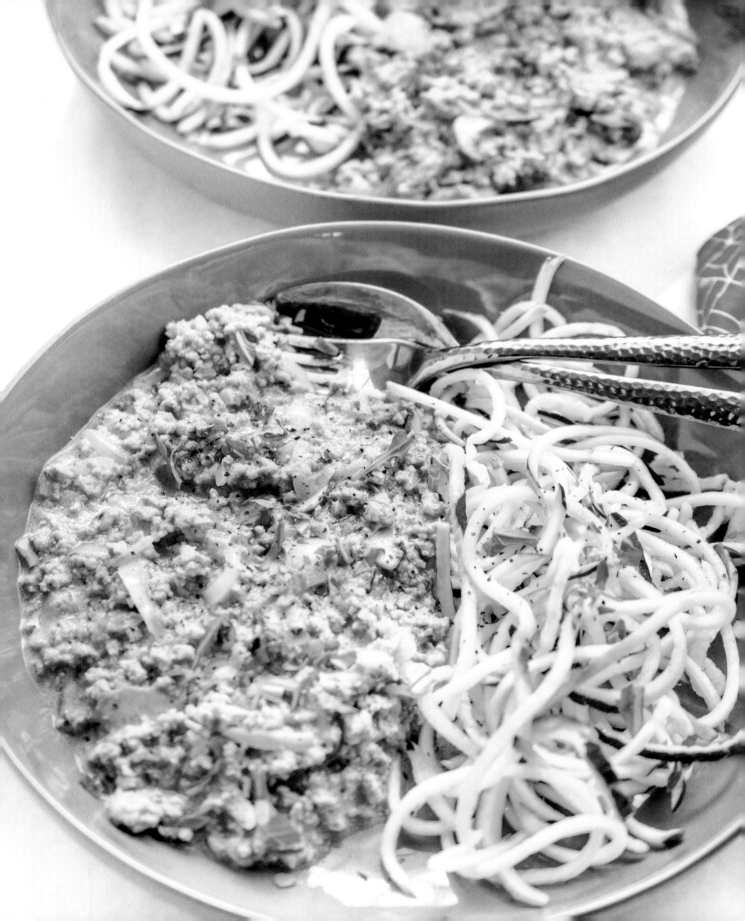

Sumac Braised Pork Chops with Creamy Spinach + Noodles

Serves 4 ◦ Prep Time: 5 minutes ◦ Cook Time: 20 minutes

This powerhouse meal has it all: nutrient-rich lean pork, iodine-rich kelp noodles, vitamin C–rich cauliflower, iron-rich spinach, and sumac, a potent anti-inflammatory and antioxidant. As an added bonus, this restaurant-worthy meal comes together in one skillet. Who knew "medicine" could taste this good? (I did.)

For the pork chops:

4 thick-cut boneless pork chops (about 2 pounds)

2 teaspoons fine salt

2 teaspoons ground sumac

1 teaspoon garlic powder

1 teaspoon ginger powder

1 teaspoon ground cumin

2 tablespoons extra-virgin olive oil, for the pan

1 cup bone broth

For the noodles:

2 packages kelp noodles (about 1 pound)

1 tablespoon extra-virgin olive oil

3 cups baby spinach

½ cup Cauliflower Sour Cream (page 74)

◦ Set the pork chops on a cutting board or large plate. Mix the salt and spices in a small bowl and liberally rub the mixture all over the chops.

◦ Cook the pork chops: Heat a large skillet with a tight-fitting lid over medium heat. When it's hot, drizzle the olive oil into the skillet. Put the pork chops in the skillet, making sure they are not touching. Sear the chops without moving them for 5 minutes, then flip them over and sear for 5 minutes, again without moving them. Turn the heat down to low and pour in the broth. Cover with the lid and cook for 5 minutes.

◦ While the pork chops cook, soak the kelp noodles in warm water for 5 minutes, then drain them.

◦ When the pork chops are done, remove them to a plate and cover with aluminum foil to keep them warm.

◦ Cook the noodles: Drizzle the olive oil into the skillet and add the drained noodles. Sauté until softened, about 3 minutes. Add the spinach and cook until wilted, about 2 minutes, then stir in the sour cream.

◦ Serve right away, or place the pork chops on top of the noodles, cover with the lid, and keep warm over very low heat until you're ready to eat.

◦ Store leftovers in the fridge for up to 4 days. To reheat, slice the pork chops and stir-fry with the noodles in a large skillet over medium heat.

modifications: *To make this dish coconut-free, use the coconut-free version of the sour cream.*

Per serving: Calories **406** · Fat **18.2g** · Total Carbs **5.1g** · Fiber **1.9g** · Protein **53.8g**

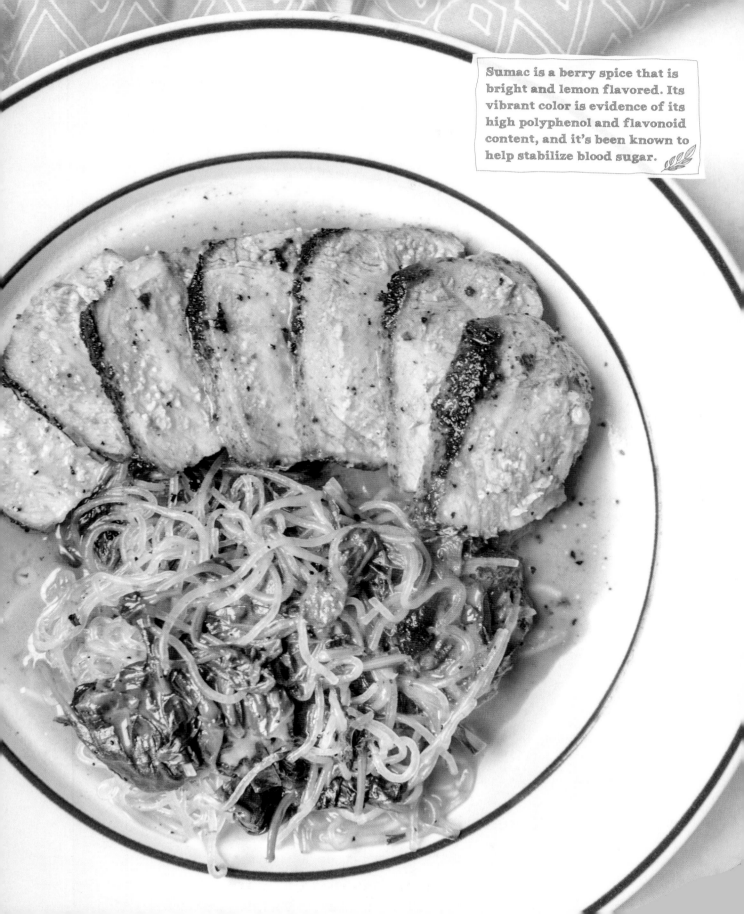

Sumac is a berry spice that is bright and lemon flavored. Its vibrant color is evidence of its high polyphenol and flavonoid content, and it's been known to help stabilize blood sugar.

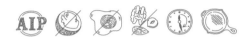

South Florida Stir-Fry

Serves 4 ◦ Prep Time: 5 minutes ◦ Cook Time: 20 minutes

This dish reminds me of home because it's made with ingredients that grow there, like lime and okra. It's also got a little picadillo action going on. It makes this Cuban American Miami girl very happy. Packed with choline, thiamine, selenium, and monounsaturated fats, it will make your body happy too!

2 tablespoons extra-virgin oil olive

2 pounds ground pork

1 tablespoon grated lime zest

4 cloves garlic, minced

Leaves from 2 sprigs fresh thyme, plus more sprigs for garnish if desired

1 (10-ounce) bag frozen riced cauliflower

1 (10-ounce) bag frozen sliced okra

2 teaspoons fine salt

2 tablespoons aged balsamic vinegar (see notes, page 90)

◦ Heat a 15-inch skillet over medium heat. When it's hot, drizzle in the olive oil, then crumble in the ground pork. Mix in the lime zest, garlic, and thyme. Cook, stirring often, until the pork is mostly browned, about 8 minutes.

◦ Mix in the frozen vegetables and salt and cook, stirring often, for another 10 minutes, or until everything is heated through and lightly browned.

◦ Stir in the vinegar and continue stirring as you bring the mixture to a simmer over high heat; continue stirring and simmering for 2 minutes. Remove from the heat. Serve in bowls, garnished with thyme sprigs if desired.

awesome additions: *Top the bowls with diced avocado. If you happen to be in South Florida, try the local avocados!*

Per serving: Calories **567** · Fat **40.3g** · Total Carbs **7.5g** · Fiber **2.4g** · Protein **44.8g**

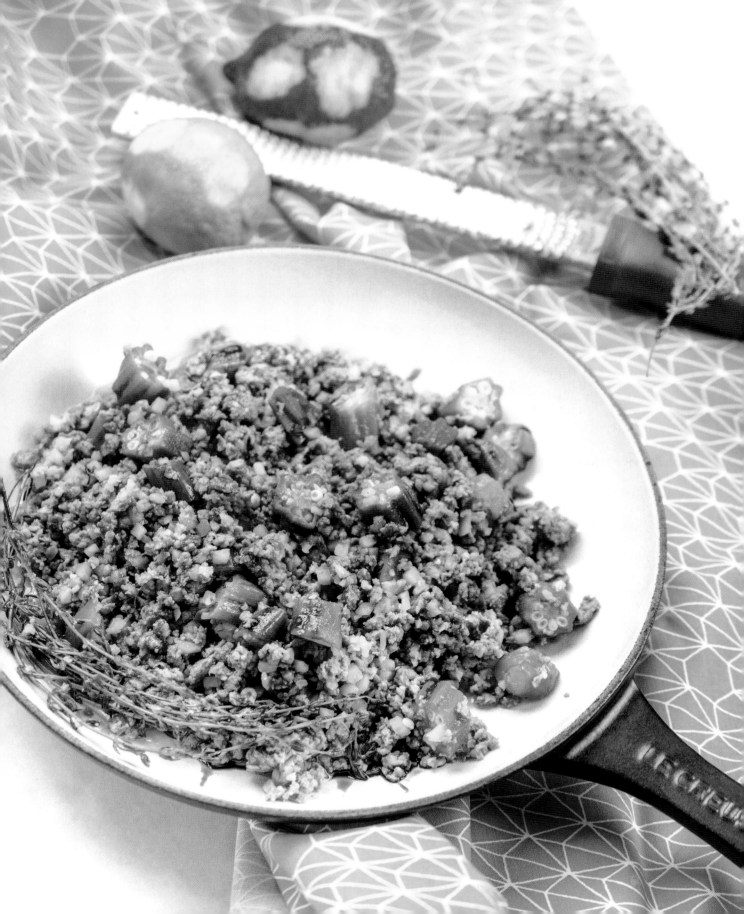

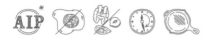

Coconut Lime Spiced Meatballs

Serves 5 ◦ Prep Time: 10 minutes ◦ Cook Time: 20 minutes

She put the lime in the coconut... It's not mandatory to sing the Harry Nilsson song while you make this dish, but it's definitely suggested. If you don't eat pork, remember that ground dark meat turkey works well in these recipes too! I love serving these meatballs over Spicy Yellow Rice (page 320) to complement the tropical flavors of the dish.

2 pounds ground pork

2 teaspoons grated lime zest

2 teaspoons fine salt

1 teaspoon ginger powder

1 teaspoon ground coriander

1 teaspoon onion powder

2 tablespoons unflavored grass-fed beef gelatin or flaxseed meal

1 tablespoon coconut oil

1 small onion, diced (about ½ cup)

Juice of 3 limes

1 (13.5-ounce) can unsweetened full-fat coconut milk

1 lime, thinly sliced, for serving (optional)

○ Heat a 15-inch skillet over medium heat. While it heats, form the meatballs.

○ Put the ground pork, lime zest, salt, ginger powder, coriander, onion powder, and gelatin in a large bowl. Mix well and shape into 15 meatballs that are about 1½ inches in diameter.

○ Melt the coconut oil in the skillet, then arrange the meatballs in the pan so they're not touching. Brown the meatballs for 3 minutes on each side, turning them over 3 times with tongs, 12 minutes total.

○ Sprinkle the diced onion among the browned meatballs and add the lime juice. Use a wooden spoon to move everything around gently.

○ Pour in the coconut milk and let the mixture simmer, gently stirring and turning over the meatballs once or twice, for 8 minutes, or until the meatballs are cooked through. (The internal temperature should reach 150°F.) Remove from the heat, nestle the lime slices (if using) in between the meatballs, and serve!

modifications: *To make this dish AIP compliant, omit the coriander and use gelatin, not flaxseed meal.*

Per serving: Calories **536** · Fat **41.6g** · Total Carbs **5.9g** · Fiber **0.5g** · Protein **35.2g**

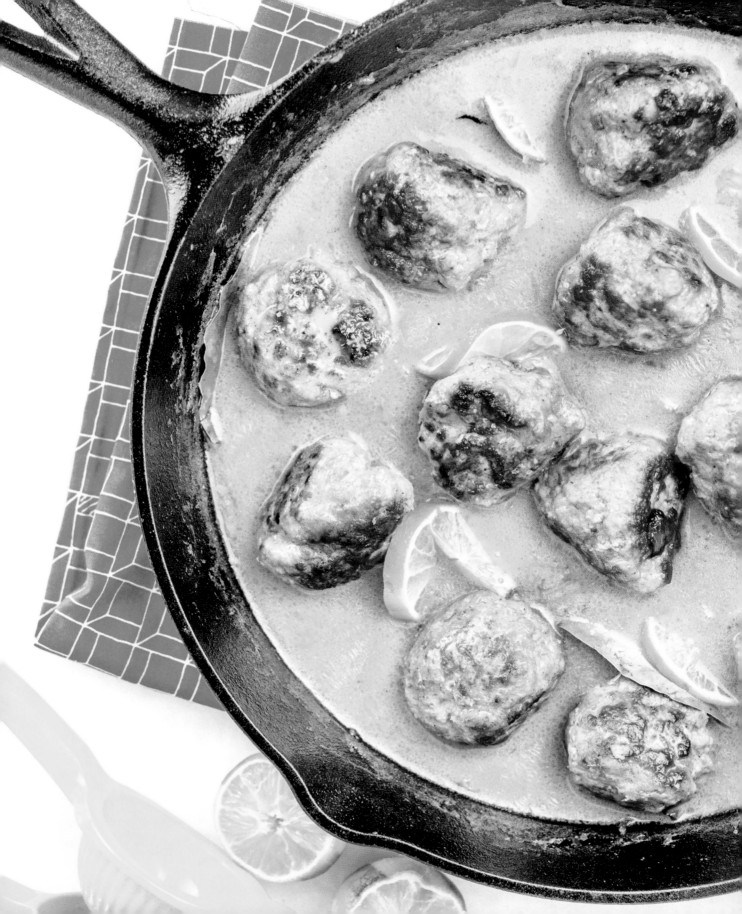

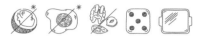

Crispy Brats + Cabbage

Serves 2 ◦ Prep Time: 5 minutes ◦ Cook Time: 30 minutes

I am obsessed with crispy bratwurst. When I found the nightshade-free brats from Niman Ranch, I was hooked. We keep them in the house at all times; these crispy, fatty, and flavorful sausages grace our table at least once a week. In this dish, the sweetness of soft and charred cabbage pairs perfectly with mustard seeds. To take the meal to the next level, I recommend drizzling some Everything Sauce on top. It's a three-ingredient sauce that would bring the total number of ingredients up to eight. It's optional, but totally worth it.

2 tablespoons extra-virgin olive oil, divided

3 cups shredded red cabbage

4 fully cooked bratwursts (about 12 ounces)

1 teaspoon mustard seeds

½ teaspoon fine salt

Everything Sauce (page 72), for drizzling (optional)

- Place an oven rack in the middle position. Preheat the oven to 400°F.

- Drizzle 1 tablespoon of the olive oil on a sheet pan. Distribute the cabbage evenly all over the sheet pan, then make 4 spaces in the cabbage and place the bratwursts in those spaces, directly on the sheet pan.

- Sprinkle the mustard seeds and salt all over the cabbage. Drizzle the remaining tablespoon of olive oil over the entire sheet pan.

- Place the sheet pan in the oven on the middle rack and roast for 30 minutes, until the brats are wrinkly and crispy and the cabbage is tender. Remove from the oven and use a spatula to scrape up the crispy bratwurst and cabbage.

- Divide the bratwursts and cabbage evenly between 2 plates and drizzle with Everything Sauce, if desired. Enjoy!

- This dish stores well, and it's great for meal prep; you can cook 2 sheet pans of this recipe simultaneously. Store the cabbage with the bratwursts on top or on the side in the fridge for up to 5 days. If you store the leftovers in a baking dish, just bring it to room temperature before you pop it in the oven to reheat at 350°F for 10 minutes.

note: *You can use green cabbage instead of red, or use a mixture of the two. Broccoli florets also would work, as would any kind of vegetable slaw! Either beef or pork bratwursts can be used for this recipe.*

modifications: *To make this dish coconut-free, use the coconut-free version of the Everything Sauce or omit the sauce altogether. To make it egg-free, use the egg-free version of the Everything Sauce or skip the sauce.*

Per serving: Calories **641** · Fat **52.3g** · Total Carbs **10.6g** · Fiber **3.3g** · Protein **30.1g**

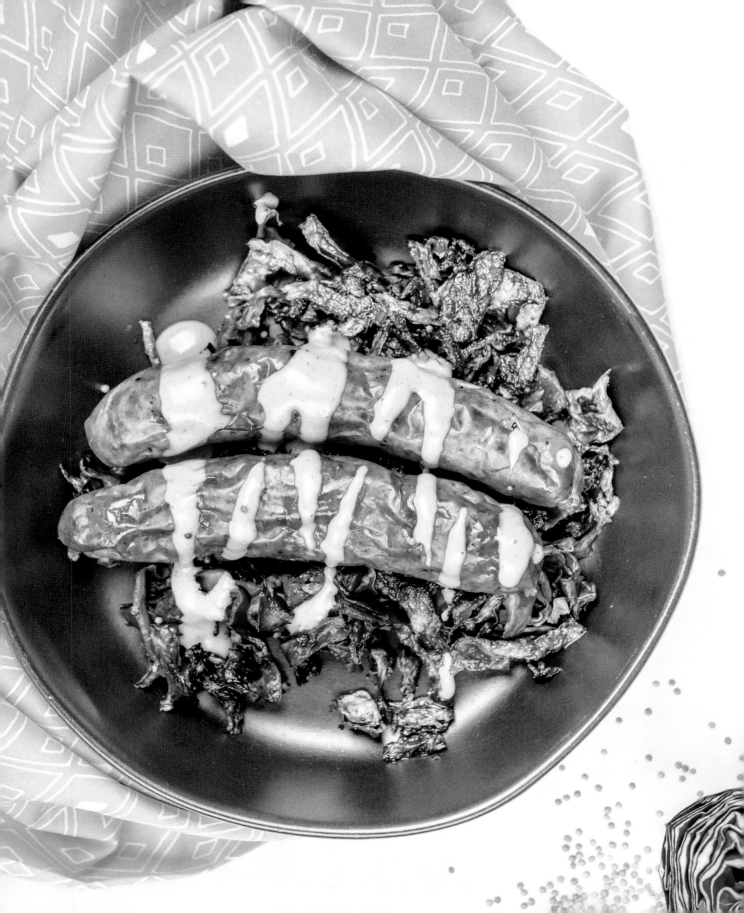

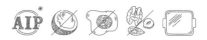

Spaghetti Squash Bratwurst Boats

Serves 4 ◦ Prep Time: 10 minutes ◦ Cook Time: 40 minutes

Spaghetti squash is a great real-food alternative to pasta. It's a little higher in carbs than zucchini or kelp noodles, but at 10 grams of carbs per cup, it won't spike your blood sugar—plus, it's delicious and perfect for post-workout meals! I like to buy small spaghetti squash (about 4 pounds) so that each half yields the perfect single serving. However, if you encounter a massive squash, it can feed quite a few people, so you can serve this meal in bowls instead of boats.

2 small spaghetti squash (about 4 pounds each)

2 tablespoons avocado oil or extra-virgin olive oil, divided

5 fully cooked bratwursts or smoked sausages (about 15 ounces), sliced

½ cup Briny Arugula Pesto (page 90) or Green Onion Relish (page 98)

1 teaspoon fine salt

notes: *I like Niman Ranch pork bratwursts because they are nightshade-free and good quality. US Wellness Meats also has great AIP-friendly options. f you don't eat pork, you may use beef bratwursts.*

You may use any sauce you like in place of the pesto. Here are some suggestions from my first book, Made Whole: *Pistou, Beet Marinara, or Cauliflower Alfredo. You may also use Cauliflower Sour Cream (page 74) or Salted Cashew Cream (page 76) with nutritional yeast for a white sauce.*

◦ Place one oven rack in the middle position and another in the bottom position. Cut the squash in half horizontally or vertically; either works as long as the halves are even. Coat the squash halves all over with 1 tablespoon of the oil and place them cut side down on a sheet pan. Put the sheet pan in the oven on the middle rack and set the oven temperature to 400°F.

◦ Arrange the bratwurst slices on another sheet pan and drizzle them with the remaining tablespoon of oil. When the oven reaches temperature, put this second sheet pan on the bottom rack and roast everything for 30 minutes, until you can easily pierce the squash with a fork.

◦ Take both pans out of the oven. Use tongs or a spatula to turn over the squash and use a spoon to carefully remove the seeds. Use a fork to shred the insides of the squash into a large bowl and toss it with the pesto, salt, and bratwurst slices.

◦ Scoop the mixture into the squash shells and return them to the oven to roast for another 10 minutes. Remove from the oven and dig in!

◦ Store leftovers in the fridge for up to 5 days. To reheat, sauté the contents of the boats in a skillet over medium heat for 5 minutes.

modifications: *To make this dish AIP compliant, use an AIP-friendly bratwurst or other sausage. Even precooked ground sausage will work.*

awesome additions: *Top each squash boat with a fried egg!*

Per serving: Calories **584** · Fat **50.1g** · Total Carbs **15.5g** · Fiber **3g** · Protein **19.2g**

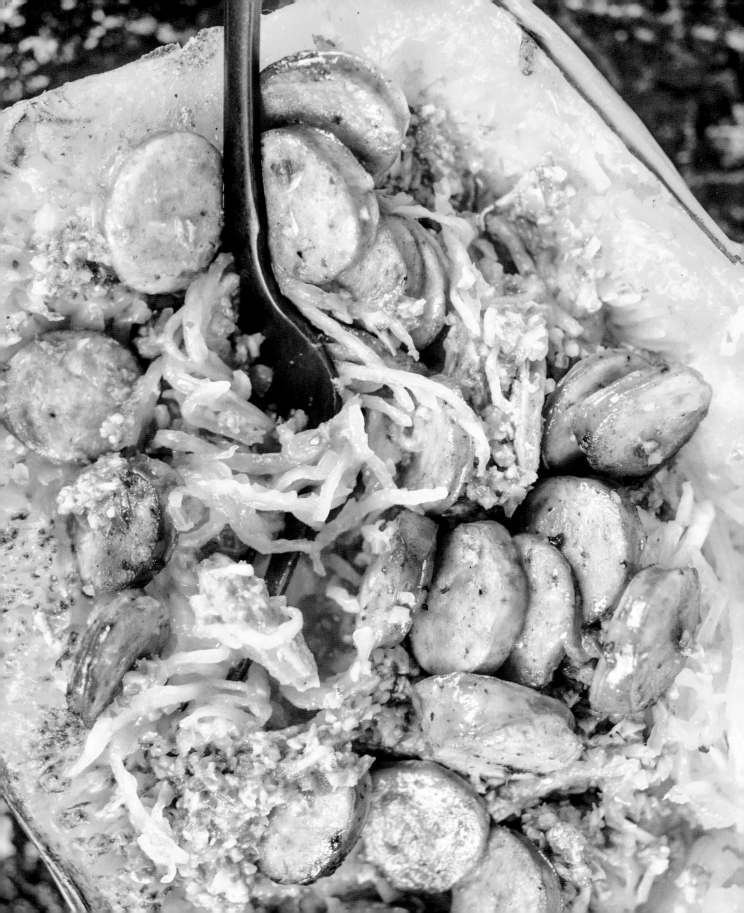

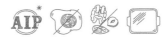

BBQ Spare Ribs

Serves 4 ◦ Prep Time: 10 minutes ◦ Cook Time: 3 hours

My blueberry BBQ sauce comes alive in this rib recipe. I went traditional with the cooking method, swapping out aluminum foil for nontoxic parchment paper. A simple dry rub, a low-and-slow roast, a nice layer of sauce, and then some heat to really bring home the caramelization, and boom! You have sugar-free, nightshade-free, antioxidant-rich, anti-inflammatory barbecued ribs that are nothing short of magical.

2½ pounds St. Louis spare ribs

1 teaspoon fine salt

1 teaspoon ground black pepper

1 teaspoon onion powder

6 tablespoons Slow Cooker Blueberry BBQ Sauce (page 100), divided

◦ Place an oven rack in the middle position. Preheat the oven to 250°F.

◦ Cut the rack of ribs in half—2 smaller slabs will be easier to handle. Rub the ribs with the salt, pepper, and onion powder. Wrap each piece in parchment paper and place on a sheet pan. Put the pan in the oven on the middle rack and bake for 2 hours.

◦ Remove the sheet pan from the oven and carefully unwrap the ribs. Increase the oven temperature to 375°F.

◦ Put a fresh sheet of parchment paper on the sheet pan. Set aside 1 tablespoon of the BBQ sauce and brush the remaining 5 tablespoons of sauce all over the ribs. Place the ribs meat side up on the parchment paper and lightly cover with a second sheet of parchment. Use wooden spoons to weight down the paper on either side.

◦ Put the ribs back in the oven and bake for 45 minutes. Remove the top piece of parchment paper and the wooden spoons, then bake for another 10 minutes. Remove the ribs from the oven; they will have a lovely brown color on them.

◦ Let the rib racks cool for a few minutes before cutting them into single ribs. Drizzle with the BBQ sauce from the sheet pan.

modifications: *To make this dish AIP compliant, omit the black pepper and use the AIP version of the BBQ sauce.*

awesome additions: *Serve with Not Yo' Momma's Coleslaw (page 330) or Warm Garlic Herb Radish Salad (page 298).*

Per serving (about 4 ribs): Calories **571** · Fat **42.5g** · Total Carbs **3.3g** · Fiber **0.5g** · Protein **40.9g**

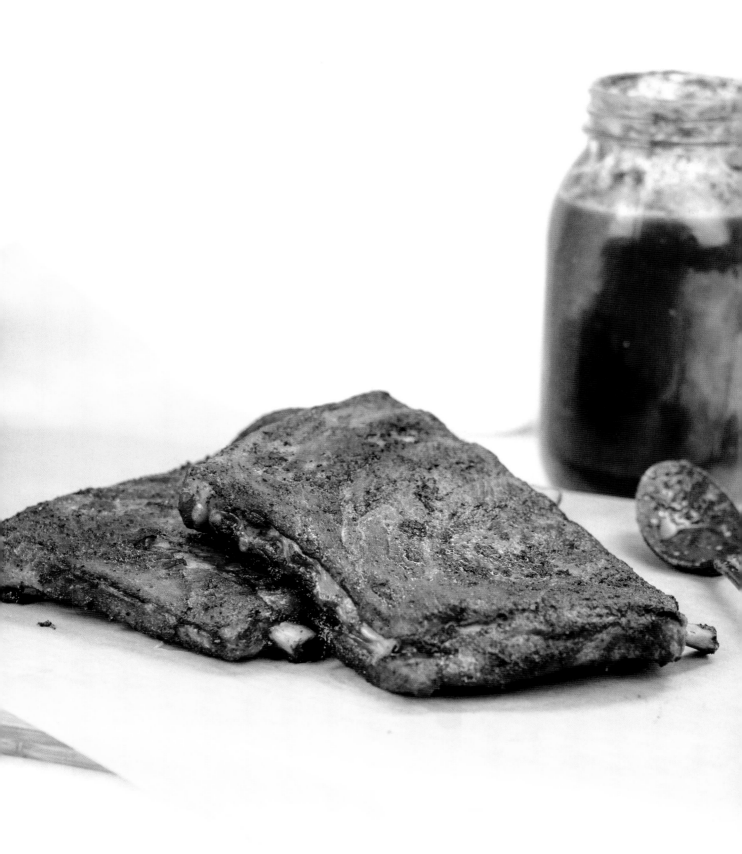

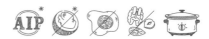

Tasty Mojo Pork

Serves 8 ◦ Prep Time: 10 minutes, plus 12 hours to marinate ◦ Cook Time: 10 hours

This is my go-to recipe for slow cooker pork. When I cook pork, I usually default to lechón asado (Cuban roast pork) flavors—why mess with perfection, right? If you want a shortcut for this recipe, replace the marinade with 2 cups of The New Primal Citrus Herb Marinade; it is essentially Cuban mojo, which is the traditional marinade for lechón asado. But if you want to make the marinade the old-fashioned way, let's go—I'll show you how!

For the marinade:

¼ cup extra-virgin olive oil

3 tablespoons coconut aminos

Juice of 2 oranges

Juice of 1 grapefruit

1 large onion, sliced

4 cloves garlic, smashed with the side of a knife and peeled

1 tablespoon fine salt

1 tablespoon garlic powder

2 teaspoons dried oregano leaves

2 teaspoons ground cumin

2 teaspoons turmeric powder

1 teaspoon ground black pepper

2 bay leaves

1 (3-pound) boneless pork shoulder

2 cups bone broth

◦ In a large bowl, whisk together all of the marinade ingredients. Put the pork shoulder in the bowl and turn it over several times to coat it with the marinade, then place some of the onion slices on top. Cover the bowl and put it in the fridge to marinate for 12 hours, turning the pork shoulder over at least once.

◦ Set the bowl out at room temperature for 1 hour before cooking.

◦ Put the pork shoulder in a slow cooker with the fat cap side up. Pour the marinade and onions all over the pork and pour the broth around it. Cover and cook on low for 10 hours, until you can easily pull the meat apart with a fork.

◦ When the pork is done, transfer it to a casserole dish or sheet pan and use 2 forks to shred it. Place it under the broiler for 4 minutes before serving.

modifications: *To make this dish AIP compliant, omit the cumin and black pepper. To make it coconut-free, use low-sodium gluten-free tamari or aged balsamic vinegar instead of the coconut aminos.*

Per serving: Calories **489** · Fat **29.5g** · Total Carbs **4.8g** · Fiber **0.6g** · Protein **48g**

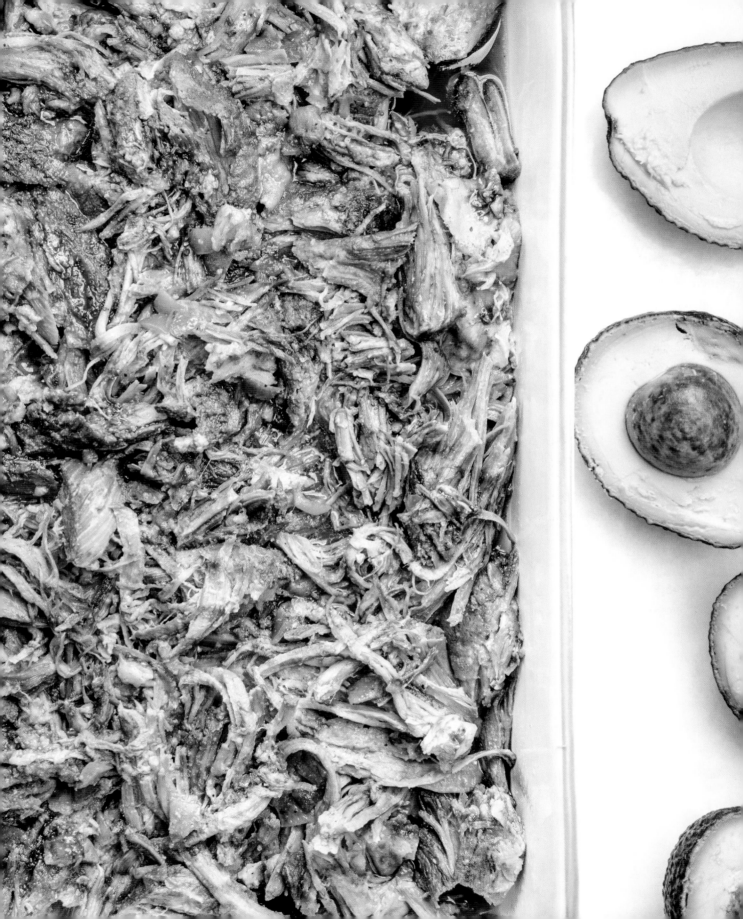

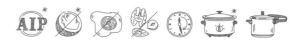

Pressure Cooker Ribs

Serves 5 ○ Prep Time: 5 minutes ○ Cook Time: 25 minutes

Fall-off-the-bone ribs are good and all, but you can't eat them with your hands. The truly perfect doneness point is right *before* they fall off the bone, when the meat is juicy, your teeth sink right into it, and it's melt-in-your-mouth good. This recipe gets ribs to that exact point, and it won't take hours! It's so simple, but the flavors are so good. I love serving these ribs with my Cauliflower "Fried" Rice (page 316).

1 rack baby back ribs (about 2 pounds)

1 teaspoon fine salt

1 tablespoon Castaway Seed Blend (page 82)

2 cups filtered water

2 tablespoons apple cider vinegar

¼ cup coconut aminos

2 tablespoons melted lard

modifications: *To make the ribs AIP compliant, replace the seed blend with ½ teaspoon ginger powder, ½ teaspoon ground cinnamon, ½ teaspoon garlic powder, and ½ teaspoon onion powder. To make them coconut-free, use aged balsamic vinegar instead of the coconut aminos.*

○ Cut the rack of ribs into 3 even sections, each about 6 inches wide. Rub them with the salt and seed blend.

○ Pour the water and vinegar into a pressure cooker, then place the rack accessory inside the pot.

○ Arrange the sections of ribs on the rack in the pot so that they are standing up but leaning inward and against each other to form a tepee. This way, they will cook more evenly. Seal the lid and cook on high pressure for 20 minutes.

○ While the ribs cook, put an oven rack in the top position, under the broiler. Place a cooling rack on a sheet pan or line the pan with aluminum foil.

○ When the ribs are done, release the pressure manually. Set the oven's broil setting to high (550°F).

○ Open the pressure cooker lid and use tongs to carefully transfer the ribs to the prepared sheet pan. Use a brush to coat them with the coconut aminos and lard.

○ Broil the ribs for 5 minutes, or until they get very toasty and browned with charred bits. Remove from the oven and use a knife to cut the ribs apart. Serve hot!

○ Store leftovers wrapped up tightly in the fridge. To reheat, place the ribs on a sheet pan, cover them with aluminum foil, and bake in a preheated 300°F oven for 20 minutes.

Slow Cooker Method: Pour the water and vinegar into a slow cooker and put the seasoned ribs directly in the liquid. Cook on low for 8 hours or on high for 4 hours, then continue the recipe as written.

Per serving: Calories **684** · Fat **54.6g** · Total Carbs **3.1g** · Fiber **0.1g** · Protein **43.3g**

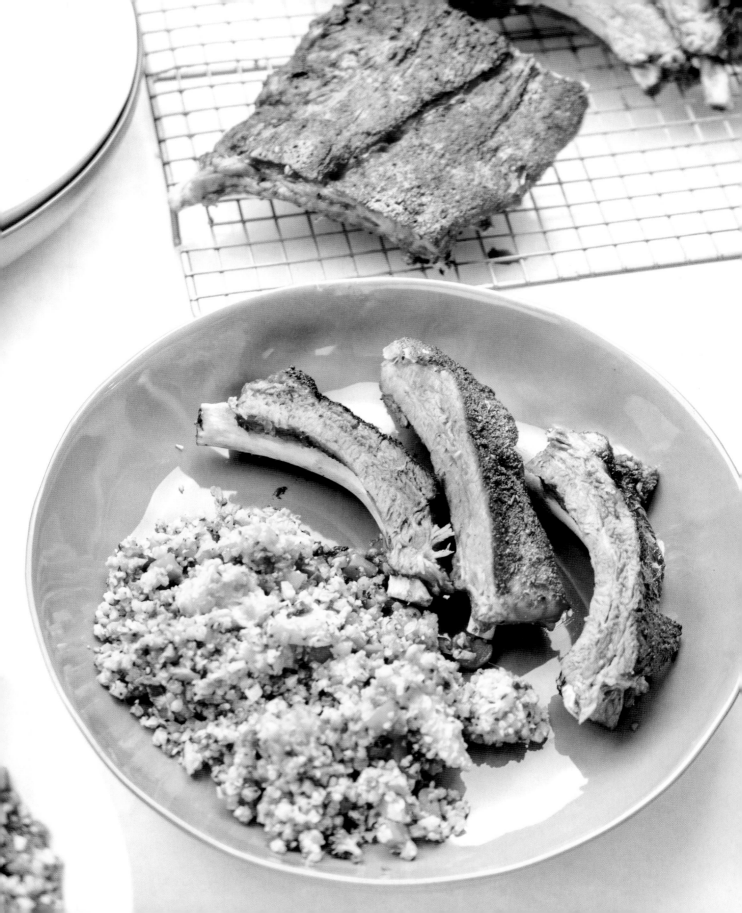

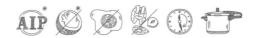

Curried Pork Chops with Cabbage

Serves 4 ◦ Prep Time: 10 minutes ◦ Cook Time: 20 minutes

If you tend to have a hard time with cruciferous vegetables, try pressure cooking them! A pressure cooker is great for cooking foods that can be hard to digest because it breaks down antinutrients, fiber, and cellulose, which can cause gut irritation or gas. This recipe has it all: antioxidants, anti-inflammatory compounds, and a delicious curry flavor. It's a seriously feel-good meal. For the best flavor, don't skip the gremolata!

4 thick-cut boneless pork chops (about 2 pounds)

1 tablespoon Citrus Curry Powder (page 82)

2 teaspoons fine salt

2 tablespoons ghee or coconut oil

4 cups shredded red cabbage

½ cup bone broth

1 tablespoon coconut aminos

¼ cup Gremolata with Olive Oil (page 86)

◦ Put a pressure cooker in sauté mode. While it heats, season the pork chops with the curry powder and salt. Melt the ghee in the cooker, then sear the chops, 2 at a time, for 2 minutes on each side. Remove the pork chops from the cooker and cancel the sauté function.

◦ Put the cabbage, broth, and coconut aminos in the pressure cooker. Stir well, then place the chops on top of the cabbage. Seal the lid and cook on high pressure for 10 minutes, then release the pressure manually.

◦ Open the lid and use tongs to remove the pork chops from the pot. Scoop out the cabbage with a spoon. To serve, pour the gremolata over the chops and spoon the cabbage on the side. I like to thinly slice my chops with a chef's knife before serving.

◦ Store leftovers in the fridge for up to 4 days. To reheat, sauté in a skillet over medium heat for 5 minutes.

modifications: *To make this dish AIP compliant, use the AIP version of the curry powder. To make it coconut-free, use aged balsamic vinegar or gluten-free tamari instead of the coconut aminos.*

Per serving: Calories **528** · Fat **25.4g** · Total Carbs **11.4g** · Fiber **4g** · Protein **60.2g**

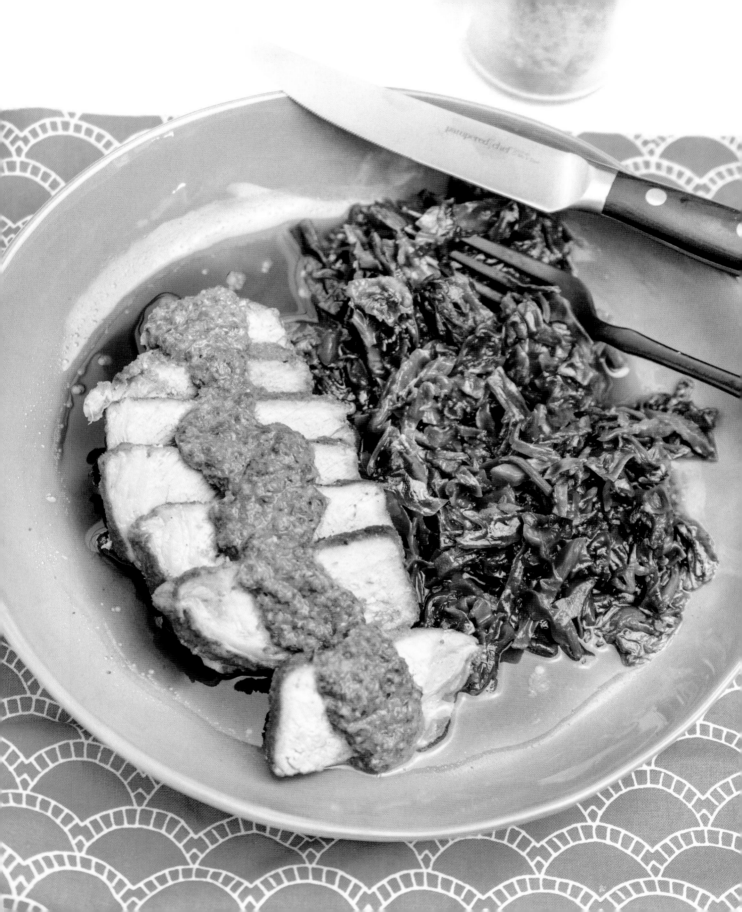

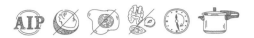

Pork + Kale in an Instant

Serves 5 ○ Prep Time: 10 minutes ○ Cook Time: 15 minutes

I love cooking with fresh herbs—hence the Frozen Herb Blocks on page 109. If you're out of fresh herbs, I hope you have some of those blocks in the freezer to use here. This is a great one-pot recipe that comes together super fast in a pressure cooker. Serve it as is or over cauliflower rice for a weeknight meal the entire family can get into!

2 tablespoons extra-virgin olive oil or avocado oil

2 pounds ground pork

2 teaspoons fine salt

2 teaspoons minced fresh chives

2 teaspoons minced fresh rosemary

2 teaspoons minced fresh thyme

2 teaspoons garlic powder

2 teaspoons ginger powder

5 cups chopped dinosaur kale, coarse stems removed (about 2 bunches)

Juice of 2 lemons

2 tablespoons aged balsamic vinegar (see notes, page 90)

○ Put a pressure cooker in sauté mode. Once it's hot, drizzle in the oil. Crumble in the ground pork and use a wire whisk to break it up and stir until it begins to brown. Switch to a rubber spatula and stir in the salt, fresh herbs, and spices.

○ Add the kale, lemon juice, and vinegar and stir until well combined. Cancel the sauté function. Seal the lid and cook on low pressure for 8 minutes. Let the pressure release naturally, then open the lid. Mix well and serve hot.

○ Store leftovers in the fridge for up to 5 days. To reheat, sauté in a skillet over medium heat for 5 to 6 minutes.

Per serving: Calories **466** · Fat **32.3g** · Total Carbs **9.4g** · Fiber **1.6g** · Protein **36.3g**

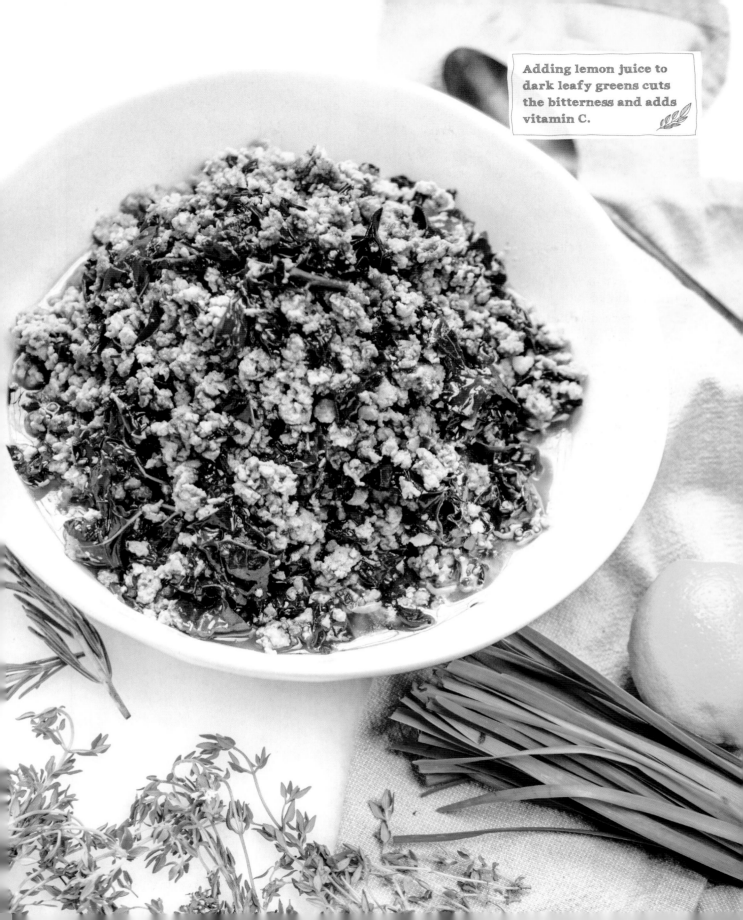

Adding lemon juice to
dark leafy greens cuts
the bitterness and adds
vitamin C.

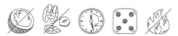

Prosciutto Wraps

Serves 1 ○ Prep Time: 10 minutes

This light dish pairs well with a cup of bone broth or some hard-boiled eggs if you have them. If not, this is a great, quick no-cook recipe to tide you over!

4 slices prosciutto di Parma or thinly sliced cured beef

2 tablespoons Horseradish Mayo (page 94)

1 cup arugula

4 fresh basil leaves

½ ripe Hass avocado, peeled and cut into 4 slices

○ Lay the prosciutto slices flat on a cutting board. Gently smear them with the mayo.

○ Evenly pile the arugula, basil leaves, and avocado slices in the center of the prosciutto slices and roll them up, using the mayo to glue them shut.

○ Plate and eat! Make sure you have a napkin—you're going to need it.

awesome additions: *I love sneaking in green onions and seasoning the arugula with olive oil, aged balsamic vinegar, and salt—but none of that is needed.*

Per serving: Calories **409** · Fat **36.6g** · Total Carbs **6.7g** · Fiber **5g** · Protein **1.9g**

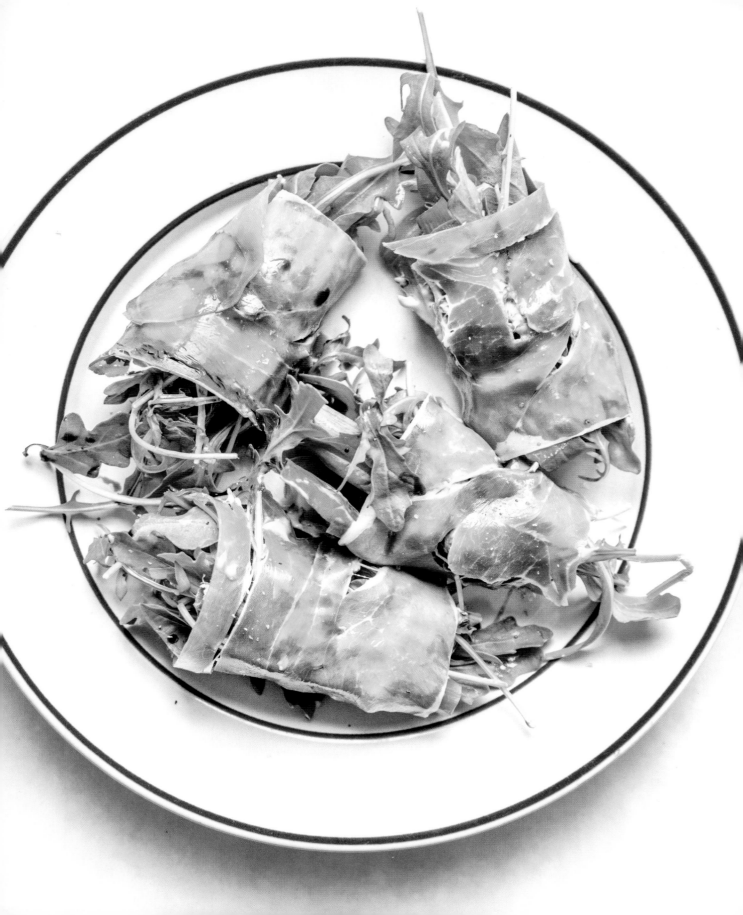

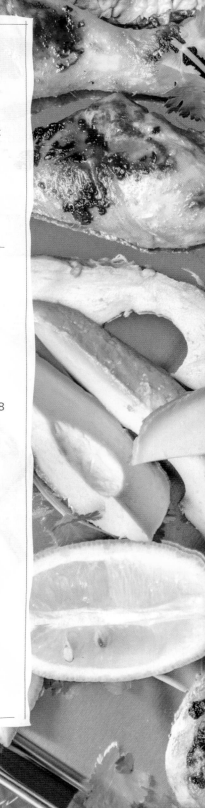

POULTRY

Everything tastes like chicken, unless you cook chicken like I do! Chicken is rich in niacin, which helps the body process carbohydrates for energy and is important for cardiovascular health. While turkey isn't as high in niacin, it does contain tryptophan, which your body converts to niacin.

You can't beat chicken breasts for their versatility and ability to take on the flavor of any dish. But I love using affordable chicken thighs and ground dark meat turkey even more—dark meat has so much flavor!

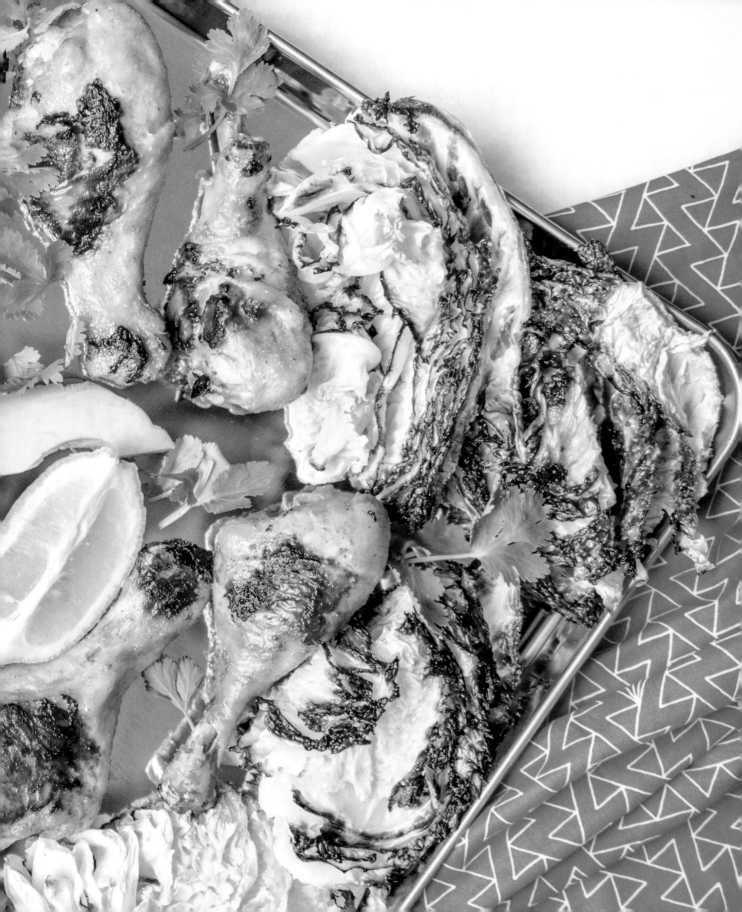

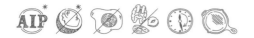

Teriyaki Noodle Bowl

Serves 3 ○ Prep Time: 10 minutes ○ Cook Time: 20 minutes

Forget takeout—this one-pot meal has all the bright flavors of Japanese cuisine, and it'll ready before your order could be delivered. Savory, tangy, sweet, and salty, this balanced stir-fry satisfies the palate and the gut. Pro tip: cook up some extra chicken breast while you're at it and set it aside for other meals. You can sneak batch cooking into everyday recipes like this one to save time and stock up on flavorful dishes.

1½ pounds boneless, skinless chicken breasts

2 teaspoons fine salt, divided

1 teaspoon garlic powder

1 teaspoon ginger powder

2 tablespoons coconut oil or ghee, divided

6 baby bok choy, halved lengthwise

1 cup sliced shiitake mushrooms (about 4 ounces)

4 cloves garlic, sliced

2 (7-ounce) packages shirataki noodles

1 tablespoon apple cider vinegar

2 tablespoons toasted sesame oil

⅔ cup Gut-Healing Teriyaki Sauce (page 70)

1 teaspoon sesame seeds, for garnish

2 green onions, sliced on the bias, for garnish

○ Heat a 15-inch skillet over medium heat. Season the chicken breasts with 1½ teaspoons of the salt, the garlic powder, and ginger powder. Once the pan is hot, melt 1 tablespoon of the coconut oil in the skillet, then add the chicken and cook for 4 minutes on each side, or until cooked through (the internal temperature of the chicken should reach 165°F). Remove the chicken from the skillet and set it aside.

○ Melt the remaining tablespoon of coconut oil in the skillet. Add the bok choy, mushrooms, and garlic and sprinkle with the remaining ½ teaspoon of salt. Cook, stirring occasionally, until tender and lightly browned, about 10 minutes.

○ While the veggies cook, open the noodle packets and empty the noodles into a colander. Rinse with warm water for 2 to 3 minutes, then drain well. Slice the chicken into ¼-inch-wide pieces.

○ Stir the vinegar into the veggies and deglaze the skillet, scraping up the browned bits on the bottom. Move the veggies to one side of the skillet and place the noodles on the other side. Drizzle the noodles with the sesame oil and sauté for 3 minutes, until they get some color on them.

○ Add the chicken pieces and teriyaki sauce to the skillet; if the sauce has solidified because it's straight out of the fridge, stir it around the chicken until it melts.

○ To serve, you can mix it all up like a proper stir-fry or keep everything separate for a pretty presentation. Garnish with the sesame seeds and sliced green onions.

○ Store leftovers in the fridge for up to 5 days. To reheat, sauté in a skillet over medium heat for 4 minutes.

modifications: *To make this dish AIP compliant, omit the sesame oil and sesame seeds. To make it coconut-free, use the coconut-free version of the teriyaki sauce.*

Per serving: Calories **453** · Fat **25.8g** · Total Carbs **12.5g** · Fiber **5.1g** · Protein **44.6g**

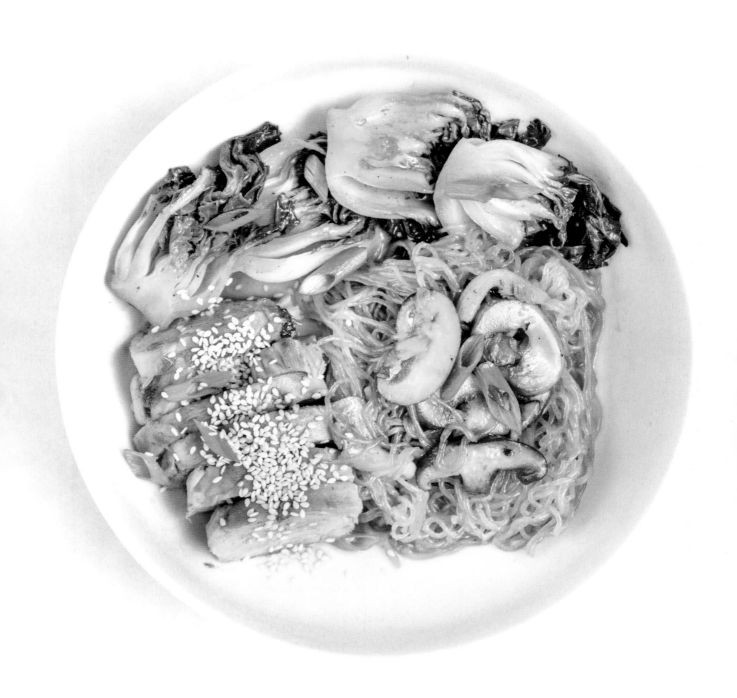

Chicken Scaloppine with Creamy Spinach + Artichokes

AIP

Serves 3 ○ Prep Time: 10 minutes ○ Cook Time: 20 minutes

The light coating of coconut flour on the chicken adds a subtle sweetness to this dish that plays really well with the creamy spinach and tangy artichoke hearts. It's a wonderful medley of flavors and textures that delivers immune-boosting antioxidant goodness and satiating lean protein!

3 small boneless, skinless chicken breast halves (about 12 ounces)

1½ teaspoons fine salt, divided

2 teaspoons Italian herb blend

3 tablespoons coconut flour

4 tablespoons extra-virgin olive oil or ghee, divided

6 cups baby spinach

3 cloves garlic, sliced

½ cup coconut cream

2 (14-ounce) cans artichoke hearts packed in water, drained

Juice of 1 lemon

○ Heat a 15-inch skillet over medium heat. While it heats, prepare the chicken.

○ Lay the chicken breasts on a cutting board and flatten to ¼ inch thick by beating them with a kitchen mallet or rolling pin. Mix together 1 teaspoon of the salt, the Italian herb blend, and coconut flour in a small bowl, then dust the chicken with the seasoned flour.

○ Once the skillet is hot, pour 3 tablespoons of the olive oil into the pan. Pan-fry the chicken breasts for 4 to 5 minutes on each side, until golden brown and cooked through (the internal temperature of the chicken should reach 165°F). Remove the chicken from the skillet with tongs, cover it with aluminum foil to keep it warm, and set it aside.

○ Pour the remaining tablespoon of oil into the skillet. Quickly add the spinach and garlic to the skillet and season with the remaining ½ teaspoon of salt. Sauté for 3 minutes, until the spinach is tender. Stir in the coconut cream, artichoke hearts, and lemon juice and bring to a vigorous simmer, then remove from the heat.

○ Divide the creamy spinach mixture among 3 shallow bowls and top each with a chicken breast. Serve immediately.

○ Store leftover chicken and vegetables in separate containers in the fridge for up to 5 days. Reheat them in separate skillets over medium heat until warmed through.

modifications: *To make this dish coconut-free, use blanched almond flour instead of coconut flour in the breading and replace the coconut cream with Salted Cashew Cream (page 76).*

Per serving: Calories **553** · Fat **36.6g** · Total Carbs **15.1g** · Fiber **7.6g** · Protein **40.9g**

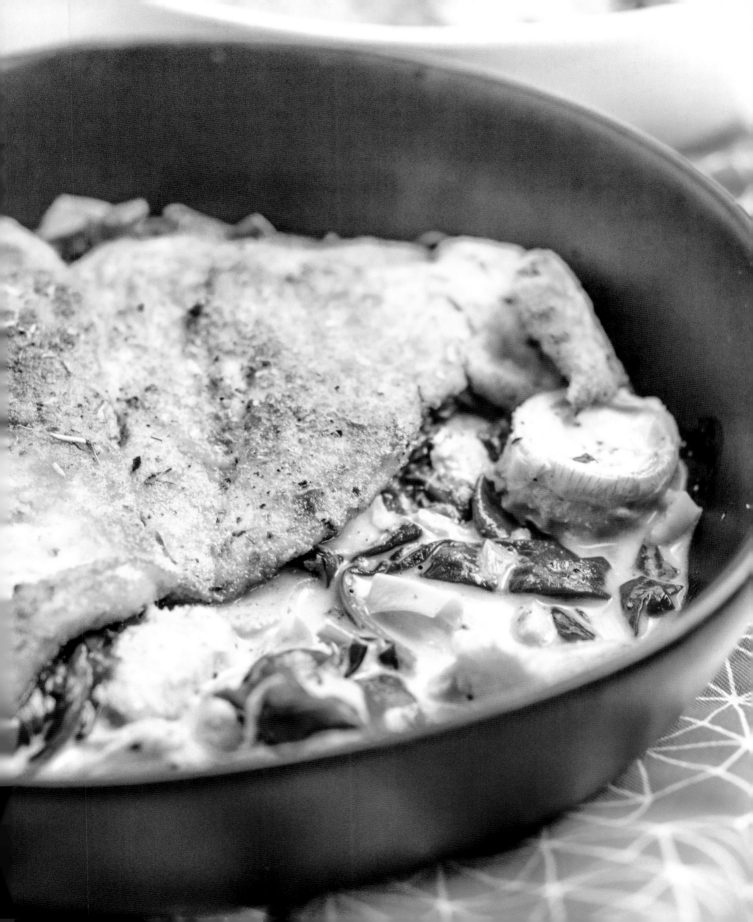

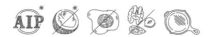

Turkey Burger Bowls

Serves 6 ◦ Prep Time: 15 minutes ◦ Cook Time: 35 minutes

If you want to know how I cook for myself almost daily, this is it: a typical Cristina meal. I made this for my friend Michele when she was visiting, and her reaction convinced me to include this recipe in this book. It's perfect for meal prep—with the cooked components ready to go in the fridge, throwing together the bowls for lunch is a breeze.

6 slices bacon

2 pounds ground dark meat turkey

¼ cup tahini

2 teaspoons fine salt

2 teaspoons onion powder

1 teaspoon garlic powder

1 teaspoon ground black pepper

8 ounces sliced cremini mushrooms (about 2 cups)

2 tablespoons coconut aminos

¼ cup bone broth

For serving:

6 cups arugula

4 ounces broccoli sprouts

3 tablespoons extra-virgin olive oil

2 tablespoons sprouted pumpkin seeds (see notes, page 178)

Fine salt

◦ Heat a 15-inch skillet over medium heat. Fry the bacon in the skillet for 5 minutes per side, or until crispy.

◦ While the bacon cooks, mix the turkey with the tahini, salt, and spices in a large bowl until well combined. With wet hands, shape the mixture into six 3-inch balls, then flatten them into patties and set aside.

◦ Use tongs to remove the bacon from the skillet and set aside. Use a large spoon to remove about 2 tablespoons of bacon fat from the skillet and set aside to use later.

◦ Add the mushrooms to the skillet and sauté for 8 minutes, or until tender and browned. Stir in the coconut aminos and broth and bring to a simmer; continue to simmer until the liquid has reduced by half and the mushrooms are glazed, about 5 minutes. Remove the mushrooms from the skillet and set aside.

◦ Return the reserved bacon fat to the skillet and add the turkey patties one by one, making sure they're not touching. Fry for 6 minutes per side, or until they have nice dark crust on both sides and are cooked through (the internal temperature should reach 165°F). While the burgers are cooking, chop the bacon into ½-inch pieces.

◦ To assemble the bowls, place a spoonful of glazed mushrooms in each bowl and top with a burger and bacon pieces. Place the arugula and broccoli sprouts next to the burger and top the greens with the olive oil, pumpkin seeds, and a sprinkle of salt.

◦ Store leftover bowl components separately in the fridge for up to 4 days. The bowls are great cold, or you can reheat the burgers before adding them to the bowls by baking them for 10 minutes in a preheated 350°F oven.

modifications: *To make this dish AIP compliant, use coconut butter instead of the tahini and omit the black pepper and pumpkin seeds. To make it coconut-free, use aged balsamic vinegar instead of the coconut aminos.*

Per bowl: Calories **418** · Fat **28g** · Total Carbs **6.1g** · Fiber **2g** · Protein **36.9g**

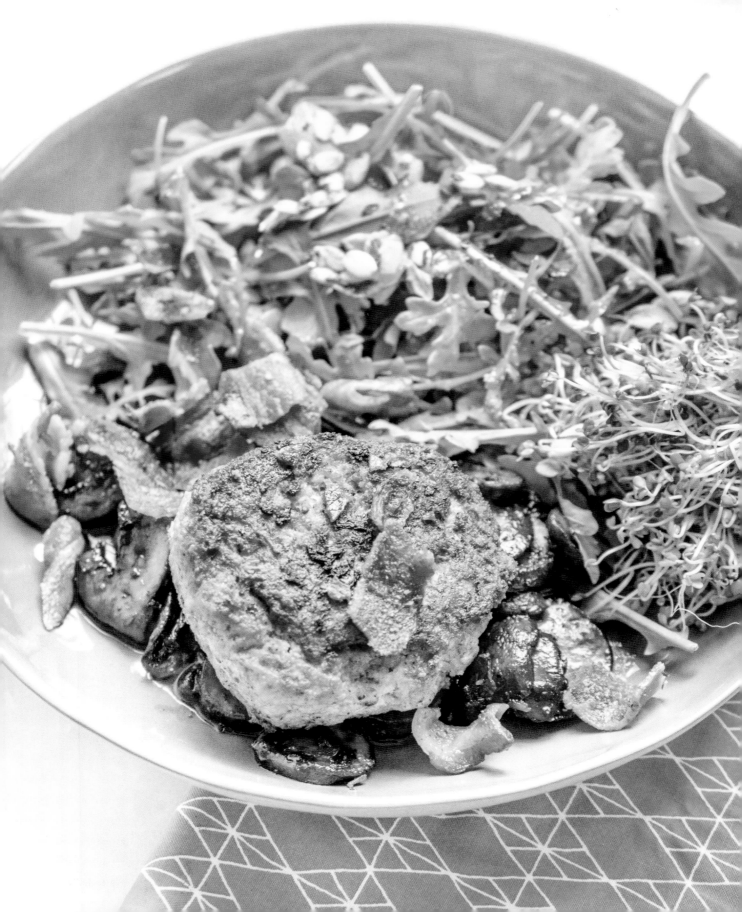

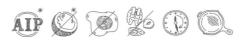

Crispy Chicken + Strawberry Balsamic Salad

Serves 3 ◦ Prep Time: 10 minutes ◦ Cook Time: 15 minutes

Crispy food is my favorite, and entrée salads are up there too! Put them together and you get this dish: almost-fried chicken paired with a simple Mediterranean-inspired salad. These classic flavors come together in a new way to create a combo that's a surefire winner.

For the chicken:

½ cup pork panko, store-bought or homemade (page 80)

1 teaspoon fine salt

1 teaspoon onion powder

6 boneless, skinless chicken thighs (about 1½ pounds)

¼ cup coconut oil or lard, for the pan

For the salad:

5 cups arugula

9 medium strawberries, hulled and halved

1 small red onion, thinly sliced

6 tablespoons Balsamic Mustard Vinaigrette (page 96)

◦ Heat a large skillet over medium heat. While it heats, combine the pork panko, salt, and onion powder in a medium-sized bowl. Toss the chicken thighs in the panko mixture to evenly coat them.

◦ Heat the coconut oil in the skillet; you'll know it's ready when the end of a wooden spoon handle sizzles when dipped into the oil. Lay the coated chicken thighs flat in the oil and pour any coating that remains in the bowl on top of the chicken. Fry for 5 to 7 minutes, then flip the thighs and fry for another 5 to 7 minutes, until browned, crispy, and cooked through.

◦ While the chicken cooks, make the salad: Place the arugula in a large bowl and toss with the strawberries and onion slices. Divide the salad among 3 plates.

◦ When the chicken is done, remove it from the skillet with tongs or a slotted spoon and place 2 crispy thighs alongside each portion of salad. Drizzle 2 tablespoons of the vinaigrette over the salad.

◦ If you have leftovers or are making this dish ahead, store the components separately in the fridge for up to 4 days and combine them only when ready to serve.

modifications: *To make this dish AIP compliant, use the AIP version of the vinaigrette. To make it coconut-free, cook the chicken in lard and use the coconut-free version of the vinaigrette.*

Per serving: Calories **557** · Fat **43.4g** · Total Carbs **6.8g** · Fiber **1.7g** · Protein **34.8g**

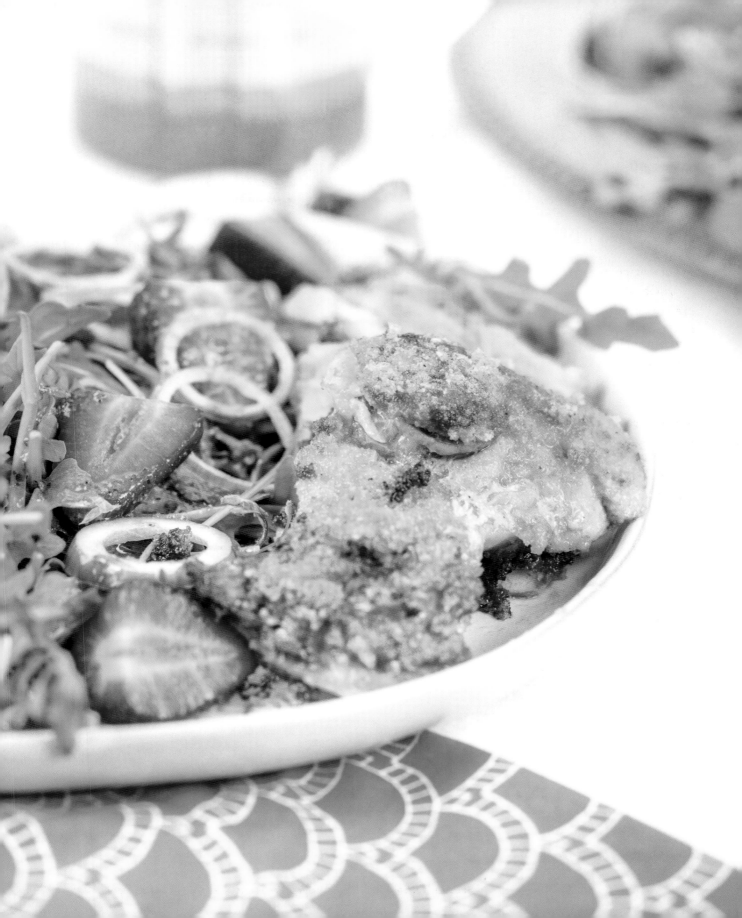

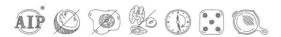

Victoria's Pollo Encebollado

Serves 2 ◦ Prep Time: 10 minutes ◦ Cook Time: 15 minutes

Pollo encebollado translates to "onion-smothered chicken." When I was growing up, my abuela liked to make this delicious traditional Cuban dish. When I visited her in the hospital toward the end of her life, we'd talk about food, and she reminded me of this recipe. The instructions here are for the version my abuela made when I was a kid. It's already easy and quick, but as she got older, my abuela was really hip to easy cooking hacks, and she created the no-standing-by-the-stove sheet pan version that appears below the recipe.

2 tablespoons extra-virgin olive oil

1 large onion, sliced

2 teaspoons fine salt, divided

2 boneless, skinless chicken breast halves (about 12 ounces), butterflied

2 teaspoons Cuban Sazón (page 83) or adobo seasoning

2 lime wedges, for serving

◦ Heat a 15-inch skillet over medium heat. Pour in the olive oil, then add the onion and ½ teaspoon of the salt and cook for about 5 minutes.

◦ While the onion cooks, use a meat mallet to pound the chicken breasts until they're about ¼ inch thick. In a small bowl, combine the remaining 1½ teaspoons of salt and the seasoning blend. Pat the seasoning all over the chicken.

◦ Use a spatula to move the onion to one side of the skillet, then lay the chicken breasts flat on the other side and cover them with the onion. Cook for 4 minutes, then flip the breasts over and again cover them with the onion. Cook for another 4 minutes, or until the chicken is cooked through (the internal temperature should reach 165°F). Serve the chicken breasts piled high with the sautéed onion, with a lime wedge on the side.

Variation: To make this a sheet pan meal, place the pounded and seasoned chicken on a sheet pan, cover with the onion, and roast in a preheated 400°F oven for 25 minutes.

modifications: *To make this dish AIP compliant, use the AIP version of the Cuban Sazón.*

Per serving: Calories **367** · Fat **19.4g** · Total Carbs **8.8g** · Fiber **1.3g** · Protein **38.3g**

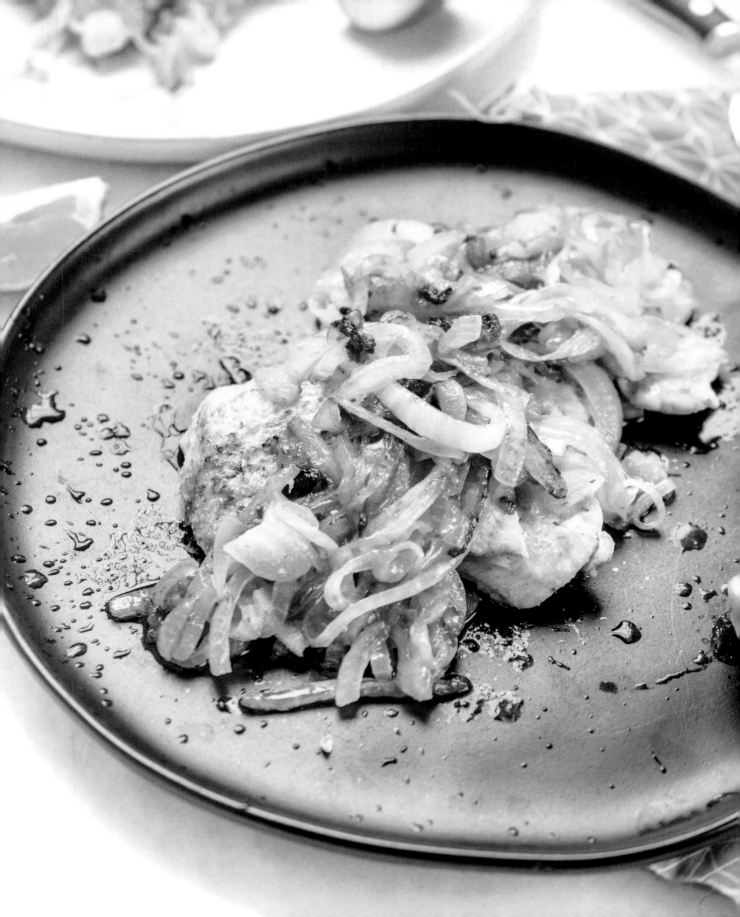

Panko Turkey Meatballs with Bok Choy

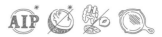

Serves 3 ○ Prep Time: 15 minutes ○ Cook Time: 20 minutes

You have been warned: these meatballs are so addictive that there may be quarrels over who gets the last bite. This is crispy, salty, savory goodness that can't be beat, especially because it's just so darn good for you. The serving suggestion for using the Green Onion Relish is just that—a suggestion. You may omit it or use Gut-Healing Teriyaki Sauce (page 70) or Horseradish Mayo (page 94) instead.

For the meatballs:

1 pound ground dark meat turkey or 93% lean ground turkey

1 large egg

½ cup pork panko, store-bought or homemade (page 80)

1 teaspoon fine salt

1 teaspoon ginger powder

1 teaspoon ground white pepper

½ teaspoon fish sauce

1 tablespoon coconut oil, for the pan

For the bok choy:

1 tablespoon coconut oil, for the pan

6 baby bok choy, leaves pulled apart

¼ teaspoon fine salt

2 teaspoons coconut aminos

1 teaspoon sesame seeds

3 tablespoons Green Onion Relish (page 98), for serving

• Prepare the meatballs: Heat a 15-inch skillet over medium heat. In a large bowl, mix the ground turkey with the egg, pork panko, salt, ginger, pepper, and fish sauce until well combined. Shape the mixture into 12 small meatballs about 1½ inches in diameter.

• Melt the coconut oil in the hot skillet and arrange the meatballs in it so they are not touching. Brown for 10 minutes, turning every 2 minutes. Transfer the browned meatballs to a plate and cover with aluminum foil to keep warm.

• Prepare the bok choy: Melt the coconut oil in the skillet. Add the bok choy leaves and season with the salt. Sauté until tender and wilted, about 8 minutes, then stir in the coconut aminos and sesame seeds.

• Return the meatballs to the skillet, cover, and cook for 2 minutes. Top with the relish and serve immediately.

• Store leftovers in the fridge for up to 5 days. To reheat, sauté in a skillet over medium heat for 10 minutes.

modifications: *To make this dish AIP compliant, omit the white pepper and sesame seeds and replace the egg with 1 tablespoon unflavored grass-fed beef gelatin. To make it coconut-free, replace the coconut oil with lard or ghee and replace the coconut aminos with liquid aminos or low-sodium gluten-free tamari.*

If you don't eat pork, blanched almond flour would work instead of the pork panko.

Per serving: Calories **621** · Fat **43.9g** · Total Carbs **5.2g** · Fiber **2.3g** · Protein **55.9g**

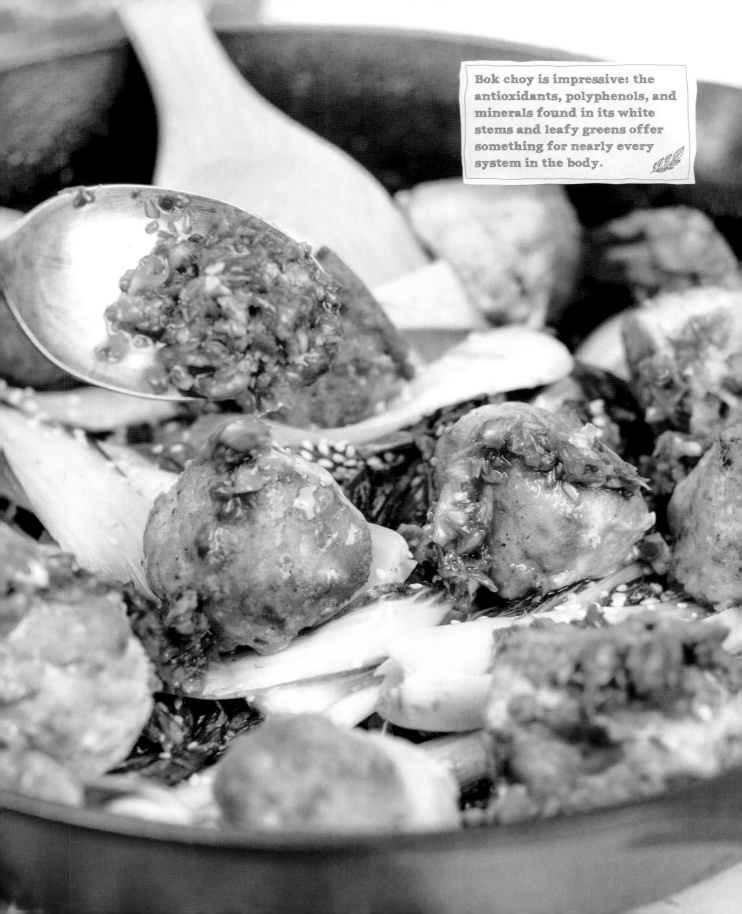

Bok choy is impressive: the antioxidants, polyphenols, and minerals found in its white stems and leafy greens offer something for nearly every system in the body.

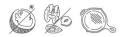

Legit Fried Chicken Tenders

Serves 5 ○ Prep Time: 15 minutes ○ Cook Time: 30 minutes

These are real deal: crispy tenders that fulfill all your cravings for fried chicken—and for fish sticks too! This breading and frying method also works perfectly with center-cut mahi-mahi fillets. Pair these with Slow Cooker Blueberry BBQ Sauce (page 100), Perfect Roasted Brussels Sprouts (page 304), and Pickled Radishes (page 84) for a comfort food spread that will convince anyone to leave processed foods behind.

---

1 cup coconut oil, tallow, or lard, for frying

2 pounds chicken breast tenders

¼ cup coconut flour

2 teaspoons fine salt

2 teaspoons garlic powder

2 teaspoons ground black pepper

2 teaspoons ground cumin

2 teaspoons onion powder

3 large eggs

2 tablespoons apple cider vinegar

3 cups pork panko, store-bought or homemade (page 80)

○ In a 15-inch skillet with at least a 2-inch rim, heat the coconut oil over medium heat. While it comes to frying temperature, bread the chicken.

○ Start by patting the chicken tenders dry; you want them bone dry. Mix together the coconut flour, salt, and spices in a shallow bowl. In a second shallow bowl, whisk the eggs with the vinegar. Put the pork panko in a third shallow bowl.

○ Check the temperature of the oil by inserting the end of a wooden spoon handle into the oil. If it sizzles loudly, it's ready.

○ Working in batches of 5 or 6 tenders, dredge the chicken tenders in the seasoned flour, then in the egg, and lastly in the panko to get a nice thick coating. Fry them for 4 minutes per side, flipping only once and using tongs. Do not overcrowd the skillet; it will result in soggy breading that falls off.

○ Once the tenders are golden brown and crispy, remove them from the pan using tongs and place them on a wire rack or sheet pan while you fry the rest of the chicken in the same way. It will take 3 or 4 batches total. If you like, you can put a wire rack on a sheet pan and place the pan in a 250°F oven to keep the tenders warm until you're ready to serve them.

○ Store leftover tenders in the fridge for up to 5 days. To reheat, bake on a wire rack in a preheated 400°F oven for 5 to 8 minutes, until heated through and crispy again.

modifications: *To make this dish coconut-free, use cassava flour, tigernut flour, or tapioca starch instead of the coconut flour. Almond flour isn't fine enough for a base coat.*

There is an AIP-friendly and egg-free chicken tender recipe on page 234.

awesome additions: *Add a little Turn Up the Heat Spice Blend (page 83) to the coconut flour mixture in step 2 to give these tenders a little kick.*

Per serving: Calories **498** · Fat **24.7g** · Total Carbs **9.7g** · Fiber **1.3g** · Protein **61g**

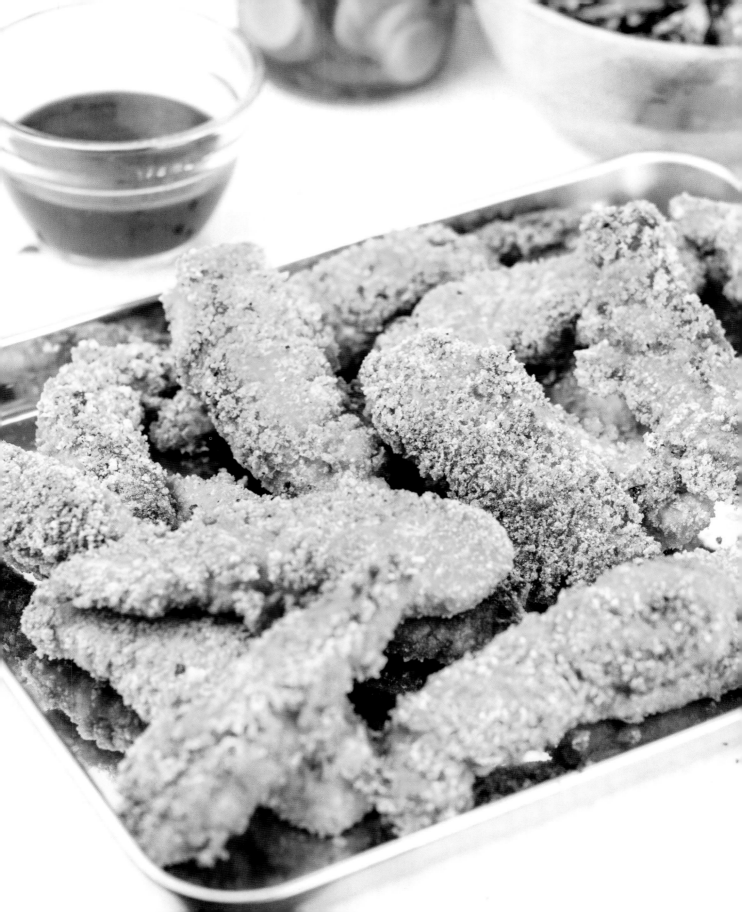

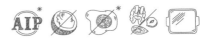

"Cheesy" Mushroom Meatzas

Serves 4 ◦ Prep Time: 20 minutes ◦ Cook Time: 30 minutes

Pizza is not one of those meals you typically walk away from feeling amazing...until now! These crispy, thin-crust meatzas are topped with mayo and nutritional yeast, which bakes up into a creamy cheesy topping. The umami flavor is amped up to eleven with a combination of roasted mushrooms and garlic. This is a truly delicious, real-food-based pizzalike creation that hits the spot!

2 pounds ground dark meat turkey or 93% lean ground turkey

2 tablespoons flaxseed meal

2 teaspoons fine salt, divided

2 teaspoons Italian herb blend, divided

1 teaspoon garlic powder

3 tablespoons extra-virgin olive oil, divided

½ cup avocado oil mayonnaise

1 tablespoon nutritional yeast

8 ounces sliced mushrooms of choice (about 2 cups; see notes)

1 small onion, sliced

4 cloves garlic, sliced

◦ Place one oven rack in the middle position and another in the bottom position. Preheat the oven to 400°F.

◦ In large bowl, mix the ground turkey with the flaxseed meal, 1½ teaspoons of the salt, 1 teaspoon of the Italian herb blend, the garlic powder, and 2 tablespoons of the olive oil until thoroughly combined. Shape the mixture into 4 evenly sized balls, like 4 giant meatballs.

◦ Line 2 sheet pans with parchment paper or silicone baking mats. Place 2 meatballs on each sheet pan and shape them into 6-inch rounds.

◦ Smear 2 tablespoons of mayo on each round and sprinkle them with the nutritional yeast. Evenly divide the sliced mushrooms, onion slices, and garlic among the rounds.

◦ Finish off the rounds by sprinkling them with the remaining ½ teaspoon of salt and remaining teaspoon of Italian herb blend and drizzling them with the remaining tablespoon of oil. Bake for 30 minutes. Remove from the oven and plate.

◦ Wrap leftovers in foil and store in the fridge for up to 4 days. To reheat, bake in a preheated 325°F oven for 10 minutes.

notes: *If you can't do flaxseed meal, you can use 1 large egg and 2 teaspoons coconut flour or psyllium husk powder.*

I love using a mixture of shiitake, cremini, and oyster mushrooms; my local grocer sells these in 4-ounce packages.

If you don't have parchment paper or silicone mats, you can make these meatzas directly on lightly oiled sheet pans.

modifications: *To make this dish egg-free, use your favorite egg-free mayo or replace the mayo with Cauliflower Sour Cream (page 74). To make it AIP compliant, follow the egg-free modifications and use 1 tablespoon coconut flour instead of the flaxseed meal.*

awesome additions: *Try sliced black olives, crispy bacon crumbles, a drizzle of aged balsamic vinegar or coconut aminos, or mustard seeds!*

Per serving: Calories **636** · Fat **50.3** · Total Carbs **5.6g** · Fiber **1.9g** · Protein **45.7g**

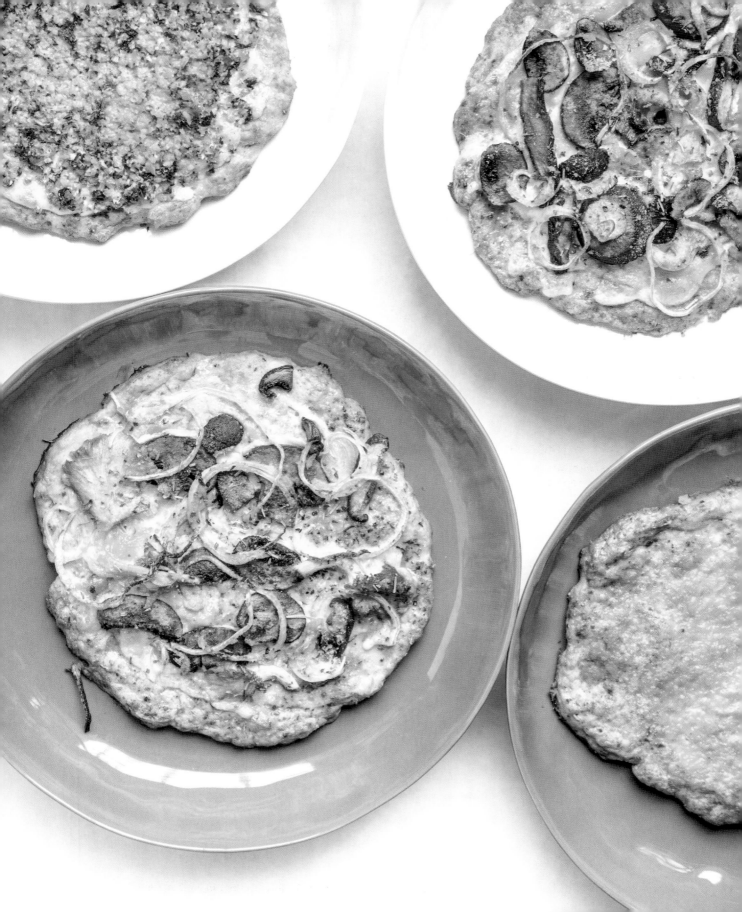

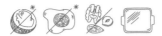

Curried Drumsticks with Burnt Cabbage

Serves 3 ◦ Prep Time: 15 minutes ◦ Cook Time: 35 minutes

These drumsticks are marinated in Everything Sauce and amped up with seasonings. The cabbage wedges are cooked along with the drumsticks, and if you think you can overcook cabbage wedges in the oven, then clearly you haven't tried, because this vegetable just gets better and better the longer it cooks. The crispy outside leaves envelop soft, sweet inner leaves. I've been known to go through an entire head of cabbage like this.

1 tablespoon extra-virgin olive oil or avocado oil, for the pan

For the drumsticks:

6 chicken drumsticks

3 tablespoons Everything Sauce (page 72)

2 teaspoons coconut aminos

1 teaspoon Citrus Curry Powder (page 82)

½ teaspoon fine salt

½ teaspoon garlic powder

For the cabbage:

1 head green cabbage (about 1½ pounds)

2 tablespoons extra-virgin olive oil

1 teaspoon fine salt

½ cup fresh cilantro leaves, for garnish

½ ripe Hass avocado, peeled, pitted, and cut into thin wedges, for serving

3 lemon wedges, for serving

- Place an oven rack in the middle position. Preheat the oven to 425°F. Lightly grease a sheet pan with 1 tablespoon of oil.

- Prepare the drumsticks: In a large bowl, toss the drumsticks with the sauce, coconut aminos, curry powder, salt, and garlic powder. Set aside to marinate for 10 minutes.

- While the chicken marinates, prepare the cabbage: Slice the head of cabbage in half, remove the core, and place both halves cut side down on the cutting board. Cut the cabbage halves diagonally from top to bottom, cutting each half into thirds.

- Place the cabbage wedges flat side down on one side of a sheet pan. Drizzle 2 tablespoons of olive oil over the wedges and sprinkle them with 1 teaspoon of salt.

- Arrange the drumsticks on the other side of the sheet pan; you want them close together but not touching.

- Put the sheet pan in the oven on the middle rack and roast for 20 minutes, then use tongs to carefully turn over the drumsticks. Roast for another 15 minutes, until the drumsticks are cooked through and tender with a nice brown color and the cabbage is tender in the center with charred and crispy outer leaves.

- Remove the chicken and cabbage from the oven and garnish with the cilantro. Serve with the avocado and lemon wedges.

- Store leftovers in the fridge for up to 4 days. To reheat, place in a skillet, cover with a tight-fitting lid, and heat over medium-low heat for 10 minutes.

modifications: *To make this dish coconut-free, use the coconut-free version of the Everything Sauce and replace the coconut aminos with low-sodium gluten-free tamari or aged balsamic vinegar. To make it egg-free, use the egg-free version of the Everything Sauce.*

Per serving: Calories **482.4** · Fat **31.4g** · Total Carbs **16.6g** · Fiber **5.8g** · Protein **35g**

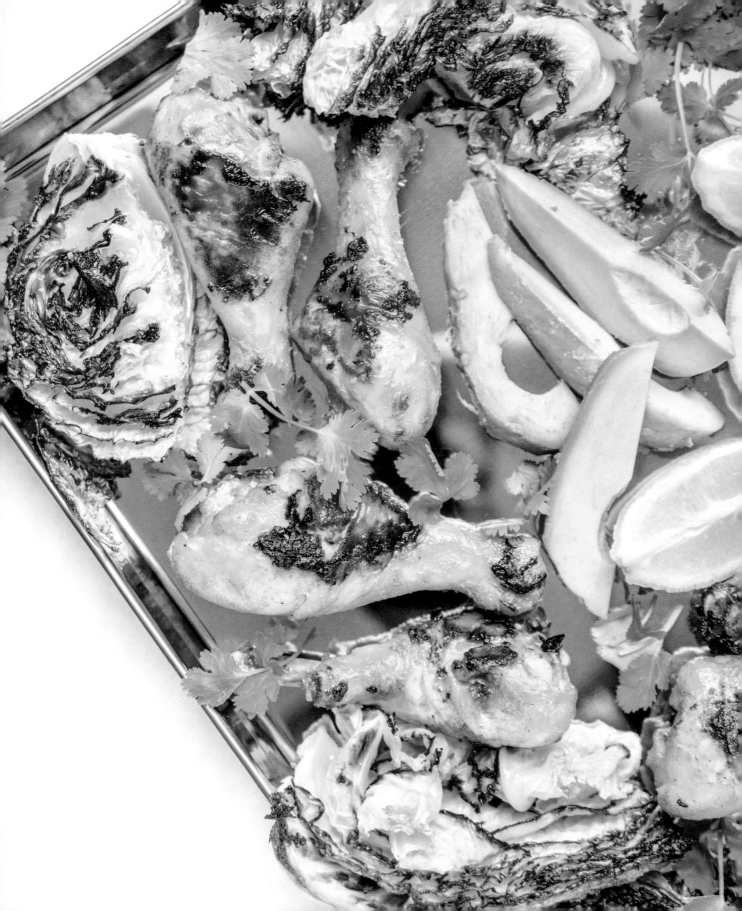

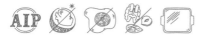

Baked Chicken Tenders with Celery Fries

Serves 3 ◦ Prep Time: 20 minutes ◦ Cook Time: 30 minutes

There are a lot of low-carb breaded chicken recipes out there, but here I've created one that is also allergen-free—and still hits the spot! This egg-free breading uses melted ghee and pork rinds, and I can't think of a more keto-friendly combination than that. I like to pair these tenders with celery fries, which are totally a thing; just ask Christina Rice of Christina Rice Wellness. She's the celery fry queen.

2 cups pork panko, store-bought or homemade (page 80)

1 tablespoon garlic powder

1 teaspoon baking powder (see note, page 148)

1 pound chicken breast tenders (see notes)

½ teaspoon fine salt, divided

⅓ cup melted ghee, coconut oil, or lard

8 long celery ribs with leaves, cut in half crosswise

Everything Sauce (page 72) or other dipping sauce of choice, for serving (optional)

◦ Place one oven rack in the middle position and another in the bottom position. Preheat the oven to 400°F.

◦ Put the pork panko in a shallow bowl. Add the garlic powder and baking powder and mix well.

◦ Pat the chicken dry and sprinkle it with ¼ teaspoon of the salt.

◦ Pour the melted ghee into a shallow bowl. One piece at a time, dip the seasoned chicken tenders in the ghee, then dredge them in the panko mixture and place them on a sheet pan.

◦ On a separate sheet pan, toss the celery with any remaining melted ghee and the remaining ¼ teaspoon of salt. Spread out the celery sticks so they are not overlapping.

◦ Place the tenders in the oven on the middle rack and the celery on the bottom rack. Roast for 30 minutes, turning the chicken tenders over halfway through cooking, until the tenders are golden brown and the celery is crispy.

◦ Remove everything from the oven and let the tenders cool for a few minutes before serving with your preferred dipping sauce, if desired.

◦ Store leftovers in the fridge for up to 4 days. To reheat, place on a sheet pan and bake in a preheated 350°F oven for 10 minutes.

note: *This recipe works best with thin pieces of chicken. If the tenders are thick, use a knife to slice them horizontally to create two slender pieces.*

modifications: *To make this dish coconut-free, use the coconut-free version of the Everything Sauce, or use another dipping sauce that does not contain coconut.*

Per serving (without sauce): Calories **499** · Fat **31.3g** · Total Carbs **3.9g** · Fiber **1.3g** · Protein **48.5g**

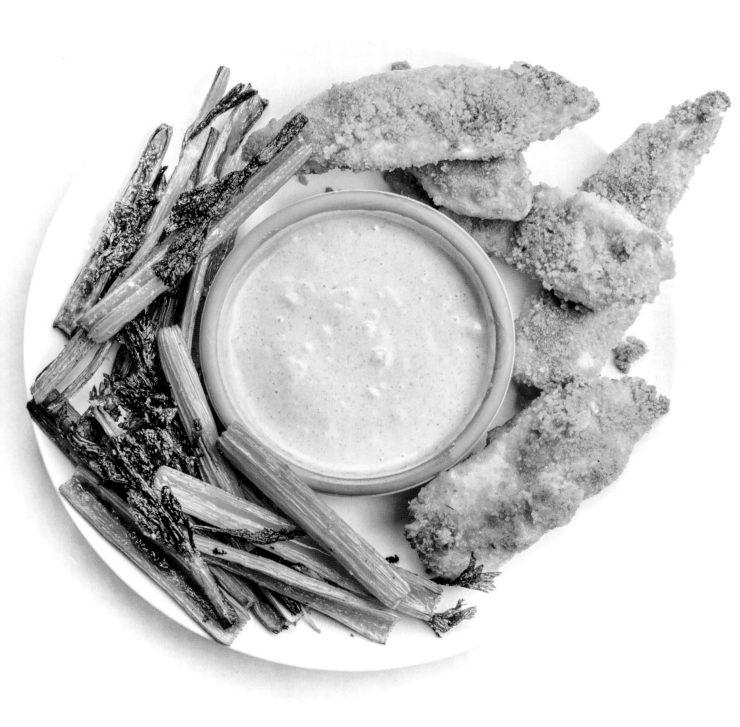

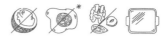

Hasselback Sausage Boats

Serves 2 ◦ Prep Time: 10 minutes ◦ Cook Time: 25 minutes

Lectins are proteins found in some plants, and they can be difficult to digest and may cause autoimmune or inflammatory symptoms in some folks. However, removing the seeds or skin from vegetables and fruits can greatly reduce their lectin content and make these foods enjoyable again. Take this recipe, for example: you scoop the seeds out of the zucchini to make room for the sausage. It's a win-win situation—no more unpleasant side effects from lectins, and you can enjoy the benefits of summer squash, which include high amounts of vitamin B6, riboflavin, and vitamin C. Slicing the sausage Hasselback style—cutting it into thin slices without cutting all the way through so that you end up with something that looks like an accordion—makes these zucchini boats delicious *and* nice to look at!

---

2 medium zucchini

½ teaspoon fine salt

4 tablespoons avocado oil mayonnaise

4 teaspoons spicy brown or Dijon mustard

4 chicken sausages (see note)

½ teaspoon Castaway Seed Blend (page 82) or your preferred all-purpose seasoning (optional)

◦ Place an oven rack in the middle position. Preheat the oven to 400°F.

◦ Slice the zucchini in half lengthwise. Use a spoon to scoop out the seeds.

◦ Line up the zucchini boats on a sheet pan, cut side up, and sprinkle them with the salt. Smear a tablespoon of mayo on each boat, followed by a teaspoon of mustard.

◦ Hasselback the sausages: Working crosswise, slice into them without cutting all the way through. Place the sausages on the boats—you can use a toothpick to secure them to the zucchini.

◦ Sprinkle the sausages with the seed blend, if using. Place the sheet pan in the oven on the middle rack and roast for 25 minutes, until the tops of the sausages are crispy and the zucchini are tender. Remove from the oven and serve right away.

◦ Store leftovers in the fridge for up to 4 days. To reheat, place on a sheet pan, cover with aluminum foil, and bake in a preheated 350°F oven for 10 minutes.

note: *This dish also makes a great appetizer or snack. Bratwursts work well in place of the chicken sausages!*

modifications: *To make these boats egg-free, replace the mayo with Cauliflower Sour Cream (page 74) or Salted Cashew Cream (page 76).*

awesome additions: *I love serving these boats with Everything Sauce (page 72) or sliced avocado.*

Per serving: Calories **513** · Fat **38.6g** · Total Carbs **12.1g** · Fiber **2g** · Protein **32.4g**

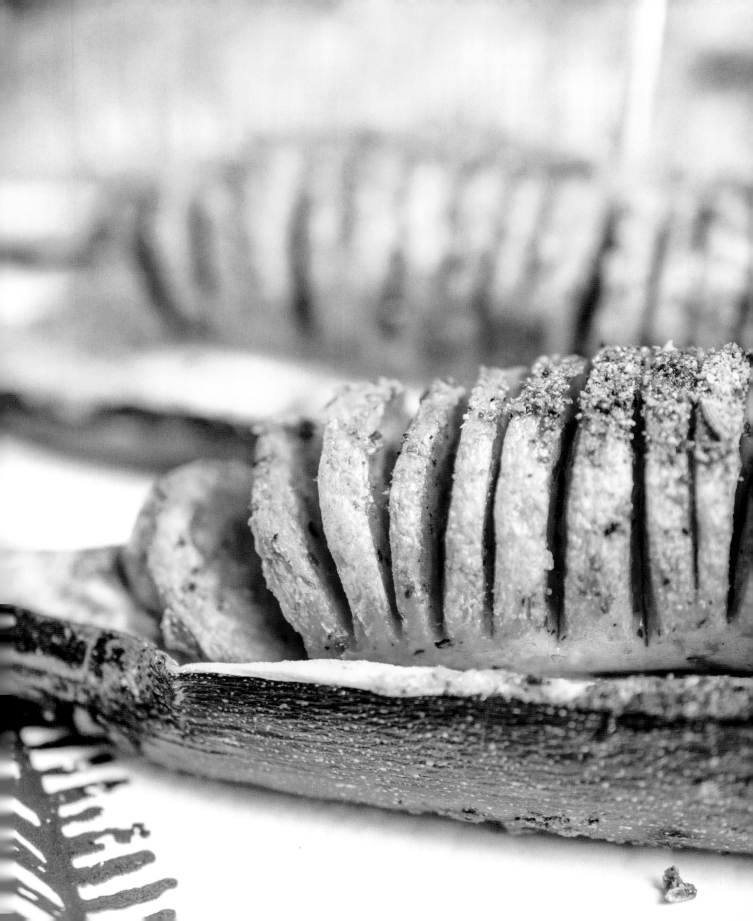

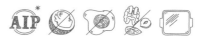

Crispy Curry Chicken Thighs

Serves 6 ○ Prep Time: 5 minutes ○ Cook Time: 40 minutes

Did you know that the curcumin in turmeric powder is most bioavailable when it's consumed alongside fats? That is why I prefer to cook with it rather than take it as a supplement. Coating these fatty chicken thighs in copious amounts of my Citrus Curry Powder is the perfect way to get this clinically proven anti-inflammatory polyphenol into your diet. It's crazy delicious too!

3 pounds boneless, skinless chicken thighs

1 tablespoon plus 1 teaspoon Citrus Curry Powder (page 82)

2½ teaspoons fine salt

3 tablespoons extra-virgin olive oil

For serving:

Leaves from 3 sprigs fresh cilantro

3 ripe Hass avocados, halved

1 lemon, cut into 6 wedges (optional)

○ Place one oven rack in the middle position and another in the bottom position. Preheat the oven to 400°F.

○ In a large bowl, combine the chicken thighs, curry powder, salt, and olive oil. Wearing gloves or using a rubber spatula so you don't stain your hands, mix well to combine and coat the chicken.

○ Put the chicken thighs smooth side down on a sheet pan. Line them up so they are not overlapping or too close together. Use 2 sheet pans if you need to.

○ Place the sheet pan in the oven on the middle rack (and bottom rack if you're using a second sheet pan) and roast for 40 minutes, until the thighs are browned, crispy, and cooked through. Remove from the oven and use a spatula to scrape the crispy thighs from the pan.

○ Garnish with the cilantro and serve each portion with half an avocado and a lemon wedge, if desired.

○ Store leftovers in the fridge for up to 4 days. To reheat, sear in a hot skillet for 3 minutes per side.

modifications: *To make this dish AIP compliant, use the AIP version of the curry powder.*

awesome additions: *This chicken is delicious with Crispy Garlic Rice (page 318) on the side.*

Per serving: Calories **479** · Fat **27.7g** · Total Carbs **6.8g** · Fiber **5.5g** · Protein **50.5g**

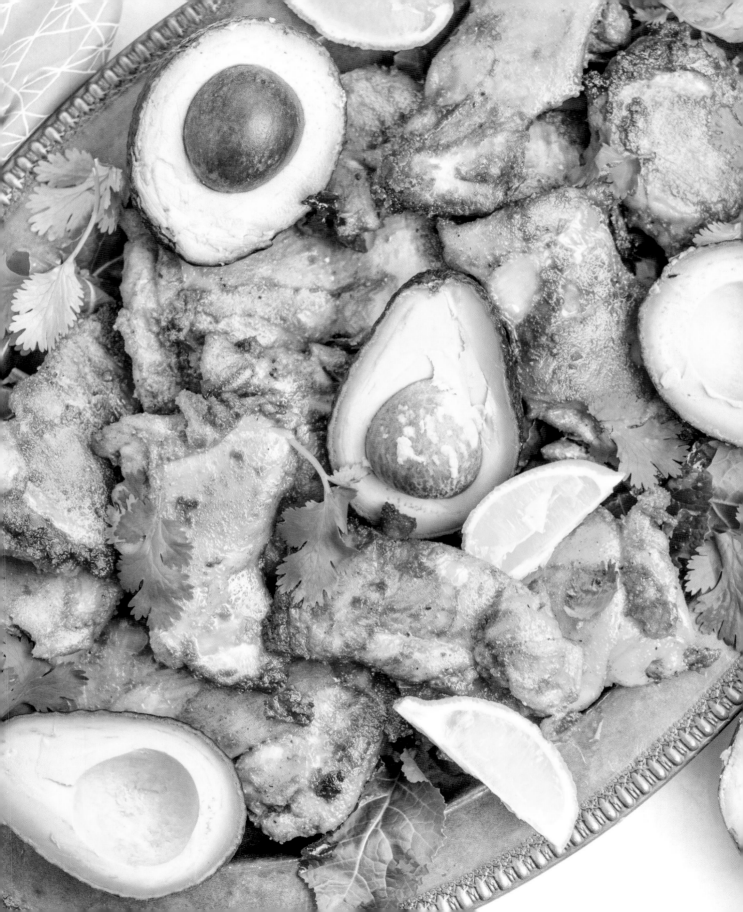

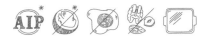

Spring Chicken with Baby Zucchini

Serves 4 ◦ Prep Time: 15 minutes ◦ Cook Time: 25 minutes

This dish may appear difficult, but it's exceptionally simple. My favorite combination: pretty to look at and easy to make! The chicken breasts are soaked in a lovely marinade and layered with cured meat and slices of lemon. The flavors are fresh and light and remind me of spring.

4 boneless, skinless chicken breast halves (about 1½ pounds)

¼ cup minced fresh cilantro or parsley

2 tablespoons extra-virgin olive oil, divided

2 tablespoons spicy brown or Dijon mustard

1 tablespoon coconut aminos

1 tablespoon garlic powder

2 teaspoons fine salt, divided

8 slices prosciutto or coppa

1 lemon, thinly sliced

1 pound baby zucchini .

◦ Preheat the oven to 400°F.

◦ Cut the chicken breasts into cutlets: Lay a breast flat on a cutting board and place one hand flat on top of the breast to keep it from moving. With a sharp knife positioned parallel to the cutting board, cut though the breast horizontally to make 2 thin cutlets. Use a meat mallet to pound the cutlets to an even ¼-inch thickness. Repeat with the remaining breasts to make 8 cutlets.

◦ Put the chicken cutlets in a large bowl. Add the cilantro, 1 tablespoon of the olive oil, the mustard, coconut aminos, garlic powder, and 1½ teaspoons of the salt. Toss well to combine and evenly coat the chicken in the marinade.

◦ Lay the chicken cutlets flat on a sheet pan, making sure not to overcrowd them—use 2 sheet pans if necessary. Top each cutlet with a slice of prosciutto and a slice of lemon.

◦ In another bowl, toss the zucchini with the remaining tablespoon of oil and remaining ½ teaspoon of salt. Arrange the zucchini on a separate sheet pan or around the chicken if there is room.

◦ Roast the chicken and zucchini for 25 minutes, until the cutlets are cooked through and the zucchini is browned and tender. Remove from the oven and serve!

◦ Store leftovers in the fridge for up to 4 days. Reheat in a skillet covered with a tight-fitting lid over medium heat for 8 minutes.

modifications: *To make this dish AIP compliant, replace the mustard in the marinade with 1 tablespoon coconut cream, 1 teaspoon coconut flour, and 1 teaspoon apple cider vinegar. To make it coconut-free, simply omit the coconut aminos or use low-sodium gluten-free tamari instead.*

awesome additions: *If you want to load this dish up with more calories, add 2 tablespoons nut or seed butter to the marinade; it will give the chicken an almost breaded texture.*

Per serving: Calories **468** · Fat **20g** · Total Carbs **7g** · Fiber **1.7g** · Protein **54.5g**

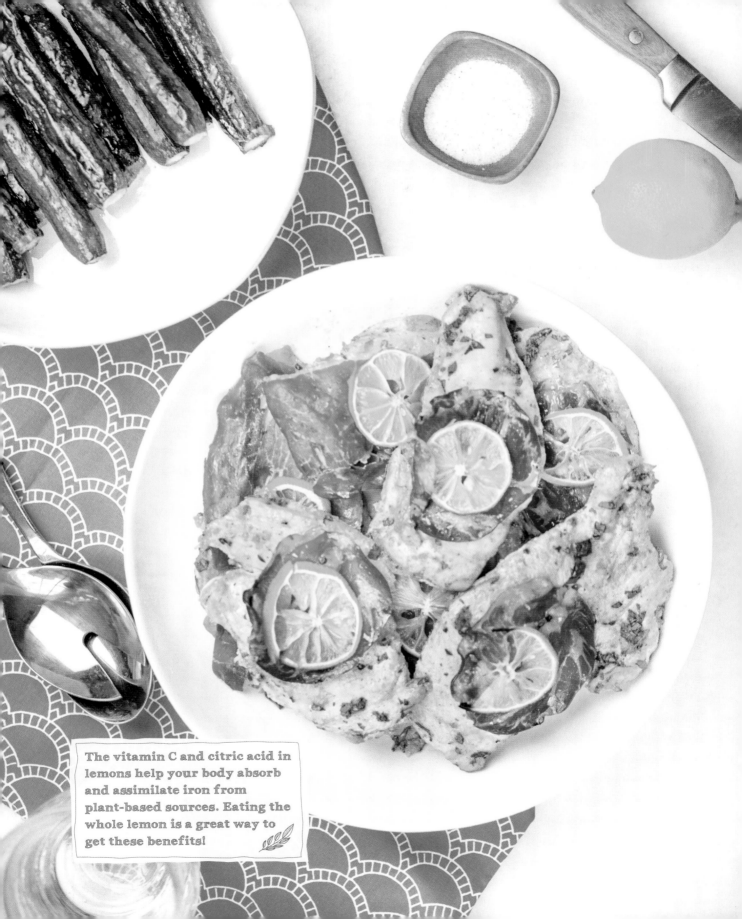

The vitamin C and citric acid in lemons help your body absorb and assimilate iron from plant-based sources. Eating the whole lemon is a great way to get these benefits!

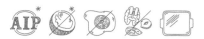

Crispy Ranch Wings

Serves 4 ◦ Prep Time: 10 minutes ◦ Cook Time: 60 minutes

I love chicken wings because they make a great protein-packed meal and double as a crispy, salty, craving-crushing snack. Throw some powerhouse veggies like broccoli sprouts, Homemade Kraut (page 102), or Pickled Asparagus (page 84) on the side for a super easy dinner.

3 pounds chicken wings, separated into wingettes and drumettes

1 tablespoon baking powder (see note, page 148)

1 tablespoon fine salt

1 tablespoon dried dill weed

1 teaspoon dried parsley

2 teaspoons garlic powder

1 teaspoon onion powder

1 teaspoon ground black pepper

3 tablespoons melted ghee or coconut oil

2 tablespoons apple cider vinegar or pickle juice

◦ Preheat the oven to 250°F.

◦ Pat the wings dry and put them in a large bowl. Toss with the baking powder to coat. Add the salt, dried herbs, and spices and toss again to coat.

◦ Lightly brush a sheet pan with some of the melted ghee and arrange the wingettes and drumettes without overlapping or crowding them—use 2 sheet pans if necessary. Lightly brush the tops of the wings with the remaining ghee and then the vinegar.

◦ Roast at 250°F for 30 minutes, then raise the oven temperature to 475°F and roast for another 30 minutes, until the chicken is cooked through and the skin is crispy. Remove from the oven and use a spatula to lift the wings from the pan.

◦ Store leftovers in the fridge for up to 4 days. To reheat, broil for 5 minutes.

note: *Switch things up by changing the herbs and spices. Use any of the seasoning blends in the Meal Makers chapter!*

modifications: *To make these wings AIP compliant, omit the black pepper.*

awesome additions: *Try dipping these wings in Cilantro Aioli (page 108) or Everything Sauce (page 72)!*

Per serving (about 8 pieces): Calories **641** · Fat **39.8g** · Total Carbs **2.9g** · Fiber **0.3g** · Protein **66.5g**

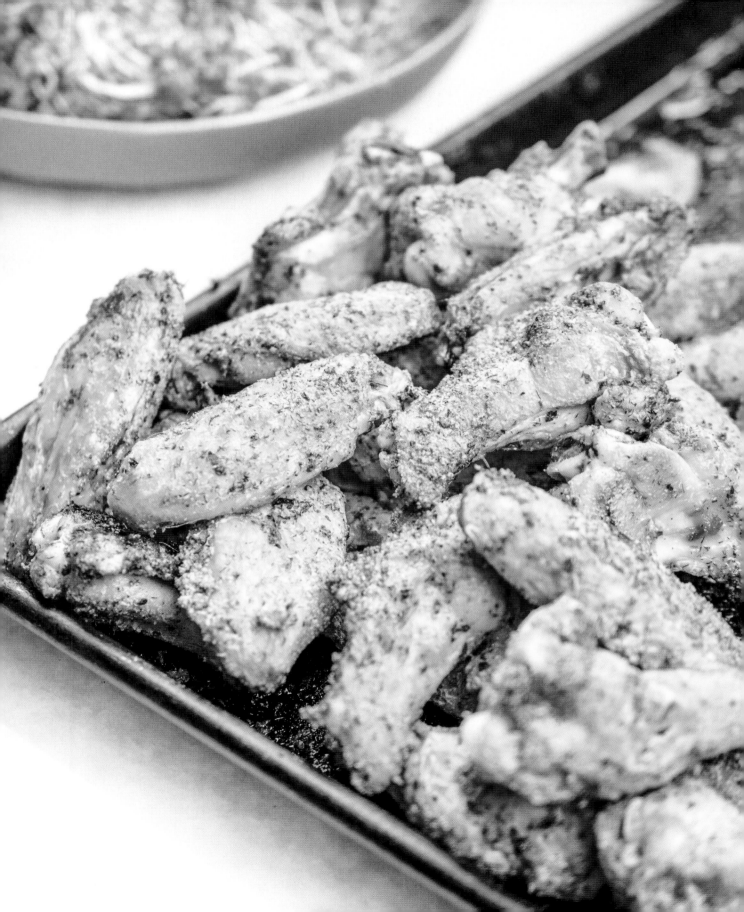

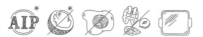

Tarragon + Spice Chicken Wings

Serves 4 ◦ Prep Time: 10 minutes ◦ Cook Time: 1 hour

Tarragon is a lovely bittersweet herb with an aniselike aroma. It's the herb that brings the classic flavor to béarnaise sauce and many a pickling brine. I love to pair tarragon with chicken, and this simple recipe is the perfect way to let this flavorful herb shine.

3 pounds chicken wings, separated into wingettes and drumettes

1 tablespoon baking powder (see note, page 148)

1 tablespoon dried tarragon leaves

1 tablespoon fine salt

1 teaspoon garlic powder

1 teaspoon ground cumin

1 teaspoon ground white pepper

½ teaspoon ginger powder

½ teaspoon ground mustard seeds

3 tablespoons melted ghee or coconut oil

◦ Preheat the oven to 250°F.

◦ Pat the wings dry and put them in a large bowl. Toss with the baking powder to coat. Add the tarragon, salt, and spices and toss again to coat.

◦ Lightly brush a sheet pan with some of the melted ghee and arrange the wingettes and drumettes without overlapping or crowding them—use 2 sheet pans if necessary. Lightly brush the tops of the wings with the remaining ghee.

◦ Roast at 250°F for 30 minutes, then raise the oven temperature to 475°F and roast for another 30 minutes, until the chicken is cooked through and the skin is crispy. Remove from the oven and use a spatula to lift the wings from the pan.

◦ Store leftovers in the fridge for up to 4 days. To reheat, broil for 5 minutes.

modifications: *To make these wings AIP compliant, omit the cumin, white pepper, and ground mustard seeds and double the garlic powder and ginger.*

awesome additions: *Toss the cooked chicken in Gut-Healing Teriyaki Sauce (page 70) for spicy and sticky wings that are finger-licking good!*

Per serving (about 8 pieces): Calories 638 · Fat 38.1g · Total Carbs 2g · Fiber 0.1g · Protein 65.9g

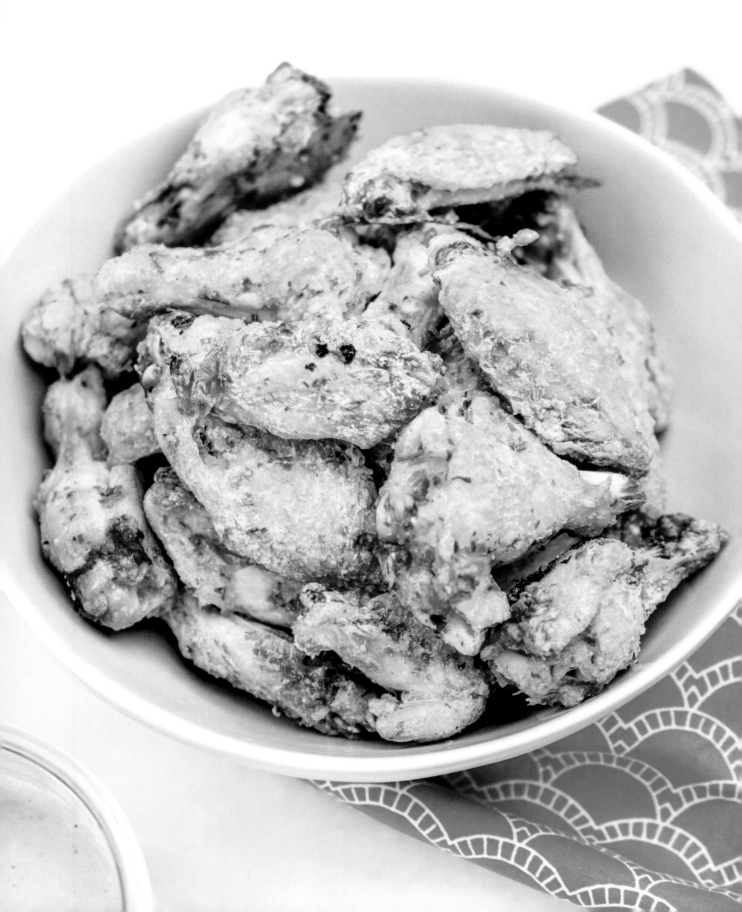

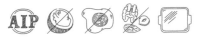

Triple Green Chicken

Serves 5 ◦ Prep Time: 10 minutes ◦ Cook Time: 40 minutes

This easy-peasy meal is jam-packed with goodness. The fresh herbs bring high doses of vitamin K to this dish, while the animal protein provides B vitamins and the broccoli is full of vitamin C!

For the chicken thighs:

3 pounds boneless, skinless chicken thighs

¼ cup extra-virgin olive oil

2 tablespoons minced fresh tarragon

2 tablespoons minced fresh thyme

1 tablespoon fine salt

2 teaspoons ginger powder

3 cloves garlic, minced

3 green onions, minced

For the broccoli rice:

6 cups fresh or frozen riced broccoli (see note, page 172)

2 tablespoons nutritional yeast (optional)

1 teaspoon fine salt

6 slices bacon, roughly chopped

◦ Place one oven rack in the middle position and another in the bottom position. Preheat the oven to 400°F.

◦ Put all of the ingredients for the chicken thighs in a large bowl. Toss well to combine and evenly coat the chicken in the marinade. Let the chicken sit while the oven preheats.

◦ In the meantime, spread the riced broccoli on a sheet pan and sprinkle it with the nutritional yeast, if using, and the salt. Distribute the bacon evenly over the broccoli.

◦ On a second sheet pan, arrange the chicken thighs so they are not overlapping. Scrape all of the marinade out of the bowl and spread it over the chicken.

◦ When the oven reaches temperature, put the chicken on the middle rack and the broccoli rice on the bottom rack. Roast everything for 40 minutes, until the chicken is cooked through and has browned edges and the broccoli rice has toasty bits.

◦ To serve, divide the broccoli rice and chicken thighs evenly among 5 plates.

◦ Store leftovers in the fridge for up to 5 days. To reheat, sauté in a skillet over medium heat for 5 minutes.

awesome additions: *Garnish the plates with some sliced avocado to make this dish even greener!*

Per serving: Calories **524** · Fat **26g** · Total Carbs **9g** · Fiber **3g** · Protein **60.6g**

Don't discount herbs when cooking! Using lots of fresh herbs is a great way to add nutrients to your plate.

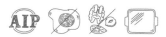

Sweet Sage Chicken Thighs

Serves 6 ⦾ Prep Time: 10 minutes ⦾ Cook Time: 40 minutes

Boneless, skinless chicken thighs have all the versatility of chicken breasts and more delicious fat and flavor! These are marinated in fresh sage, minced garlic, and diced pear for a sweet and savory roasted protein that is a treat for the senses. Not to worry, pear and all, this delectable dish has only 8 grams of total carbs per serving.

Leaves from 5 sprigs fresh sage

3 pounds boneless, skinless chicken thighs

1 ripe Bartlett pear, diced (about ½ cup)

4 cloves garlic, minced

2 tablespoons aged balsamic vinegar (see notes, page 90) or coconut aminos

2 tablespoons extra-virgin olive oil

1 tablespoon fine salt

2 teaspoons garlic powder

1 teaspoon onion powder

1 cup sliced shiitake or cremini mushrooms (about 4 ounces)

Coconut oil spray

3 cups arugula, for serving (optional)

○ Place one oven rack in the middle position and another in the bottom position. Preheat the oven to 425°F.

○ Set aside half of the whole sage leaves and mince the rest.

○ Pat the chicken dry and put it in a large bowl. Add the minced sage, pear, minced garlic, vinegar, olive oil, salt, garlic powder, and onion powder. Toss well, coating the chicken and mashing the pear chunks. Let the chicken marinate while the oven comes to temperature.

○ Lay the thighs flat on 2 sheet pans so they are not crowded, then scrape the remaining marinade all over the chicken. Distribute the mushrooms in the open spaces around the chicken. Lay the reserved whole sage leaves on the chicken thighs. Spray everything with a light coat of coconut oil spray.

○ Place one sheet pan on the middle rack and the other on the bottom rack and roast for 40 minutes, until the chicken is cooked through and nicely browned. Halfway through cooking, switch the pans, moving the bottom one to the middle and vice versa.

○ Serve hot, with the arugula on the side, if using.

○ Store leftovers in the fridge for up to 5 days. To reheat, place on a sheet pan, cover with aluminum foil, and bake in a preheated 300°F oven for 10 minutes.

note: *If you want to make this recipe with boneless, skinless chicken breasts rather than thighs, I recommend cutting them into cutlets (see page 240) and reducing the roasting time to 30 minutes.*

Per serving: Calories **276** · Fat **11g** · Total Carbs **8.1g** · Fiber **1.6g** · Protein **36.3g**

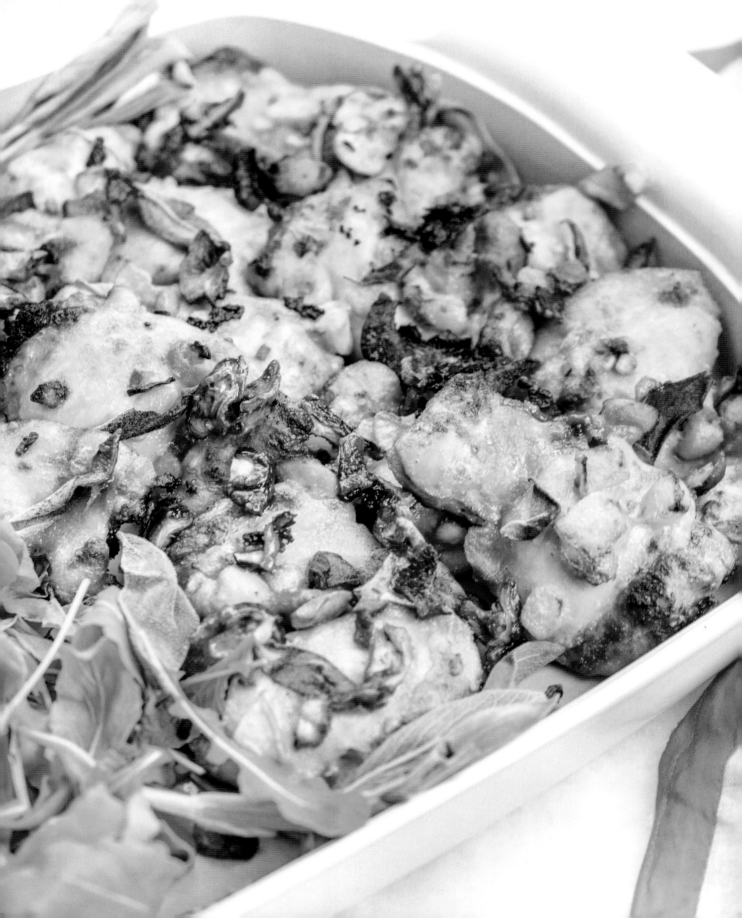

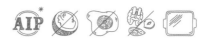

Stuffed Chicken Thighs

Serves 4 ◦ Prep Time: 20 minutes ◦ Cook Time: 35 minutes

These protein rounds might look fancy, but the recipe couldn't be easier! The trick here is butterflying the chicken thighs so you can make proper roll-ups. The stuffing is simply ground breakfast sausage mixed with minced celery, green onions, and fresh dill. The sauce is a delectable mixture of bacon fat and aged balsamic vinegar.

3 tablespoons extra-virgin olive oil, divided

8 boneless, skinless chicken thighs (about 2 pounds)

2 teaspoons fine salt

1 pound ground breakfast sausage

½ cup minced celery

¼ cup minced fresh dill

¼ cup minced green onions

2 tablespoons dried cilantro, parsley, or oregano leaves

2 tablespoons nutritional yeast

¼ cup bacon fat, room temperature

2 tablespoons aged balsamic vinegar (see notes, page 90)

Sliced green onions, for garnish (optional)

◦ Preheat the oven to 425°F. Drizzle a sheet pan with 1 tablespoon of the olive oil.

◦ Butterfly the chicken thighs: Lay a thigh flat on a cutting board, top side down, and place one hand flat on top of the thigh to keep it from moving. Holding a sharp knife parallel to the cutting board, cut into the thigh along the middle of one long side. Using a sawing motion, gradually open up the thigh like a book. Be careful not to cut all the way through. Then sprinkle the thighs with the salt.

◦ In a large bowl, mix together the sausage, celery, dill, and green onions. Scoop up 2 tablespoons of the sausage mixture and put the mound at one end of a chicken thigh, then roll up the thigh. Place the stuffed chicken seam side down on the sheet pan. Repeat with the rest of the chicken thighs and filling.

◦ Brush the thighs with the remaining 2 tablespoons of oil and sprinkle with the cilantro and nutritional yeast. Roast for 33 minutes, or until the thighs and sausage are cooked through and golden, then broil for 2 minutes to brown the tops of the roll-ups.

◦ While the chicken roasts, whisk together the bacon fat and vinegar in a small bowl, then set aside.

◦ When the chicken is ready, cut each thigh into 4 or 5 slices and brush with the bacon fat mixture before serving; serve the rest on the side. Garnish the chicken with sliced green onions, if desired.

◦ Store leftovers in the fridge for up to 3 days. To reheat, bake in a preheated 350°F oven for 10 minutes.

modifications: *To make this dish AIP compliant, use an AIP-friendly pork breakfast sausage. If you don't eat pork, use ground beef or turkey sausage and, for the sauce, use tallow instead of the bacon fat.*

Per serving: Calories **678** · Fat **50g** · Total Carbs **8.9g** · Fiber **0.5g** · Protein **44.4g**

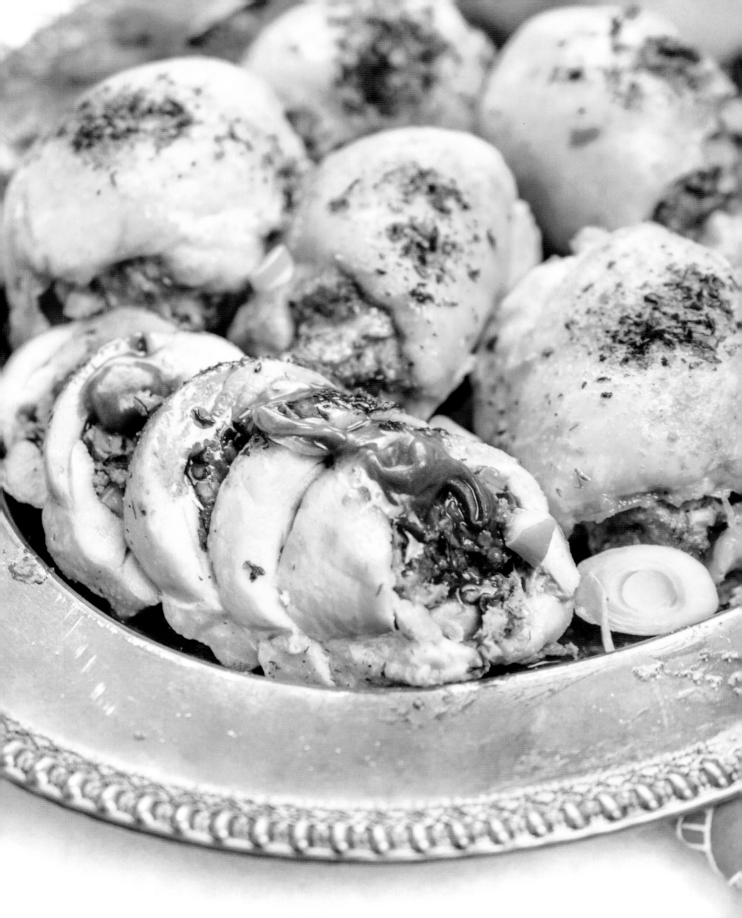

Strawberry Balsamic Baked Chicken with Kale

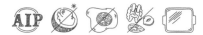

Serves 4 ◦ Prep Time: 15 minutes ◦ Cook Time: 40 minutes

If you haven't had roasted berries, you're missing out: these sweet and tender morsels add wonderful depth to dishes. This chicken is marinated in Mediterranean flavors, baked to juicy perfection over chopped kale, and topped with toasty coconut butter clumps, onions, and berries. This easy and colorful dish is perfect for when you want to impress without breaking a sweat.

6 cups chopped dinosaur kale, coarse stems removed (about 2 bunches)

3 tablespoons extra-virgin olive oil, divided

2¼ teaspoons fine salt, divided

4 large boneless, skinless chicken breast halves (about 2 pounds) (see note)

2 tablespoons aged balsamic vinegar (see notes, page 90)

1 teaspoon dried oregano leaves

1 teaspoon garlic powder

2 tablespoons coconut butter

½ cup quartered strawberries (about 5 whole strawberries)

1 small onion, diced

◦ Preheat the oven to 350°F.

◦ Toss the kale with 1 tablespoon of the olive oil and ¼ teaspoon of the salt and arrange in an even layer in an 8 by 12-inch casserole dish.

◦ In a large bowl, mix the chicken breasts with 1 tablespoon of the olive oil, the remaining 2 teaspoons of salt, the vinegar, oregano, and garlic powder. Toss well to coat the chicken and let it marinate while the oven comes to temperature.

◦ When the oven is ready, lay the chicken breasts over the kale and top them with the coconut butter by dropping clumps all over, then add the strawberries and onions. Drizzle the remaining tablespoon of olive oil over everything. Bake for 35 to 40 minutes, until the chicken is cooked through (the internal temperature should reach 165°F) and the coconut butter looks lightly toasted.

◦ Remove from the oven and serve each chicken breast with some berries and plenty of kale.

◦ Store leftovers in the fridge for up to 5 days. To reheat, dice the chicken and sauté with the kale and berries over medium heat for 5 minutes.

note: *If you prefer chicken thighs, use 8 boneless, skinless chicken thighs instead of 4 large breasts.*

modifications: *To make this dish coconut-free, use sunflower seed butter or tahini instead of the coconut butter.*

Per serving: Calories **440** · Fat **22g** · Total Carbs **9.1g** · Fiber **3.1g** · Protein **50.6g**

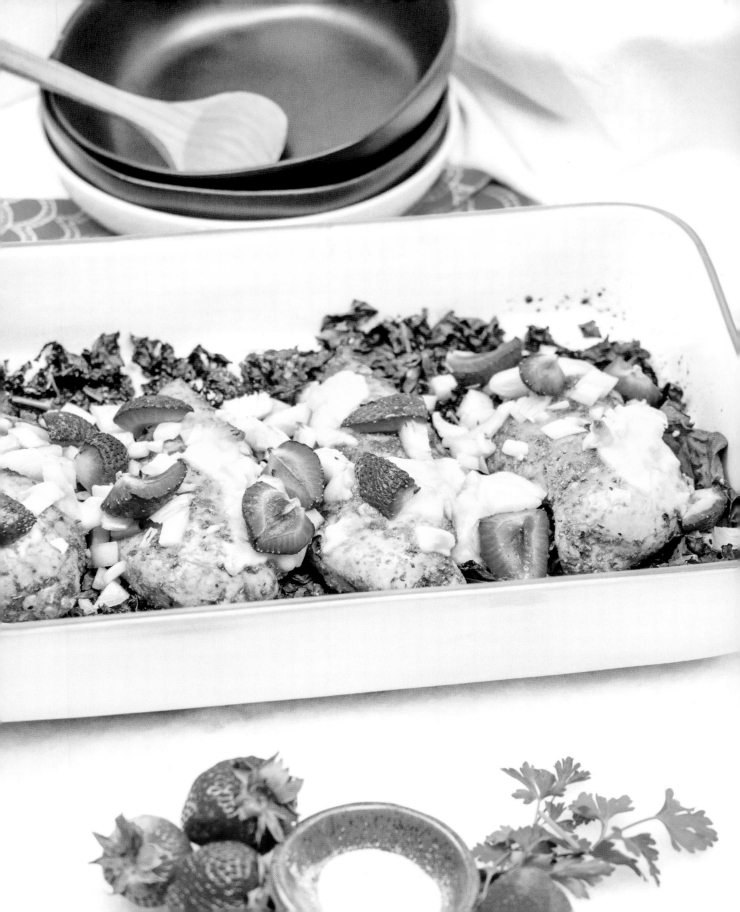

Perfect Roast Chicken with Green Beans

Serves 4 ◦ Prep Time: 30 minutes ◦ Cook Time: 70 minutes

Everyone needs a solid roast chicken recipe in their arsenal. While I usually go wild with seasonings on my birds, this version is ridiculously simple—but still addictively delicious. It's perfect for meal prep or weeknight meals. Not sure how many people your bird will feed? A rule of thumb with whole chickens is that each pound yields one serving.

1 (4-pound) whole chicken

4 Frozen Herb Blocks (page 109) (see notes)

4 teaspoons fine salt, divided

1 pound fresh green beans, trimmed

1 tablespoon melted ghee or lard

notes: *If you want to boost the flavor of this recipe, let the chicken marinate overnight! It really makes the herb flavor pop.*

I like to leave the chicken carcass sitting out after we have eaten. Then, when it's fully cooled, I shred the meat with my hands, getting every nook and cranny. The shredded chicken is great for chicken salad (see Reina Pepiada, page 262) and will keep in the fridge for up to 4 days.

If you don't have Frozen Herb Blocks on hand, make an herb-and-olive-oil paste with a combination of minced fresh herbs and garlic. You will need about ¼ cup of this paste to rub under and over the chicken skin.

◦ Remove the giblets from the chicken cavity. Rinse the chicken under cool water, then pat it dry and place it in a large bowl. Using the tips of your fingers, gently separate the skin from the meat on the breast and back of the chicken, beginning at the open end where the skin flaps over the cavity. If it feels really stuck, you can use a knife to pull it apart carefully. Try not to tear the skin.

◦ Rub an herb block all over the chicken, then put it under the skin on one side of the breast. Do the same with another herb block, placing it under the skin on the other side of the breast. Repeat with the remaining 2 blocks, placing them under the skin on either side of the back.

◦ Move the herb blocks around to spread the herb mixture all over the meat, then leave them centered in their quadrants. It will look silly, as if the chicken has implants. Salt the chicken all over, using 3½ teaspoons of the salt.

◦ At this point, you can store the chicken in the fridge to marinate for up to 12 hours. If roasting it right away, leave it out at room temperature. Preheat the oven to 375°F.

◦ Put the herbed chicken in an oven-safe 15-inch skillet. Roast for 30 minutes. Remove from the oven and arrange the green beans around the chicken. Sprinkle them with the remaining ½ teaspoon of salt and drizzle with the ghee.

◦ Return the pan to the oven and roast for another 40 minutes, or until the chicken skin is golden brown and the internal temperature reaches 165°F. Remove from the oven and serve hot!

◦ Store leftovers in the fridge for up to 4 days. To reheat, pull or dice the chicken meat and sauté with the green beans in a skillet over medium heat for 5 minutes.

modifications: *To make this dish AIP compliant, use asparagus instead of the green beans.*

Per serving: Calories **645** · Fat **51.2g** · Total Carbs **8.3g** · Fiber **3.2g** · Protein **39g**

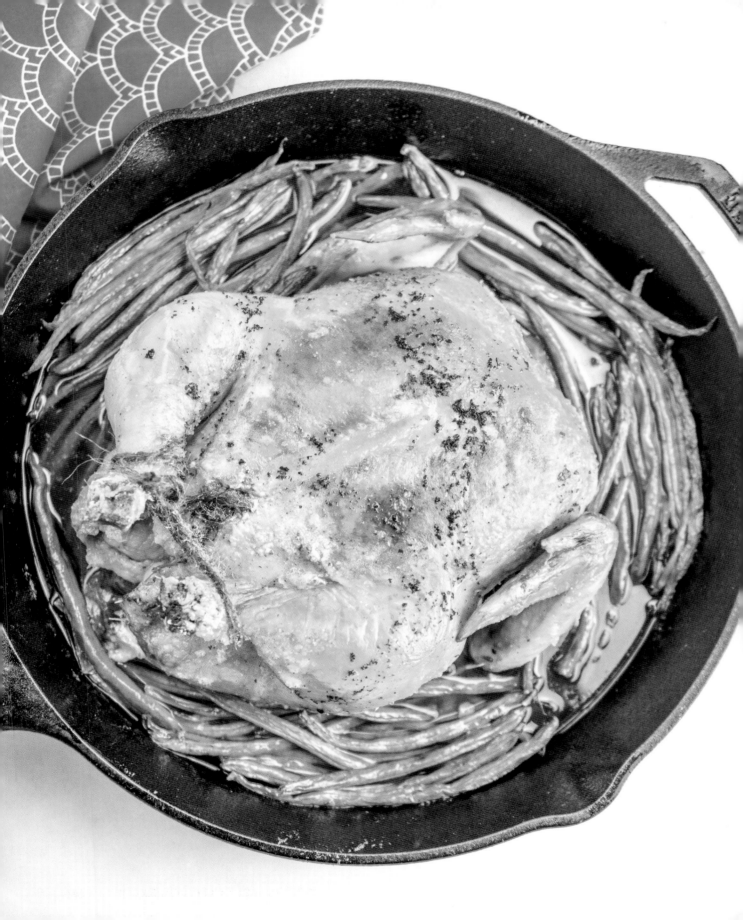

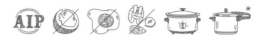

Garlic Chicken over Zoodles

Serves 4 ○ Prep Time: 15 minutes ○ Cook Time: 8 hours

There are two kinds of people: those who measure garlic with a teaspoon and those who measure garlic with their heart. This recipe is for the latter group. I love the toasty crust on this chicken, and the conservative amount of fluid used to cook it results in an almost roasted chicken texture. It's perfect over fresh zoodles!

8 boneless, skinless chicken thighs (about 2 pounds)

1½ teaspoons fine salt, divided

1 teaspoon turmeric powder

½ teaspoon onion powder

3 tablespoons extra-virgin olive oil, divided

10 cloves garlic, smashed with the side of a knife and peeled (see notes)

3 sprigs fresh thyme

1 cup bone broth (see notes)

Juice of 1 lemon

2 large zucchini or summer squash, spiral sliced into noodles

○ In a slow cooker, combine the chicken thighs, 1 teaspoon of the salt, the turmeric, onion powder, and 2 tablespoons of the olive oil. Add the garlic and mix well, then arrange the thighs so they are lying flat.

○ Top the chicken with the thyme sprigs, then pour the broth and lemon juice over everything. Cover and cook on low for 8 hours.

○ When you're ready to serve the meal, toss the zoodles with the remaining ½ teaspoon of salt and remaining tablespoon of oil. Divide the zoodles among 4 plates and top each portion with 2 chicken thighs and plenty of garlic and sauce from the slow cooker.

○ Store leftover chicken and zoodles separately in the fridge for up to 5 days. To reheat, sauté the chicken and zoodles together in a skillet over medium heat until warm.

Pressure Cooker Method: Follow the recipe as written, but cook the chicken in an electric pressure cooker on high pressure for 20 minutes, then release the pressure manually.

notes: *I find that the fastest way to peel garlic cloves is to smash them with the flat side of a knife first, which loosens the skin so you can easily remove it.*

If your slow cooker is smaller than 6 quarts, use just enough broth to cover the chicken. Leaving the tops of the thighs exposed results in a roasted texture. If you're planning to shred the chicken, however, feel free to submerge it.

Per serving: Calories **301** · Fat **15.2g** · Total Carbs **9.5g** · Fiber **2.3g** · Protein **32.6g**

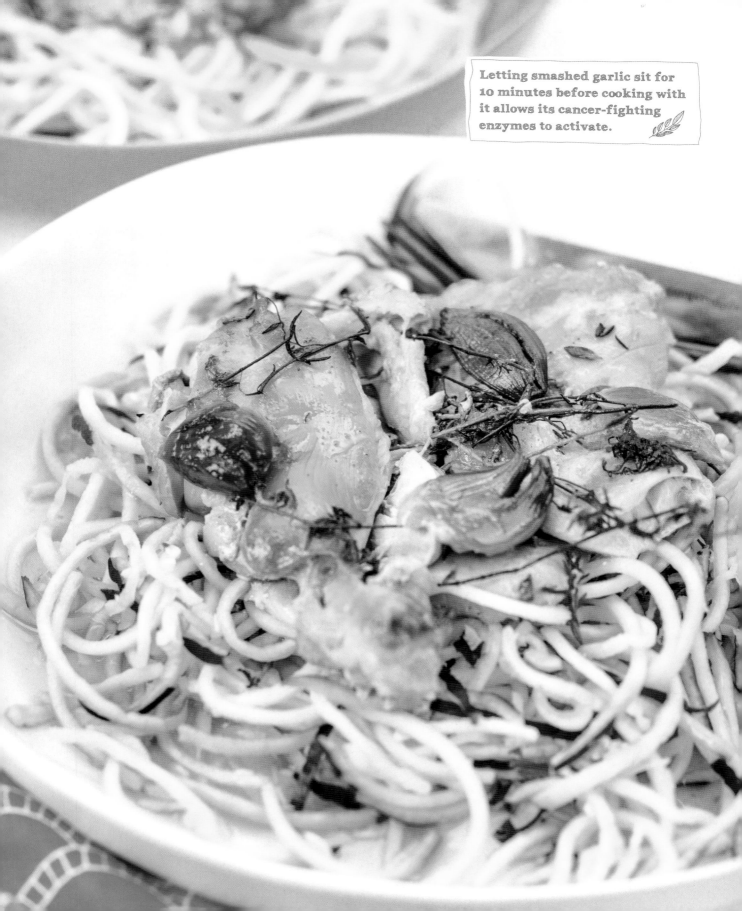

Letting smashed garlic sit for 10 minutes before cooking with it allows its cancer-fighting enzymes to activate.

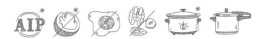

Hail Mary Chicken

Makes 2½ pounds shredded chicken (10 servings) ○ Prep Time: 5 minutes ○ Cook Time: 40 minutes

From frozen to cooked in 40 minutes, this is the chicken recipe that saves the day. I love how flexible this flavorful chicken is: it makes the perfect shredded chicken for casseroles, salad, tacos, and more. It also works in a slow cooker. This is a great weekly meal prep recipe!

3 pounds frozen boneless, skinless chicken thighs (see note)

2 teaspoons fine salt

2 teaspoons garlic powder

2 teaspoons ground cumin

2 tablespoons coconut aminos

Juice of 1 orange

3 tablespoons extra-virgin olive oil or avocado oil

note: *This recipe works equally well with boneless, skinless chicken thighs or breasts, or a mix of both.*

modifications: *To make this dish AIP compliant, omit the cumin. To make it coconut-free, use low-sodium gluten-free tamari instead of the coconut aminos.*

○ Combine the chicken, salt, garlic powder, cumin, coconut aminos, and orange juice in a pressure cooker.

○ Drizzle the olive oil over everything. Set to cook on high pressure for 40 minutes, then let the pressure release naturally.

○ Open the lid and use 2 forks to shred the chicken.

○ Store leftovers in the fridge for up to 5 days or in the freezer for up to 2 months. Reheat in a skillet with a tight-fitting lid over medium heat until warmed through.

Slow Cooker Method: Follow the recipe as written but cook the chicken in a slow cooker on high for 6 hours.

Per serving: Calories **204** · Fat **9.1g** · Total Carbs **2.1g** · Fiber **1.8g** · Protein **27.8g**

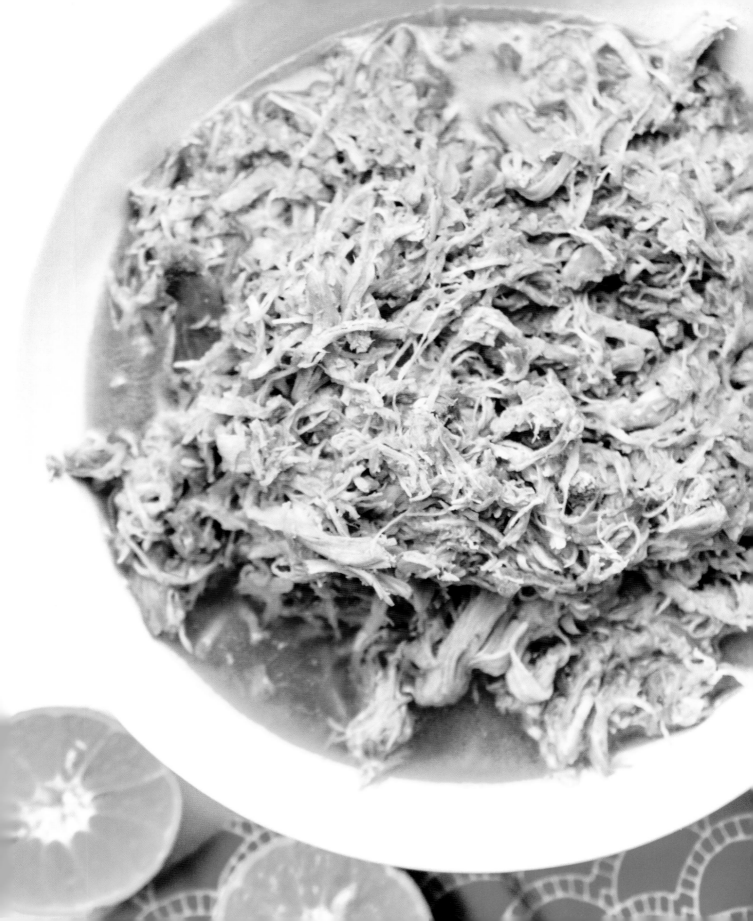

Balsamic Cashew Chicken

Serves 8 ◦ Prep Time: 10 minutes ◦ Cook Time: 30 minutes

I know we eat with our eyes first, but some tasty foods just don't look so pretty. This dish fits that bill. It's got loads of flavor, tender chicken, and soft cashews in a tangy herb sauce. You can serve the chicken breasts whole or shred them and toss everything together. This chicken is great over zoodles, thinly sliced summer squash, or arugula or with Crispy Garlic Rice (page 318).

4 tablespoons extra-virgin olive oil, divided

1 large white onion, sliced

2 cloves garlic, minced

1 cup whole raw cashews

3 tablespoons aged balsamic vinegar (see notes, page 90)

3 pounds boneless, skinless chicken breasts

1 tablespoon fine salt

2 teaspoons dried tarragon leaves

2 teaspoons ground black pepper

2 teaspoons nutritional yeast

1 cup bone broth

◦ Put a pressure cooker in sauté mode and drizzle in 2 tablespoons of the olive oil. Add the onion and garlic and sauté for 5 minutes, then add the cashews and vinegar. Cook for another 5 minutes and stir well. Transfer everything from the cooker to a platter and set aside.

◦ Drizzle the remaining 2 tablespoons of oil into the pressure cooker. Add the chicken breasts, salt, tarragon, pepper, and nutritional yeast and mix well. Cook the breasts, turning them over occasionally, until they begin to brown, about 5 minutes.

◦ Return the onion-and-cashew mixture to the pressure cooker and pour in the broth. Seal the lid and cook on high pressure for 15 minutes.

◦ Release the pressure manually. Open the lid, mix well, and serve hot!

◦ Store leftovers in the fridge for up to 4 days. To reheat, sauté in a skillet over medium heat until warm.

Slow Cooker Method: Sauté the onion and garlic and brown the chicken in a large skillet over medium heat. Once you have combined everything in the pan, transfer the mixture to a slow cooker, cover, and cook on high for 4 hours or on low for 6 hours.

Per serving: Calories **352** · Fat **17g** · Total Carbs **8.2g** · Fiber **1.1g** · Protein **44.1g**

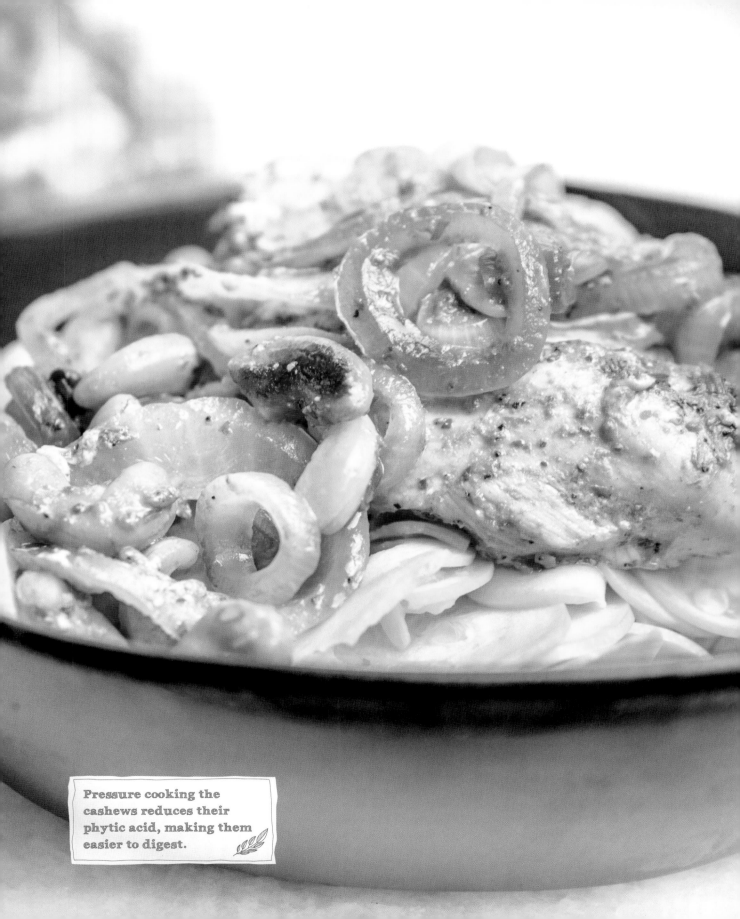

Pressure cooking the cashews reduces their phytic acid, making them easier to digest.

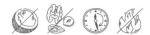

Reina Pepiada

Serves 4 ◦ Prep Time: 15 minutes

This is a Venezuelan remix on a classic that combines mayo and avocado for a super creamy chicken salad. I love using leftover Hail Mary Chicken (page 258) for this recipe, but rotisserie chicken works well too, for a great no-cook meal. This chicken salad is perfect on Fiber-Rich Naan (page 314) for an arepa-like dish.

1 pound shredded cooked chicken breasts

½ cup minced celery

¼ cup minced fresh cilantro

¼ cup minced white onions

1 ripe Hass avocado, peeled, pitted, and diced

3 tablespoons avocado oil mayonnaise

1 teaspoon fine salt

1 teaspoon lemon juice

◦ Put all of the ingredients in a large bowl and mix well.

◦ Store leftovers in the fridge for up to a week.

note: *When stored, the avocado may brown a bit, but this won't affect the flavor.*

Per serving: Calories **369** · Fat **27.9g** · Total Carbs **8.4g** · Fiber **3.9g** · Protein **24.4g**

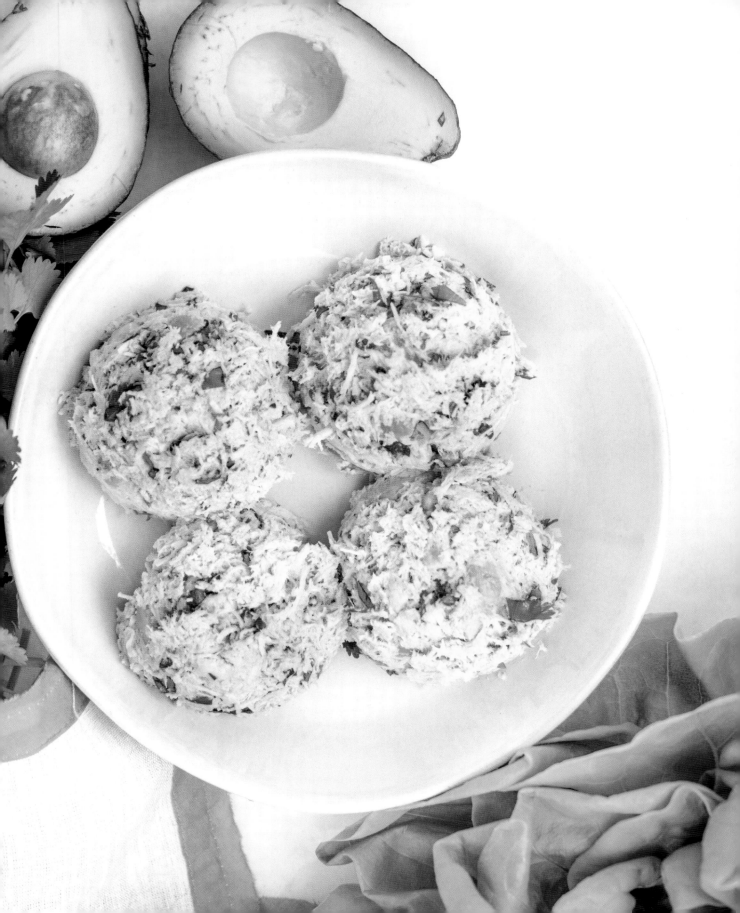

FISH + SEAFOOD

Sea life is a source of so many essential nutrients, iodine and omega-3 fatty acids being two of the big ones. I often hear from readers that they don't cook fish at home because they don't know how or are afraid of messing it up. To those readers, I say, give these recipes a try. Not only are they nutrient dense, but they're some of the quickest to make in this book. Regular and proper omega-3 consumption is life-changing, and this chapter is packed with that anti-inflammatory goodness.

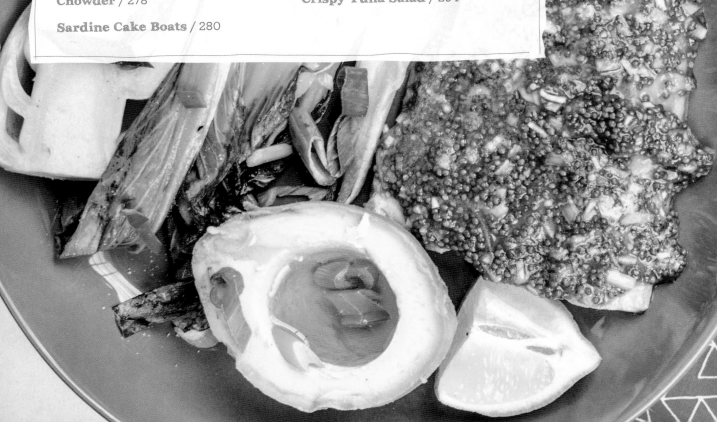

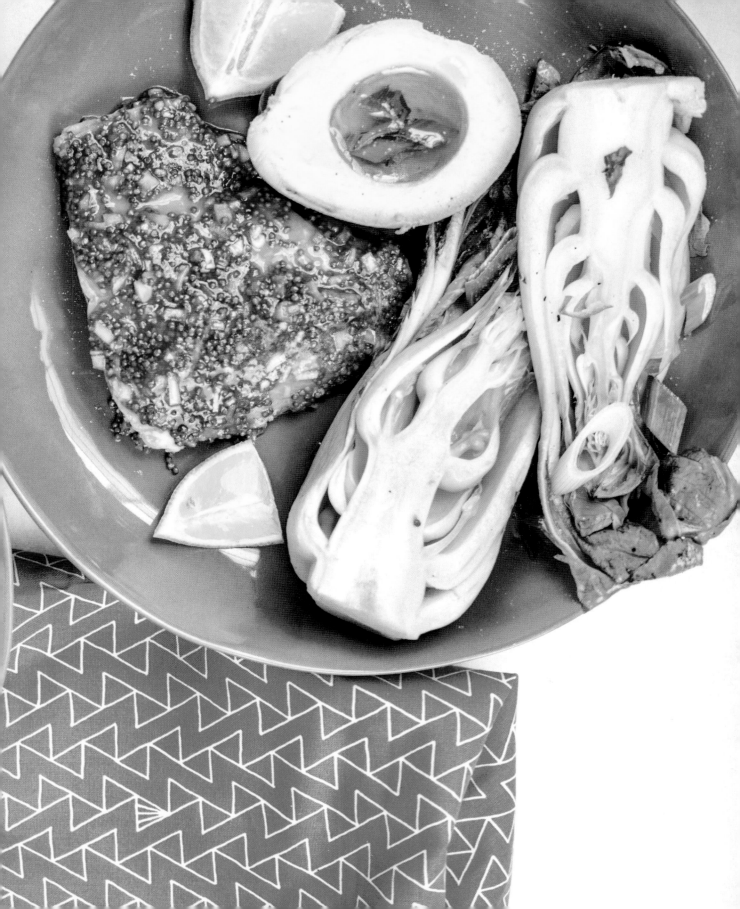

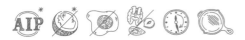

Shrimp Curry with Broccoli

Serves 2 ◦ Prep Time: 10 minutes ◦ Cook Time: 20 minutes

When I learned that nightshades were very inflammatory to my body, I mourned tomatoes the most, but curry came in a close second. However, I learned to make my own curry, and while it's lacking in nightshades, it's definitely not lacking in flavor or anti-inflammatory goodness. This beautiful curry includes sulforaphane-packed broccoli, a welcome addition.

3 tablespoons extra-virgin olive oil

1 pound large shrimp, peeled, deveined, and tails removed

2 teaspoons fine salt, divided

1 large carrot, julienned

1 large onion, thinly sliced

1 yellow squash, julienned

1 cup broccoli florets

3 cloves garlic, minced

1 tablespoon Citrus Curry Powder (page 82)

1 (13.5-ounce) can unsweetened full-fat coconut milk

1 cup bone broth

¼ cup chopped fresh cilantro, for garnish

2 lime wedges, for serving

◦ Heat a Dutch oven or large heavy-bottomed pot over medium heat. When it's hot, drizzle in the olive oil. Add the shrimp and 1 teaspoon of the salt and sauté until the shrimp coils and turns pink, about 6 minutes. Remove the shrimp from the pot and set aside.

◦ Put all of the vegetables in the pot along with the garlic, remaining teaspoon of salt, and curry powder. Sauté for 10 minutes, or until the vegetables are tender and aromatic.

◦ Stir in the coconut milk and broth and bring to a simmer. Simmer for 5 minutes, stirring well, until you have a smooth, fragrant vegetable curry. Stir in the shrimp and remove the pot from the heat.

◦ Garnish with the cilantro and serve with the lime wedges. Store leftovers in the fridge for up to 3 days. To reheat, bring to a simmer in a saucepan.

modifications: *To make this dish AIP compliant, use the AIP version of the curry powder. To make it coconut-free, use an unsweetened nut milk.*

Per serving: Calories **572** · Fat **42.7g** · Total Carbs **18g** · Fiber **3.8g** · Protein **27.2g**

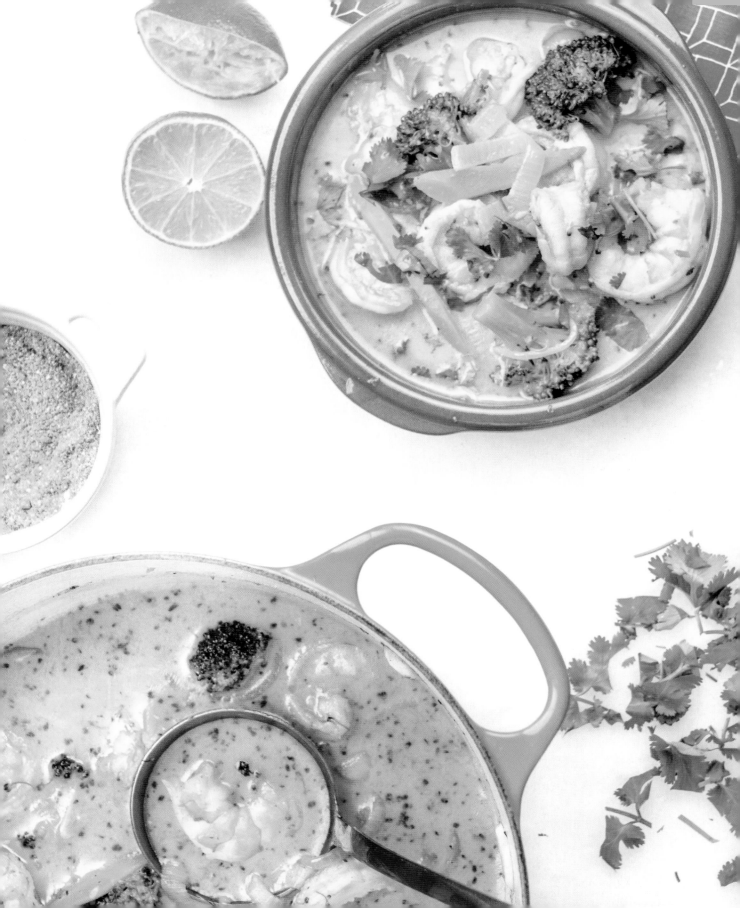

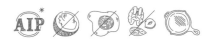

Crispy Salmon Wraps

Serves 4 ◦ Prep Time: 10 minutes, plus 12 hours to cure ◦ Cook Time: 8 minutes

This is my favorite way to cook salmon. It creates a wonderful crust on the meat and the skin gets nice and crispy, yet the center stays perfectly medium. Take the time for the curing process here—it takes only a little bit of planning, and the results are amazing. These crispy salmon wraps are going to be on your weekly rotation!

1 (1-pound) skin-on wild-caught salmon fillet, cut into 12 strips

1½ teaspoons grated lemon zest

1 teaspoon fine salt

2 tablespoons lard or extra-virgin olive oil

For serving:

12 large Bibb lettuce leaves

1 red onion, thinly sliced

½ cup Pickled Radishes (page 84)

6 fresh dill fronds

1 tablespoon everything bagel seasoning (optional)

2 teaspoons toasted sesame oil (optional)

◦ Pat the salmon strips dry all over. Lay them skin side down on a plate lined with a paper towel. Sprinkle with the zest and salt. Place the plate in the fridge, uncovered, for 12 hours.

◦ When you're ready to cook the salmon, remove it from the fridge. Heat the lard in a 15-inch skillet until hot; when the end of a wooden spoon handle sizzles when inserted in the oil, it's ready. Put the salmon strips skin side down in the hot skillet and cook undisturbed for 5 minutes.

◦ Gently flip the salmon over to show the crispy salmon skin. Cook for 1 minute, then use a spatula to quickly remove the salmon from the skillet.

◦ Set out all of the lettuce leaves and place a strip of salmon in the center of each one. Top with 1 or 2 slices of red onion and some pickled radishes. Garnish each with a few fronds of fresh dill and, if desired, the seasoning and sesame oil. Enjoy right away—these are best eaten fresh. I don't recommend making them ahead or reheating them.

modifications: *To make this dish AIP compliant, omit the everything bagel seasoning and sesame oil.*

Per serving: Calories **248** · Fat **14.2g** · Total Carbs **3.4g** · Fiber **1g** · Protein **26.3g**

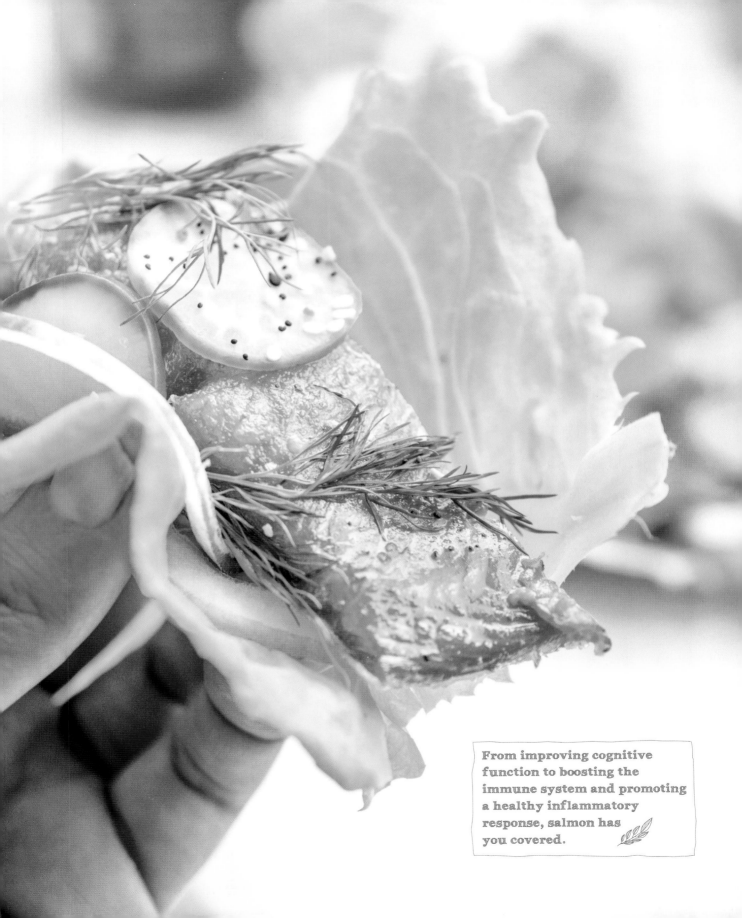

From improving cognitive function to boosting the immune system and promoting a healthy inflammatory response, salmon has you covered.

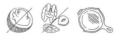

Salmon Herb Skillet Cake

Serves 4 ◦ Prep Time: 10 minutes ◦ Cook Time: 30 minutes

Fish isn't something I like to reheat, but this recipe is an exception! It's the perfect meal-prep salmon dish, so you can get your omega-3 fix all week long. This version of salmon cakes saves time by making one large cake that's baked instead of fried. Made with canned wild-caught salmon, it's also very affordable!

10 slices bacon, diced

½ red onion, finely diced

4 (6-ounce) cans wild-caught salmon, drained

½ cup minced fresh parsley

2 large eggs

½ teaspoon fine salt

Fresh parsley leaves, for garnish

◦ Preheat the oven to 350°F.

◦ Heat an oven-safe 15-inch skillet over medium heat. Put the bacon in the skillet and cook until lightly browned, then add the onion and continue cooking until the bacon is crispy, about 10 minutes total.

◦ Add the salmon to the skillet, flaking it out of the cans and breaking it up well as you mix it with the bacon and onion. Stir in the minced parsley, then spread the mixture evenly over the skillet and press it into the bottom.

◦ Whisk the eggs well and pour them evenly over the salmon. Sprinkle with the salt.

◦ Transfer the skillet to the oven and cook until the center is set and the edges are pulling away from the sides, about 15 minutes.

◦ Remove the salmon cake from the oven and let it cool a bit before slicing and serving.

◦ Store leftovers in the fridge for up to 5 days. Enjoy the leftovers cold or reheat in a preheated 350°F oven for 8 minutes.

Per serving: Calories **381** · Fat **18.3g** · Total Carbs **3.7g** · Fiber **0.6g** · Protein **49.7g**

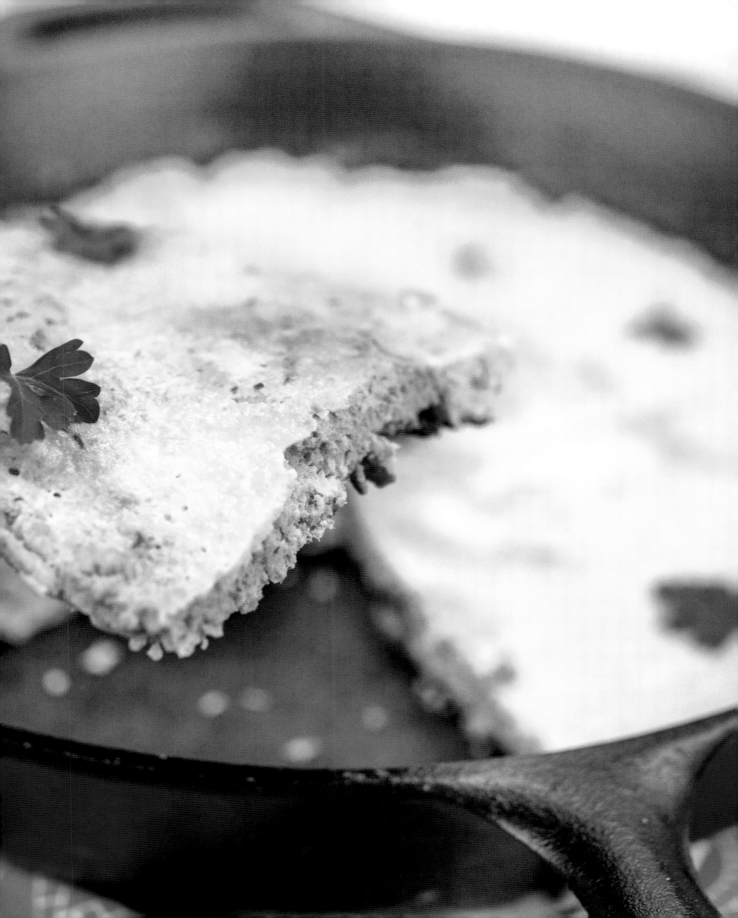

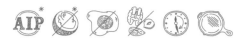

Salmon Noodle Soup

Serves 3 ◦ Prep Time: 10 minutes ◦ Cook Time: 20 minutes

This light soup is a beautiful way to use fresh salmon that goes beyond the usual broiling and pan-frying methods. It pairs well with Fiber-Rich Naan (page 314) or my recipe for nut-free keto rolls, based on a famous Diet Doctor bread, which you can find on TheCastawayKitchen.com.

1 pound wild-caught salmon fillets, skin removed

1¼ teaspoons fine salt, divided

1 teaspoon ground mustard seeds

3 tablespoons extra-virgin olive oil or avocado oil

3 cups spiral-sliced butternut squash or zucchini noodles (see note)

3 cloves garlic, minced

2 sprigs fresh thyme

3 cups bone broth

1 cup canned unsweetened full-fat coconut milk

2 cups arugula, chopped

1 tablespoon fish sauce

Squeeze of lemon juice

◦ Heat a soup pot over medium heat. Cut the salmon into 1-inch chunks, place them in a medium-sized bowl, and toss them with 1 teaspoon of the salt and the ground mustard.

◦ Drizzle the oil into the pot, then add the salmon chunks. Sauté for 5 minutes, or until lightly browned. Remove the salmon from the pot with a slotted spoon and set aside.

◦ Add the squash noodles and garlic to the pot and sauté for 8 minutes, or until the noodles are tender. Add the thyme sprigs and remaining ¼ teaspoon of salt and sauté for 2 minutes. Then pour in the broth and coconut milk and simmer for 5 minutes.

◦ Stir in the arugula, fish sauce, lemon juice, and browned salmon chunks. Serve right away!

◦ Store leftovers in the fridge for up to 4 days. To reheat, bring to a simmer in a saucepan over medium heat.

note: *You will need to purchase 1 medium butternut squash or 1 large zucchini if you are spiral slicing your own noodles. Many grocers now offer these vegetables already cut into noodles, which saves a lot of time!*

modifications: *To make this soup AIP compliant, use ginger powder instead of the ground mustard seeds. To make it coconut-free, use Salted Cashew Cream (page 76) or Cauliflower Sour Cream (page 74) instead of the coconut milk.*

   Per serving: Calories **556** · Fat **36.6g** · Total Carbs **13.7g** · Fiber **2.3g** · Protein **43.9g**

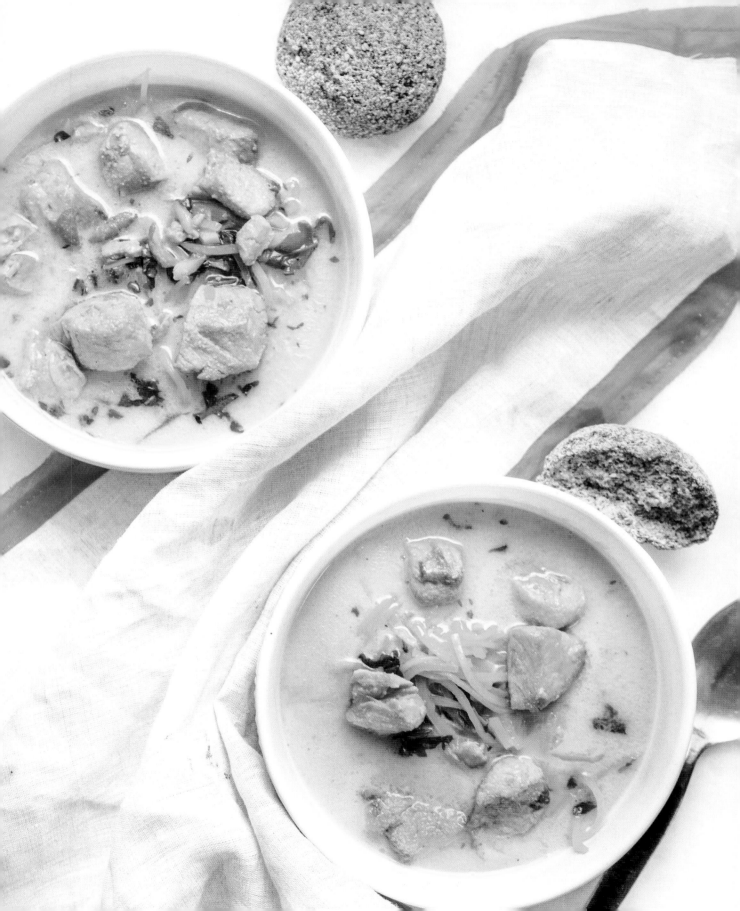

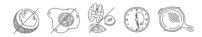

Cumin-Dusted Mahi-Mahi

Serves 4 ◦ Prep Time: 5 minutes ◦ Cook Time: 8 minutes

That crust, though! This cumin-dusted fish didn't come to play. Loaded up with warm spices and cooked in ghee, this simple yet impressive dish pairs perfectly with Berry Much Like Caprese Salad (page 334), as pictured here, but it's also legendary over Pressure Cooker Saag (page 326).

4 (4-ounce) center-cut mahi-mahi fillets

1 teaspoon fine salt

1 teaspoon ground coriander

1 teaspoon ground cumin

½ teaspoon ground white pepper

2 tablespoons ghee or lard

◦ Heat a large skillet over medium heat. While it heats, mix the dried seasonings together in a small bowl and rub the blend evenly into the mahi-mahi fillets on both sides.

◦ Melt the ghee in the skillet, then add the fillets. Sear undisturbed for 4 minutes, then flip the fillets over and sear for another 4 minutes, until a nice golden crust has formed on both sides and the fillets are cooked through.

◦ Remove the fish from the skillet with a spatula and serve right away. Store leftovers in the fridge for up to 3 days. I don't like to reheat this kind of fish—just enjoy the leftovers cold, flaked over a salad or mixed with mayo.

Per serving: Calories **164** · Fat **7.8g** · Total Carbs **0.6g** · Fiber **0.2g** · Protein **21.4g**

Cumin is a carminative spice, meaning it aids in digestion and can relieve gas.

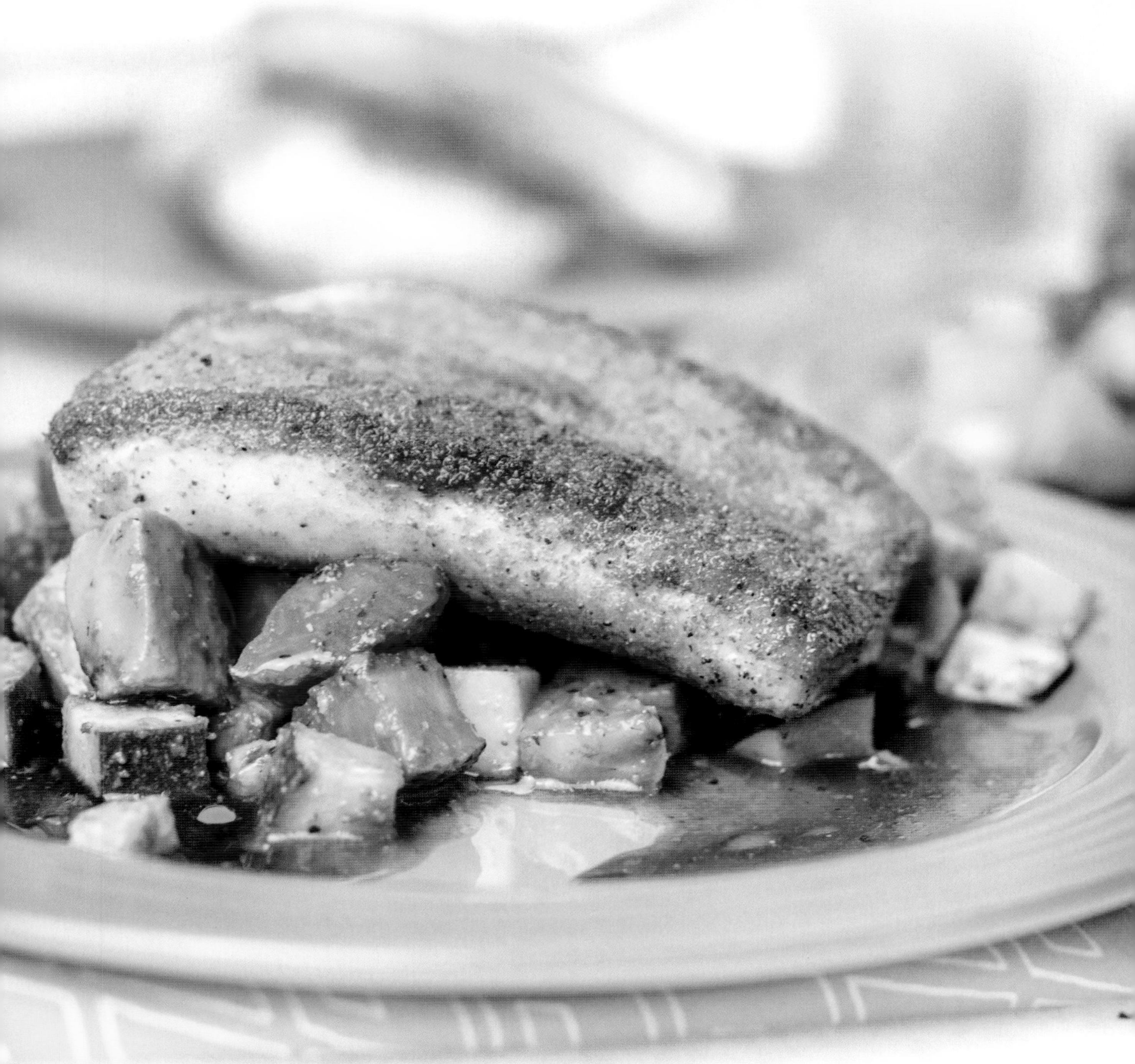

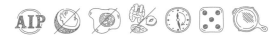

Herbed Yellowfin Tuna Steaks

Serves 3 ◦ Prep Time: 5 minutes ◦ Cook Time: 20 minutes

These pan-seared tuna steaks are the perfect fish for those who hate fish. Tuna is very meaty, not fishy at all, and very nutritious. Yellowfin is lean for tuna but high in vitamins and minerals. While mercury content is a concern for large fish, the perfect solution is to eat it every so often, not daily. This recipe makes excellent use of Frozen Herb Blocks.

3 Frozen Herb Blocks (page 109)

2 teaspoons fine salt, divided

3 (5-ounce) yellowfin tuna steaks

1 pound frozen riced cauliflower

Juice of 1 lemon

◦ Heat a 15-inch skillet with a tight-fitting lid over medium heat. When it's hot, put the herb blocks in the skillet and let them soften.

◦ Sprinkle 1 teaspoon of the salt over the tuna steaks, then place them in the skillet, moving the herb blocks aside. Sear for 4 minutes, then flip the steaks over and place one melting herb block on top of each steak. Sear the steaks for another 4 minutes, until they are golden on the outside and the edges flake easily, then remove them from the skillet.

◦ Put the frozen riced cauliflower in the skillet and add the remaining teaspoon of salt and the lemon juice. Cook, stirring occasionally, for 6 to 8 minutes, until the cauliflower is heated. Put the steaks on top of the rice and cover. Heat for 2 minutes, then serve right away.

◦ Store leftovers in the fridge for up to 4 days. To reheat, warm in a skillet with a tight-fitting lid over low heat for 10 minutes.

Per serving: Calories **363** · Fat **18.8.g** · Total Carbs **7.8g** · Fiber **3.6g** · Protein **40.6g**

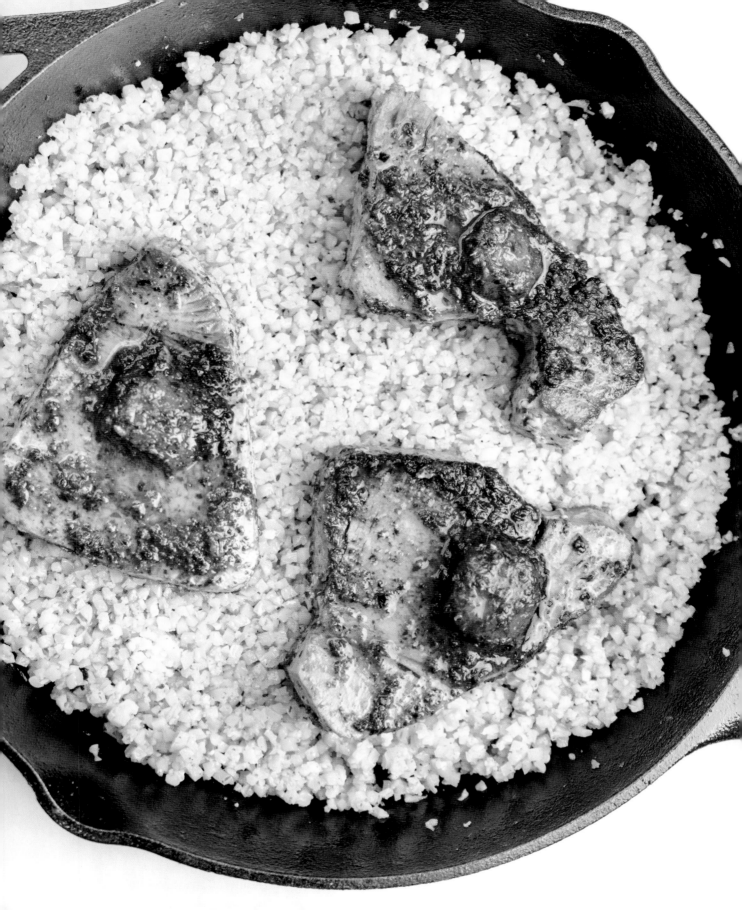

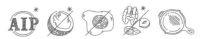

Butternut Sage Smoked Oyster Chowder

Serves 4 ◦ Prep Time: 10 minutes ◦ Cook Time: 25 minutes

Concerned about hormone health? Eat oysters. Want to support your immune system? Oysters. Managing inflammation? Oysters. Bad credit? Oysters! Just kidding about that last one. But seriously, I can't get over the powerful nutrition in these little guys. Smoked oysters packed in olive oil are an affordable and delicious way to get all the potent nutrition of oysters, even if you're landlocked. And this rich, delicious, comforting soup is the perfect vessel for oysters, especially if you're hesitant to try them. Think New England clam chowder, but better. Yes, I went there.

5 slices bacon, diced

3 small onions, diced (about 1½ cups)

3 cloves garlic, minced

2 bay leaves

1 teaspoon fine salt

1 teaspoon ground cumin

1 teaspoon ground white pepper

10 ounces frozen diced butternut squash

Leaves from 4 sprigs fresh sage, minced, divided

3 (3-ounce) cans smoked oysters packed in olive oil

2 cups bone broth

1 cup unsweetened dairy-free milk of choice

1 teaspoon fish sauce

2 tablespoons white wine vinegar

◦ Heat a Dutch oven or large heavy-bottomed pot over medium heat. Put the bacon in the pot and cook, stirring often, until it's browned and crispy, 5 to 6 minutes. Using a slotted spoon, remove the bacon from the pot and set it aside.

◦ Put the onions, garlic, bay leaves, and dried seasonings in the pot and cook until the onions are very tender and aromatic, about 8 minutes. Mix in the frozen butternut squash and half of the minced sage. Cook until the squash is thawed and tender, about 5 minutes.

◦ While the squash cooks, open the cans of oysters and drain the oil into a glass jar or small bowl. Then chop the oysters and set them and the oil aside.

◦ Transfer half of the onion-and-squash mixture to a blender, then add the broth, milk, fish sauce, and oil from the cans. Puree until smooth, creamy, and white. Pour the mixture back into the pot.

◦ Stir in the oysters, reserved bacon, and remaining sage and bring to a simmer. Simmer for 5 minutes, then stir in the vinegar. Taste and add more salt and/or pepper as desired.

◦ Store leftovers in the fridge for up to 5 days. To reheat, bring to a simmer in a saucepan.

notes: *If you don't like butternut squash, frozen riced cauliflower works well too. So would diced sweet potatoes! Make this soup your own.*

If you have fish stock made with fish heads, use it and omit the bone broth and fish sauce. Bone broth is great and all, but for seafood recipes, fish stock is a game changer. If you don't have fish stock, it's cool—that's what the fish sauce is for.

modifications: *To make this soup AIP compliant, omit the cumin and white pepper and add 1 teaspoon garlic powder and 1 teaspoon turmeric powder.*

Per serving: Calories **383** · Fat **24.8g** · Total Carbs **21.7g** · Fiber **2.1g** · Protein **20.2g**

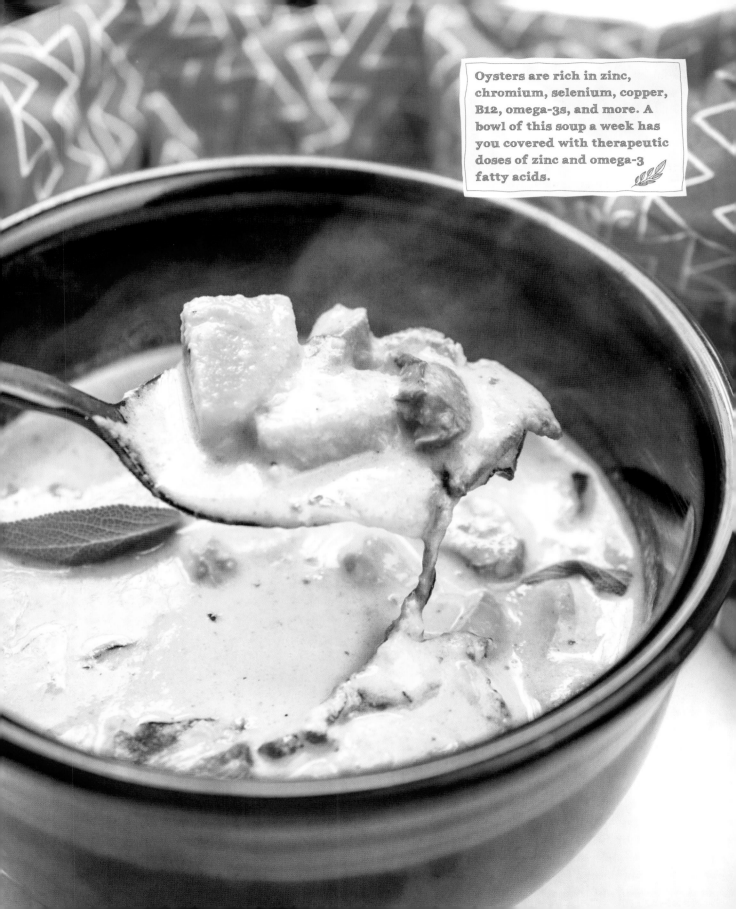

Oysters are rich in zinc, chromium, selenium, copper, B12, omega-3s, and more. A bowl of this soup a week has you covered with therapeutic doses of zinc and omega-3 fatty acids.

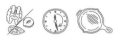

Sardine Cake Boats

Serves 2 ◦ Prep Time: 10 minutes ◦ Cook Time: 10 minutes

For this recipe, I use Wild Planet's wild sardines packed in extra-virgin olive oil with lemon. They are lightly smoked and contain 1,800 milligrams of EPA and DHA omega-3s, plus they clock in at 18 grams of protein per serving (per can). They are also scale-free, sustainably sourced, and just so good. You're going to go nuts over these sardine cakes. Even if you are hesitant to try sardines, the anti-inflammatory benefits and flavors of this recipe will make you a believer.

2 (4.4-ounce) cans sardines packed in extra-virgin olive oil with lemon

¼ cup minced fresh dill, plus more for garnish

¼ cup minced red onions

½ teaspoon fine salt

½ teaspoon garlic powder

1 large egg

3 tablespoons lard or ghee, for the pan

2 tablespoons coconut aminos

1 tablespoon spicy brown or Dijon mustard

1 teaspoon ground black pepper

For serving:

1 ripe Hass avocado, peeled, pitted, and sliced

4 romaine lettuce leaves

8 slices Pickled Radishes (page 84)

Lemon wedges

◦ Open the cans of sardines and drain the oil into a measuring cup; set the oil aside for the sauce.

◦ Crumble the sardines into a medium-sized bowl and add the dill, onions, salt, garlic powder, and egg. Mix well and shape into 8 small patties, about 2 inches in diameter.

◦ Heat a large skillet over medium heat. Heat the lard in the skillet until the end of a wooden spoon handle sizzles when inserted into it. Fry the patties for 3 minutes per side, then remove from the heat.

◦ Pour the reserved oil from the cans of sardines into a widemouthed jar, then add the coconut aminos, mustard, and black pepper. Use an immersion blender to blend the sauce until well combined. Add salt to taste.

◦ To assemble the boats, lay a few avocado slices on each lettuce leaf. Top with the sardine cakes and then the pickled radishes. Drizzle the sauce over the cakes (or serve it on the side if you prefer), garnish with dill, and serve with lemon wedges.

◦ Store leftover sardine cakes in the fridge for up to 4 days. To reheat, pan-fry in a skillet over medium heat for 3 minutes per side.

Per serving: Calories **583** · Fat **47g** · Total Carbs **12.9g** · Fiber **5.1g** · Protein **29.8g**

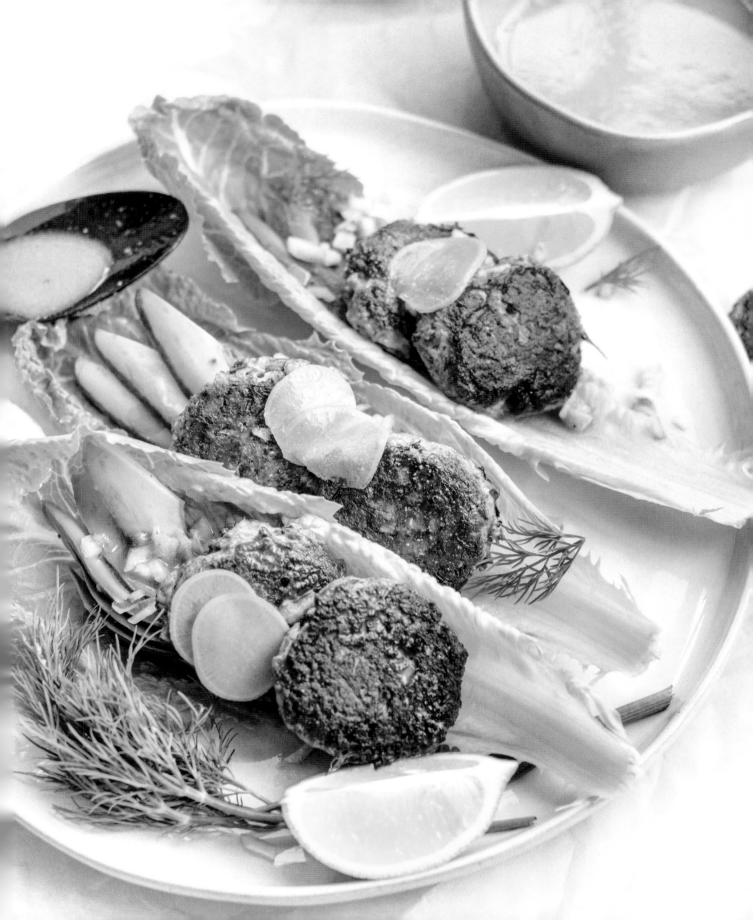

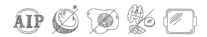

Quick Citrus Salmon

Serves 6 ◦ Prep Time: 5 minutes, plus 20 minutes to marinate ◦ Cook Time: 8 minutes

This salmon recipe is so easy, it's ridiculous! It cooks up in less than 10 minutes and is served with some fresh arugula for a simple, no-fuss meal. This fish also pairs well with Spicy Yellow Rice (page 320).

1 side skin-on wild-caught salmon, deboned (about 1½ pounds)

1 tablespoon grated orange zest

¼ cup coconut aminos

¼ cup freshly squeezed orange juice

2 tablespoons extra-virgin olive oil

1½ teaspoons fine salt

2 tablespoons minced fresh chives, for garnish

3 cups arugula, for serving

Lemon wedges, for serving

◦ Put an oven rack just below the broiler. Set the oven to broil on high (550°F). Line a sheet pan with parchment paper.

◦ Pat the salmon dry and place it skin side down in a casserole dish large enough to allow it to lie flat. Sprinkle the orange zest over the fish, then drizzle it with the coconut aminos and orange juice. Flip the fish over and let it rest skin side up in the marinade for 20 minutes.

◦ Transfer the salmon to the lined sheet pan, skin side down. Gently rub the olive oil into the fish and sprinkle the salt evenly over it. Pour the marinade over the salmon. Set the salmon just beneath the broiler and broil for 8 minutes, until it has a bright pink color and flakes easily.

◦ If the salmon is more than 2 inches thick, use a fork to check the thickest part of the fish at the 8-minute mark: if it flakes easily, the fish is ready; if not, cook it longer and check it for doneness every minute until it's ready.

◦ Remove the salmon from the oven, garnish with the chives, and serve with the arugula and lemon wedges.

◦ This perfectly cooked broiled salmon will become dry if reheated, so don't do it. Store leftovers in the fridge for up to 2 days and enjoy them cold, or use them to make the Salmon Herb Skillet Cake (page 270).

notes: *Always choose in-season, wild-caught salmon. Look for a smooth, even fillet.*

modifications: *To make this dish coconut-free, use low-sodium gluten-free tamari instead of the coconut aminos.*

Per serving: Calories **240** · Fat **12.8g** · Total Carbs **5.4g** · Fiber **0.2g** · Protein **25.2g**

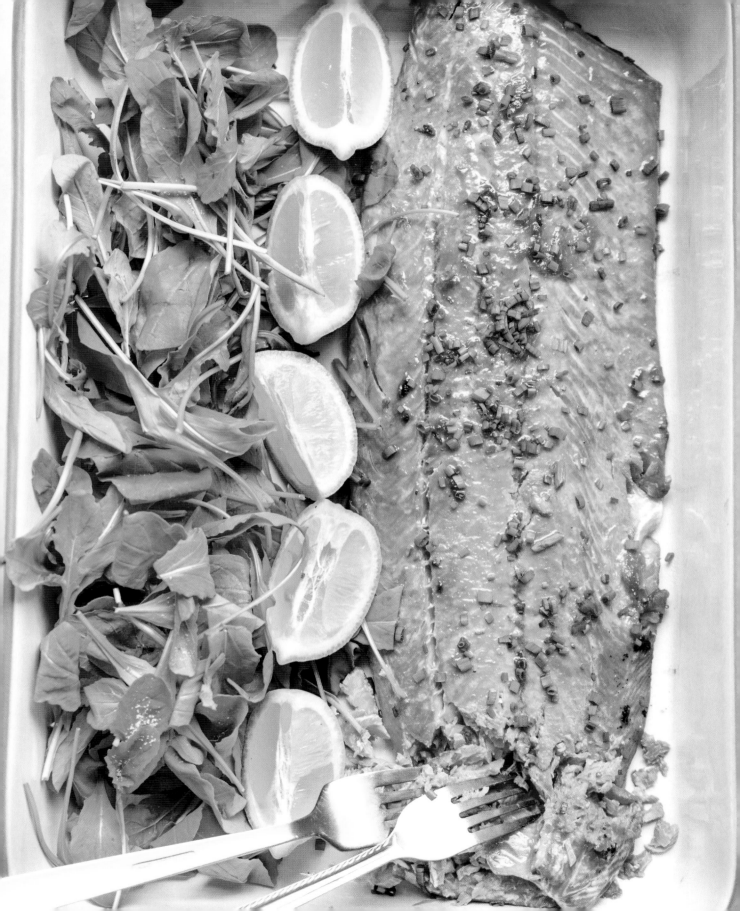

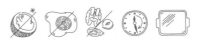

Mustard Salmon + Bok Choy

Serves 4 ○ Prep Time: 10 minutes ○ Cook Time: 10 minutes

Salmon takes no time to cook—it truly is the perfect meal for a busy night. Plus, it comes with the added bonus of being delicious and rich in omega-3 fatty acids. If you use frozen fish, always remember to unwrap it from the vacuum-sealed packs before thawing!

4 (4-ounce) skin-on wild-caught salmon fillets

3 tablespoons whole-seed mustard (see notes)

1½ tablespoons coconut aminos

2 tablespoons minced shallots

4 baby bok choy

4 tablespoons extra-virgin olive oil, divided

1 teaspoon fine salt, divided

2 ripe Hass avocados, peeled, halved, and pitted

1 green onion, sliced on the bias

○ Place one oven rack in the middle position and another in the bottom position. Preheat the oven to 400°F. Line a sheet pan with parchment paper and place the salmon fillets on it.

○ In a small bowl, mix together the mustard, coconut aminos, and shallots. Spoon the mixture over the salmon.

○ Cut the bok choy in half lengthwise. Give them a rinse, especially near the root, where debris hangs out. Dry them and lay them cut side down on a separate sheet pan. Drizzle them with 2 tablespoons of the olive oil and sprinkle them with ½ teaspoon of the salt.

○ Put both sheet pans in the oven, with the salmon in the middle and the bok choy on the bottom. Roast everything for 8 minutes. Remove the salmon from the oven and move the bok choy to underneath the broiler. Broil for 2 minutes, then remove from the oven.

○ Serve each piece of salmon with 2 bok choy halves and an avocado half. Drizzle the avocado halves with the remaining 2 tablespoons of oil and sprinkle them with the remaining ½ teaspoon of salt. Garnish the plates with the sliced green onion.

○ Store leftovers in the fridge for up to 4 days. To reheat the bok choy, sauté it in a skillet over medium heat for 5 minutes, then flake in the leftover salmon and stir for 1 minute.

notes: *If you don't have whole-seed (aka whole-grain) mustard, use spicy brown or Dijon mustard. For a different flavor profile, replace the mustard with coconut butter.*

I'm not a fan of reheating leftover fish, which tends to overcook it. However, you can crumble the cold leftovers into a salad.

modifications: *To make this dish coconut-free, use low-sodium gluten-free tamari instead of the coconut aminos.*

Per serving: Calories **452** · Fat **33.9g** · Total Carbs **12.4g** · Fiber **5.6g** · Protein **27.4g**

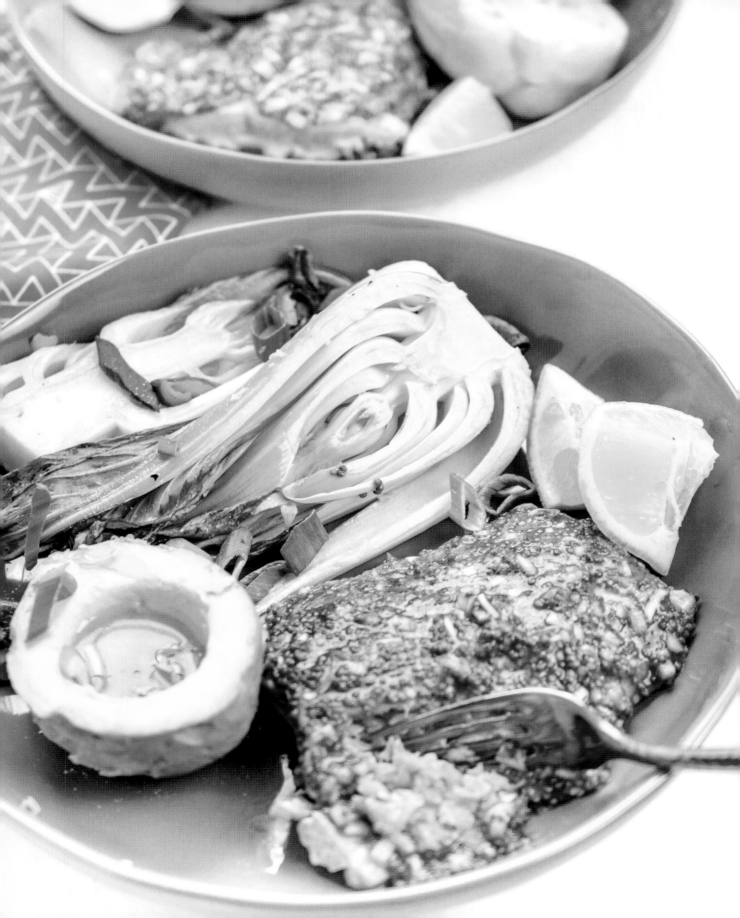

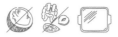

Tuna-Stuffed Mushrooms

Serves 3 ○ Prep Time: 10 minutes ○ Cook Time: 35 minutes

A delicious, vegetable-packed, curry-spiked tuna mixture baked in portobello caps! Line-caught canned tuna is a great source of protein, and if you stick to skipjack—the smaller, dark meat fish—you get the protein without the mercury. Tuna is high in niacin, a B3 vitamin that acts as an antioxidant and plays an important role in repairing DNA.

3 portobello mushrooms

2 tablespoons extra-virgin olive oil, divided

2 teaspoons fine salt, divided

3 (3-ounce) ounces no-salt-added canned tuna packed in water

2 cups shredded green cabbage

2 large eggs

¼ cup avocado oil mayonnaise

¼ cup minced fresh parsley

2 tablespoons spicy brown or Dijon mustard

1 tablespoon Citrus Curry Powder (page 82)

1 lime, cut into wedges, for serving

○ Preheat the oven to 400°F.

○ Remove the stems from the mushrooms and use a spoon to scoop out the gills. Rub the mushroom caps all over with 1 tablespoon of the olive oil and sprinkle them with ¼ teaspoon of the salt. Place the mushrooms cap side down on a sheet pan and roast for 10 minutes.

○ While the mushrooms roast, prepare the filling: Drain the cans of tuna and flake the fish into a large bowl. Add the remaining tablespoon of olive oil, the remaining 1¾ teaspoons of salt, and the rest of the ingredients, except the lime wedges, to the bowl and mix well.

○ Remove the mushrooms from the oven and flip them over. Scoop the tuna mixture into the mushrooms in large mounds.

○ Bake for 25 minutes, or until the tuna mixture is golden brown. Remove from the oven and enjoy right away. Serve with lime wedges.

○ Store leftovers in the fridge for up to 3 days. To reheat, bake in a preheated 300°F oven for 15 minutes.

notes: *You can omit the cabbage and use any vegetable slaw you like. If you don't like mushrooms, you can shape the tuna mixture into nine 2-inch cakes and bake them for 25 minutes, then serve them over salad.*

awesome additions: *I love to serve these stuffed mushrooms with fresh citrus and avocado. If you do well with dairy, you can add a slice of aged cheddar on top and broil them for a tuna melt experience.*

Per serving: Calories **443** · Fat **29.5g** · Total Carbs **8.8g** · Fiber **3.4g** · Protein **41.2g**

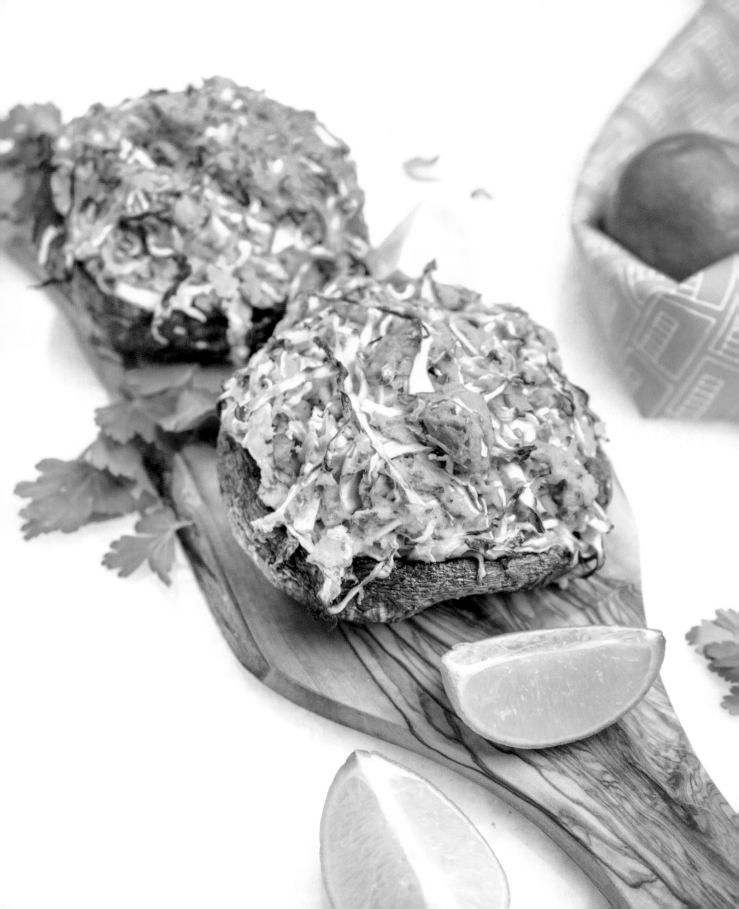

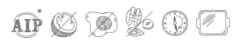

Shrimp + Sausage Sheet Pan

Serves 4 ○ Prep Time: 15 minutes ○ Cook Time: 12 minutes

This meal is for all you stir-fry lovers out there, the ones who like to mix together their food. A delicious dose of protein, selenium, and B12, this shrimp dish cooks up in 12 minutes and feeds four hungry adults. If you don't eat pork, you can leave out the sausage and double the shrimp. Full of fresh spring flavors and juicy protein, this beautiful meal was created on a stunning spring day in Alexandria, Virginia.

1 pound large shrimp, peeled, deveined, and tails removed

4 cloves garlic, minced

¼ cup minced fresh cilantro or parsley

3 tablespoons extra-virgin olive oil, divided

2 teaspoons fine salt, divided

1 pound asparagus, trimmed

12 ounces smoked sausage

1 lemon, thinly sliced

4 radishes, shaved

○ Place one oven rack in the middle position and another directly beneath the broiler. Preheat the oven to 400°F.

○ In a medium-sized bowl, toss the shrimp, garlic, cilantro, 1 tablespoon of the olive oil, and 1 teaspoon of the salt. Let the shrimp marinate while the oven preheats.

○ Drizzle 1 tablespoon of the oil on a sheet pan. Line up the asparagus on one side of the pan, then sprinkle it with ½ teaspoon of the salt. Cut the sausage on the bias into ¼-inch-thick slices and set aside.

○ Arrange the lemon slices on the other side of the sheet pan, opposite the asparagus. Place the shrimp, lying flat, in an even layer on top of the lemon slices. Scoop all of the minced garlic and cilantro out of the bowl and sprinkle it over the shrimp. Arrange the sliced sausage over the shrimp and asparagus. Drizzle everything with the remaining tablespoon of oil.

○ Place the sheet pan on the middle rack of the oven and roast for 10 minutes, then move the pan to the upper rack directly under the broiler, set the oven to broil on high (550°F), and broil for 2 minutes.

○ Remove from the oven, sprinkle with the shaved radishes and the remaining ½ teaspoon of salt, and dig in!

○ Store leftovers in the fridge for up to 4 days. To reheat, place in a skillet over medium-low heat and gently stir for 5 minutes.

notes: *I use Pederson's Natural Farms organic smoked sausage, which is nightshade-free. It's also fully cooked, so there's no need to worry about the short cook time.*

modifications: *I've yet to find an AIP-compliant smoked sausage, so to make this dish AIP, omit the sausage. You may add more shrimp or use sliced prosciutto instead.*

Per serving: Calories **402** · Fat **33.6g** · Total Carbs **6g** · Fiber **1.7g** · Protein **22.2g**

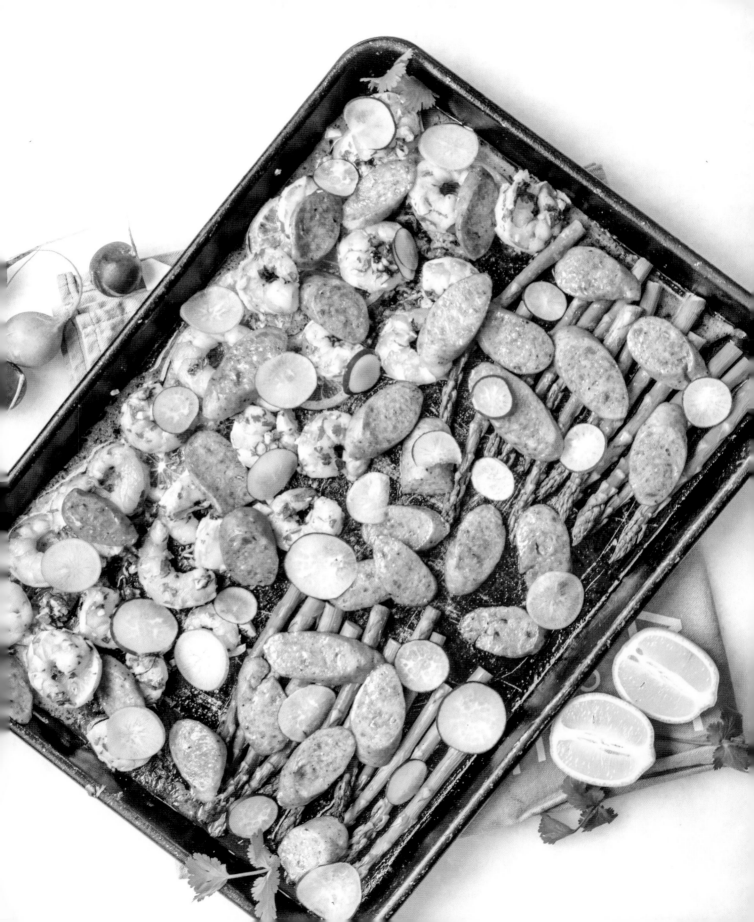

Balsamic Salmon with Toasty Vegetables

Serves 4 ◦ Prep Time: 10 minutes ◦ Cook Time: 10 minutes

When aged balsamic vinegar is cooked at high temperatures, something magical happens: it turns into a delicious glaze! Yes, it's due to the naturally occurring sugars in the vinegar, but don't despair: in the small amount used here, balsamic vinegar is not going to mess with your blood sugar. What you get is a simple, delicious meal that delivers killer flavors.

4 cups chopped dinosaur kale, coarse stems removed (1 to 2 bunches)

4 cups trimmed green beans

3 tablespoons extra-virgin olive oil or avocado oil, divided

1½ teaspoons fine salt, divided

4 (4-ounce) skin-on wild-caught salmon fillets

2 tablespoons aged balsamic vinegar (see notes, page 90)

2 tablespoons Gremolata with Olive Oil (page 86), for serving

◦ Place one oven rack in the middle position and another in the bottom position.

◦ Toss the kale, green beans, 2 tablespoons of the olive oil, and ½ teaspoon of the salt on a sheet pan, then spread the veggies evenly over the pan. Put the pan in the oven on the middle rack, then set the oven to 425°F.

◦ While the oven preheats with the veggies inside, prepare the salmon: Line a second sheet pan with parchment paper. Pat the salmon fillets dry and lay them skin side down on the lined pan. Sprinkle the fillets with the remaining teaspoon of salt and brush them with the vinegar, then drizzle the remaining tablespoon of oil over the fillets.

◦ When the oven comes to temperature, put the sheet pan with the salmon on the top rack and bake for 7 to 10 minutes, depending on how you like your salmon cooked: 7 minutes for medium or 10 minutes for well-done. (Note: These times are for 1-inch-thick fillets; if your fillets are thicker or thinner, adjust the baking time accordingly.)

◦ Remove both pans from the oven at the same time. The green beans will be nicely browned and the kale will be crispy, like kale chips! Divide the vegetables and salmon among 4 plates. Spoon the gremolata over the fish.

◦ Store leftovers in the fridge for up to 3 days. To reheat, bake in a preheated 300°F oven for 10 minutes.

note: *Instead of reheating, you can use leftover salmon to make the Salmon Herb Skillet Cake on page 270.*

modifications: *To make this dish AIP compliant, use asparagus instead of the green beans.*

Per serving: Calories **331** · Fat **20.7g** · Total Carbs **11.5g** · Fiber **3.4g** · Protein **27.5g**

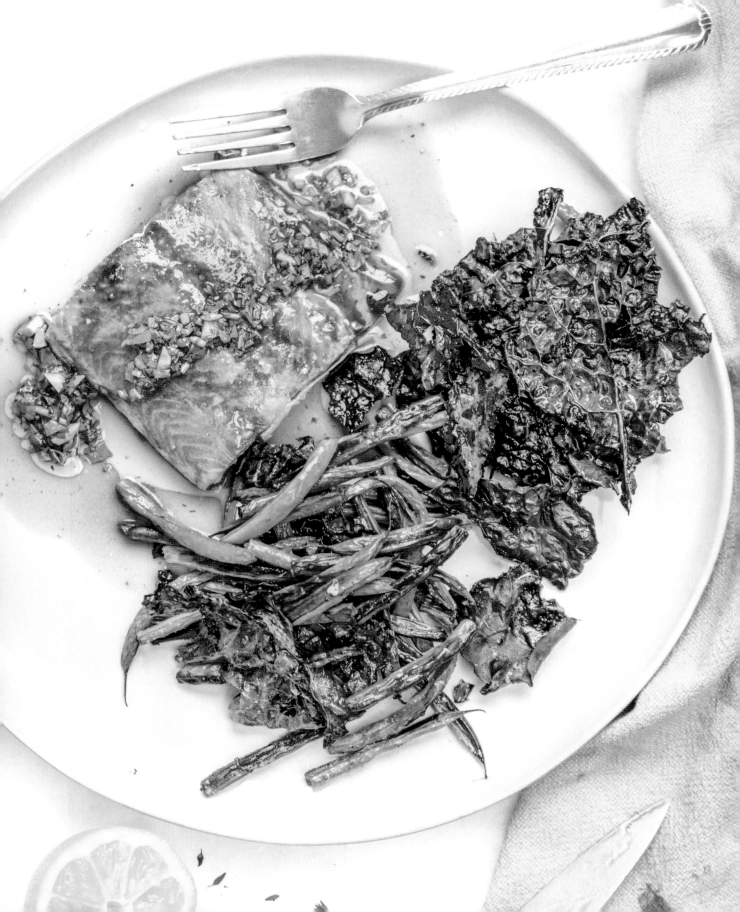

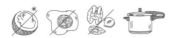

Presque Gumbo

Serves 5 ◦ Prep Time: 20 minutes ◦ Cook Time: 45 minutes

Presque means "almost" in French, and this is almost gumbo. You won't find peppers or flour in this multiprotein stew, but you will find a carnival of flavors, textures, and aromas that are pleasing to all of the senses. I recruited the pressure cooker for this recipe to create rich flavors in half the time. Don't let the long ingredient list intimidate you—most of it is dried seasonings!

For the seasoning blend:

2 teaspoons fine salt

2 teaspoons garlic powder

2 teaspoons ground black pepper

2 teaspoons onion powder

1 teaspoon dried rosemary needles

1 teaspoon dried thyme leaves

1 teaspoon ground cumin

½ teaspoon ground white pepper

½ teaspoon turmeric powder

For the gumbo:

¼ cup lard or ghee

4 celery ribs, diced (about 1 cup)

2 medium carrots, diced (about 1 cup)

1 large onion, diced (about 1 cup)

4 cloves garlic, minced

2 bay leaves

2 cups frozen sliced okra (about 10 ounces)

1 pound ground pork or ground dark meat chicken

3 cups bone broth

2 tablespoons coconut aminos

1 tablespoon apple cider vinegar

1 tablespoon fish sauce

15 jumbo shrimp, peeled, deveined, and tails removed

1 (6-ounce) can jumbo lump crabmeat

5 sprigs fresh cilantro, for garnish

2 limes, cut into wedges, for serving

◦ In a small bowl, mix together the ingredients for the seasoning blend and set aside.

◦ Put a pressure cooker in sauté mode. When it's hot, put the lard in the pot, followed by the celery, carrots, onion, garlic, and bay leaves. Sauté for 15 minutes, or until very tender and aromatic. Add 1 tablespoon of the seasoning blend and mix in the frozen okra. Sauté until the okra is completely thawed, about 8 minutes, then remove the veggies from the cooker and set aside.

◦ Put the ground pork in the pressure cooker along with another tablespoon of the seasoning blend and cook, stirring often, until browned and crumbly, about 5 minutes. Return the vegetables to the cooker and mix well.

◦ Pour in the broth, coconut aminos, vinegar, and fish sauce and stir to combine. Add the shrimp, crabmeat, and the rest of the seasoning blend. Cancel the sauté function and seal the lid. Cook on low pressure for 20 minutes.

◦ When it's done, release the pressure manually, open the lid, and stir well. Divide the gumbo among 5 bowls. Top each with a cilantro sprig and serve with a lime wedge.

◦ Store leftovers in the fridge for up to 4 days. To reheat, bring to a simmer in a saucepan over medium heat.

modifications: *To make this stew coconut-free, use low-sodium gluten-free tamari instead of the coconut aminos.*

awesome additions: *Add a little Turn Up the Heat Spice Blend (page 83) to the seasoning blend to give the gumbo a little kick.*

Per serving: Calories **414** · Fat **25.9g** · Total Carbs **16.4g** · Fiber **3.4g** · Protein **32.5g**

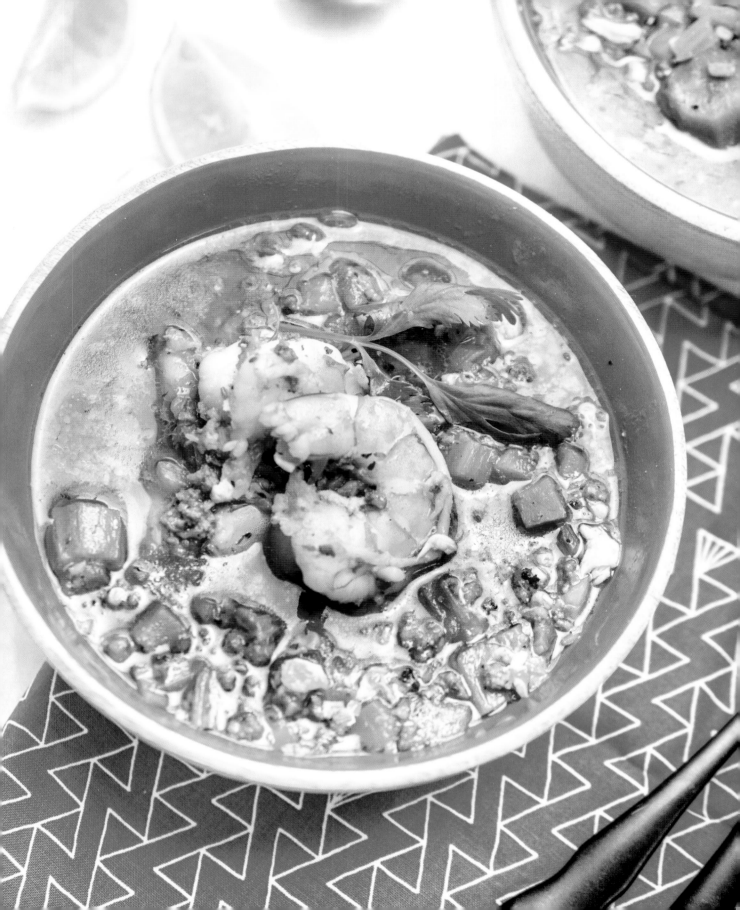

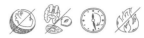

Crispy Tuna Salad

Serves 2 ○ Prep Time: 15 minutes

Tuna salad gets an upgrade! I've packed this version with loads of crunchy and crispy veggies, avocado oil mayo, and immune-boosting tarragon. It's perfect on its own, served in avocado cups, or with grain-free crackers. Double the recipe for a week's worth of grab-and-go lunches.

1 cup diced celery

3 medium radishes, shaved

2 tablespoons fresh tarragon leaves, minced

2 (5-ounce) cans tuna packed in water, drained

Juice of 1 lemon

3 tablespoons avocado oil mayonnaise

1 tablespoon Dijon mustard

2 teaspoons whole mustard seeds

½ teaspoon fine salt

½ teaspoon ground black pepper

- In a large bowl, combine the celery, radishes, and tarragon. Flake in the tuna and mix well. Add the remaining ingredients and mix well. Serve chilled.

- Store leftovers in the fridge for up to 4 days.

Per serving: Calories **324** · Fat **19.6g** · Total Carbs **3.9g** · Fiber **1.2g** · Protein **33.7g**

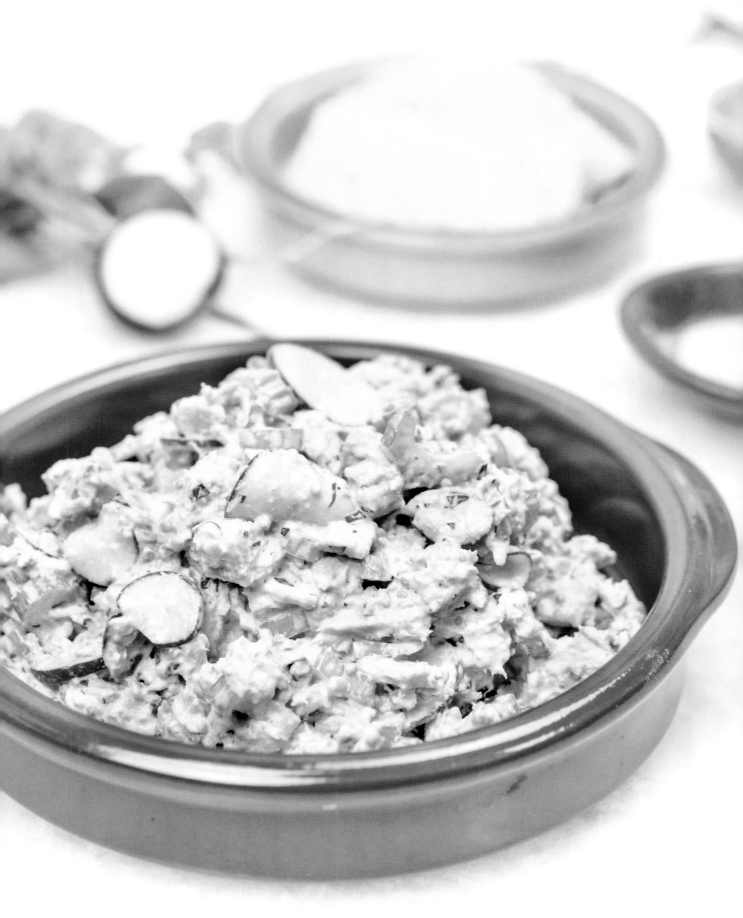

SIDES + SNACKS

Variety is the spice of life! Here is a collection of easy-to-make side dishes that are prepared on a sheet pan, in a single pan or pot, or in a pressure cooker. That way, you can pair a one-pot entrée with a hands-off side dish and have a delicious meal ready in no time. Adding a side also stretches a meal stretch further, so you can prep multiple meals in a single batch cook.

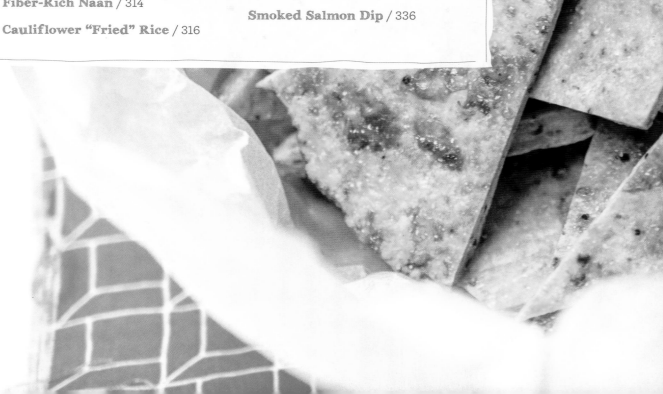

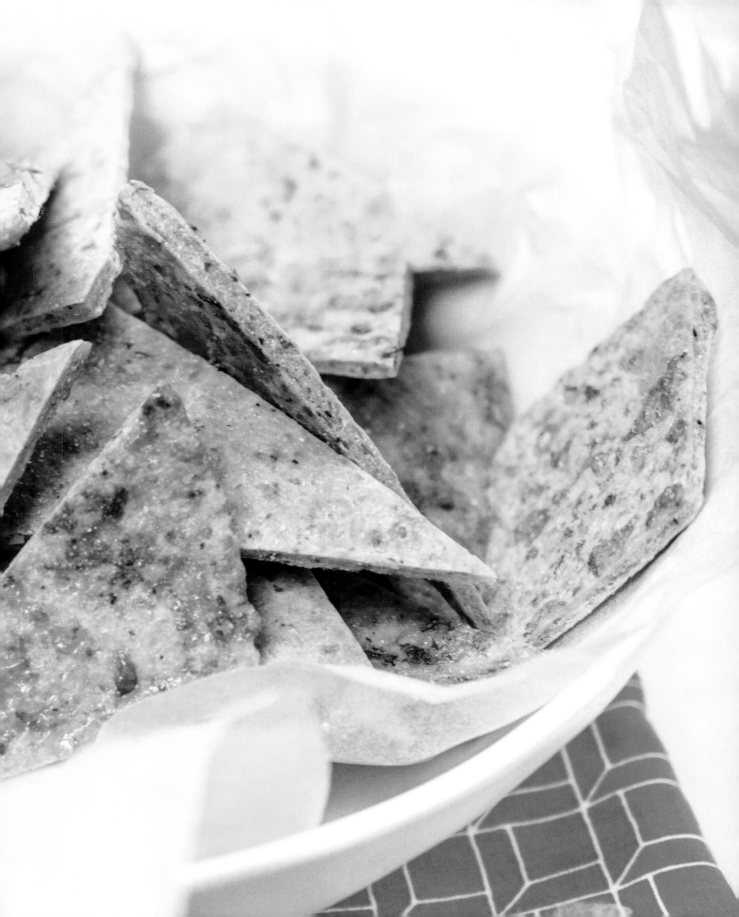

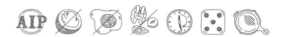

Warm Garlic Herb Radish Salad

Serves 4 ◦ Prep Time: 5 minutes ◦ Cook Time: 9 minutes

This amazing radish salad reminds me of a Spanish fava bean salad I loved as a kid—must be the loads of garlic and parsley. Here, tender radishes are tossed in a copious amount of fresh garlic, which has powerful healing properties. The garlic breath is totally worth it.

¼ cup extra-virgin olive oil

14 radishes (about 2 bunches), quartered

1 cup minced fresh parsley

6 cloves garlic, chopped

1 teaspoon fine salt

◦ Heat a large skillet over medium heat. When it's hot, drizzle in the olive oil and add the radishes. Fry them for 9 minutes, or until lightly browned, giving them a stir every few minutes.

◦ Transfer the radishes to a medium-sized bowl. Add the parsley, garlic, and salt and toss to combine. Serve warm, or chill and serve as a cold salad later.

◦ Store leftovers in the fridge for up to 4 days.

Per serving: Calories **137** · Fat **13.7g** · Total Carbs **3.6g** · Fiber **0.9g** · Protein **1g**

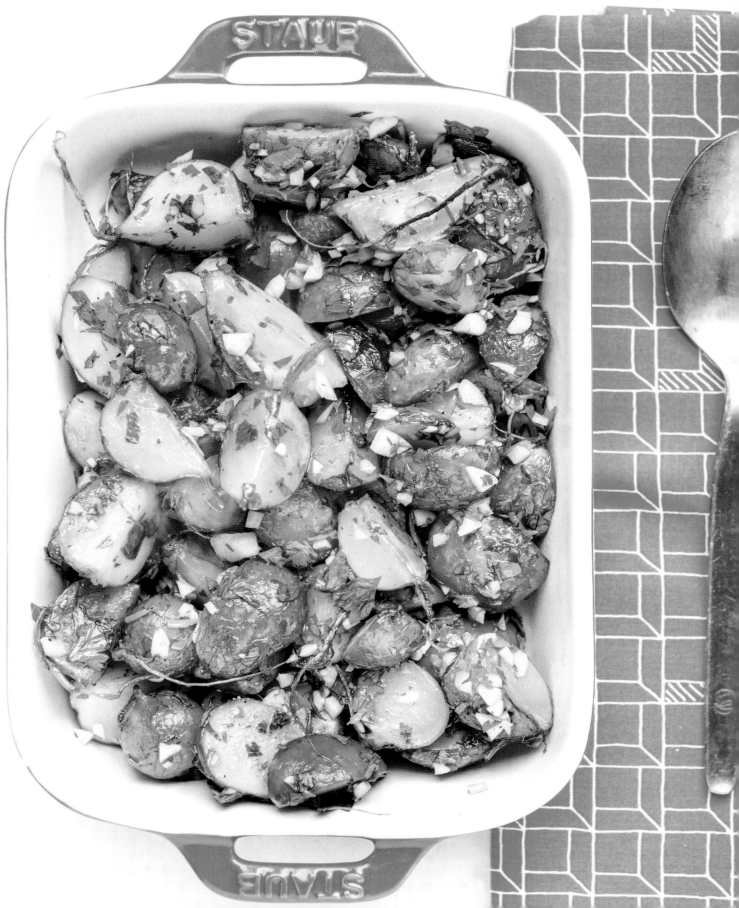

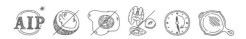

Charred Kale Soup

Serves 4 ◦ Prep Time: 10 minutes ◦ Cook Time: 18 minutes

This soup has a deep flavor thanks to smoky charred bits of greens and a bright citrus finish that cuts the bitterness. It's loaded with fiber, antioxidants, vitamin K, and iron and blended with gut-healing bone broth, hard to imagine a soup that is so good for you being so good.

3 tablespoons extra-virgin olive oil

5 cups chopped dinosaur kale, coarse stems removed (about 3 bunches)

½ teaspoon fine salt

½ teaspoon ground black pepper

2 cups bone broth, warmed

1 tablespoon nutritional yeast

1 teaspoon garlic powder

1 teaspoon grated lemon zest

- Heat a large skillet over medium heat. Drizzle the olive oil into the skillet and add the kale, salt, and pepper.

- Cook undisturbed for 5 minutes. Stir well, then leave it alone for another 5 minutes. Stir again, then leave it alone for another 5 minutes, or until the kale is tender and has dark, charred bits.

- Transfer the kale to a blender. Add the remaining ingredients and blend until smooth. Serve warm.

- Store leftovers in the fridge for up to 5 days. To reheat, bring to a simmer in a saucepan over medium heat.

notes: *You can warm the broth in the skillet with the charred kale, but the kale might lose its bright green color as the broth boils. The soup will still taste great, but it won't look as pretty.*

If you don't have nutritional yeast, you can use 1½ teaspoons fish sauce instead.

modifications: *To make this soup AIP compliant, omit the black pepper.*

Per serving: Calories **254** · Fat **20.6g** · Total Carbs **5.8g** · Fiber **2.2g** · Protein **13.5g**

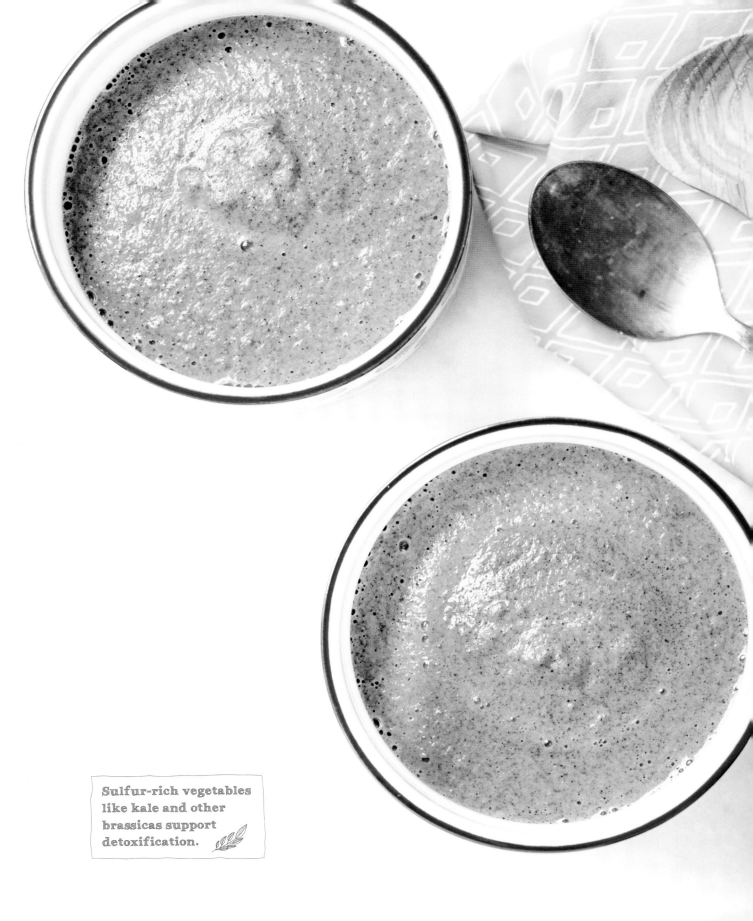

Sulfur-rich vegetables like kale and other brassicas support detoxification.

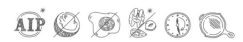

Creamy Bacon Mushroom Noodles

Serves 2 ◦ Prep Time: 10 minutes ◦ Cook Time: 20 minutes

Let's talk noodles for a second. For this recipe, you can use the healthiest option that you enjoy. For me, the top three are shirataki noodles, kelp noodles, and the very delicious Better Than brand. Better Than noodles are essentially shirataki noodles, which are made from a type of yam flour, but they also have gluten-free oat fiber, which creates a texture that more closely resembles traditional pasta. If none of these are viable options for you, use whichever noodles work best, such as zucchini noodles or spaghetti squash. This dish is ridiculously delicious no matter what type of noodle is used.

6 slices bacon, chopped

1 cup sliced cremini mushrooms (about 4 ounces)

3 cloves garlic, minced

2 servings noodles of your choice (about 7 ounces each)

2 Mozz Blocks (page 104)

¼ teaspoon fine salt

8 fresh basil leaves, sliced into ribbons

◦ Heat a large skillet over medium heat. Put the bacon in the hot skillet and cook for 8 to 10 minutes, until crispy.

◦ Add the mushrooms and garlic and sauté for 5 minutes, or until tender and aromatic.

◦ Add the noodles to the skillet (if you're using packaged noodles, prepare them as directed before using). Sauté until the noodles are heated through and combined with the mushrooms and garlic. Add the Mozz Blocks and stir until they begin to melt and get creamy. Add the salt and toss to combine.

◦ Divide the noodles between 2 bowls. Top with the fresh basil and dig in.

◦ Store leftovers in the fridge for up to 5 days. To reheat, sauté over medium heat for 5 minutes.

modifications: *To make this dish AIP compliant, use the AIP version of the Mozz Blocks. To make it nut-free, use the nut-free version of the Mozz Blocks.*

awesome additions: *I love this bowl of pasta with Cumin-Dusted Mahi-Mahi (page 274) or Hail Mary Chicken (page 258).*

Per serving: Calories **257** · Fat **17.3g** · Total Carbs **14.1g** · Fiber **7.5g** · Protein **14.9g**

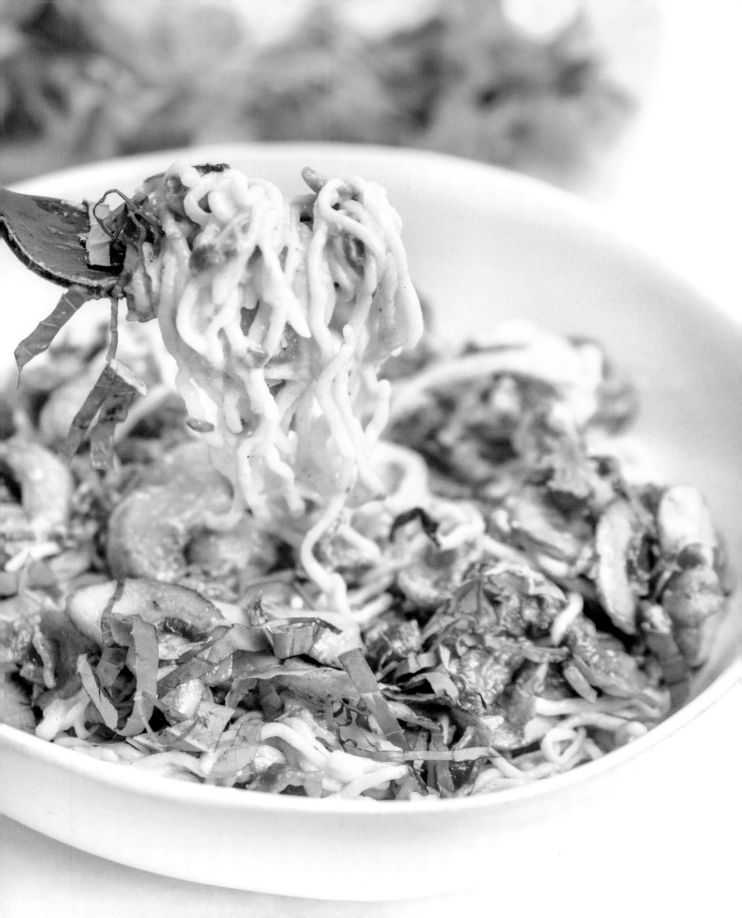

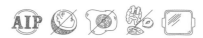

Perfect Roasted Brussels Sprouts

Serves 4 ◦ Prep Time: 10 minutes ◦ Cook Time: 35 minutes

Don't let their brown color fool you: these little sprouts have been transformed into perfectly crisp bites with a tender center. They are not the boiled, mushy Brussels sprouts you may have grown up eating; these are vegetables you want to eat! The charred lemon takes them to another level of yum.

1 pound small Brussels sprouts

3 tablespoons extra-virgin olive oil

2 cloves garlic, sliced

1 teaspoon fine salt

1 teaspoon garlic powder

2 lemons, halved

◦ Preheat the oven to 425°F.

◦ Trim any hard nubs or stems from the sprouts. Cut any big ones in half.

◦ Put the sprouts on a sheet pan and toss with the olive oil, sliced garlic, salt, and garlic powder.

◦ Spread the sprouts evenly across the pan, leaving space between them. Place the lemon halves cut side down in empty spaces among the Brussels sprouts.

◦ Roast for 35 minutes, then remove from the oven. Use tongs to pick up the tender lemon halves and squeeze the juice all over the sprouts. Use a spatula to scrape the sprouts off the sheet pan.

◦ Store leftovers in the fridge for up to 4 days. To reheat, sauté over medium heat for 5 minutes, or until warm.

Per serving: Calories **142** · Fat **10.5g** · Total Carbs **11.3g** · Fiber **4.4g** · Protein **3.9g**

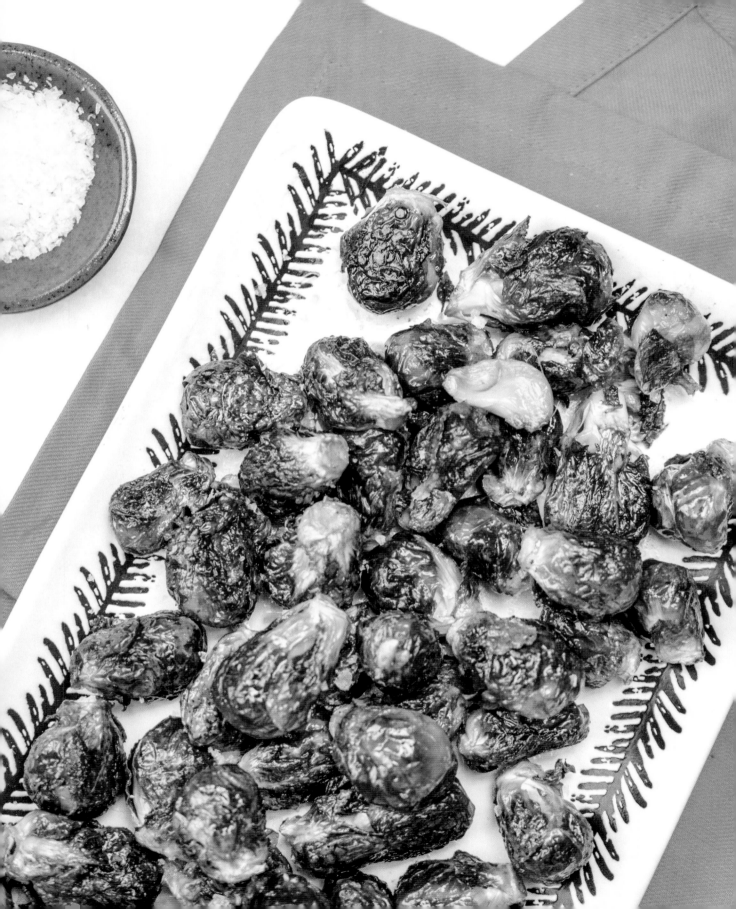

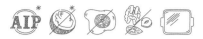

Crispy Chicken Chips

Serves 4 ◦ Prep Time: 15 minutes ◦ Cook Time: 45 minutes

I know your eyes are probably darting from the recipe photo to the recipe title, and you're scratching your head, thinking, *Chicken?* Yes, this recipe for a pita chip–like snack is made with ground chicken. Crispy snacks tend to be addictive foods for some people; once they get started, they can't stop! The benefit here is that these lean, high-protein chips, as delicious as they are, are hard to overdo. The satiating nature of protein will fill you up; just listen to your body's cues.

2 pounds ground chicken

¼ cup extra-virgin olive oil

¼ cup nutritional yeast

1 tablespoon dried oregano leaves

1 tablespoon garlic powder

1 tablespoon onion powder

1½ teaspoons ground black pepper

1½ teaspoons turmeric powder

2 teaspoons fine salt, divided

1 tablespoon coconut flour

1 tablespoon unflavored grass-fed beef gelatin

Coconut oil spray

◦ Place one oven rack in the middle position and another in the bottom position. Preheat the oven to 400°F. Cut 3 pieces of parchment paper to the size of a sheet pan.

◦ In a large bowl, combine the chicken with the olive oil, nutritional yeast, oregano, spices, and 1½ teaspoons of the salt, mixing well. Add the coconut flour and gelatin, then mix well again. Divide the chicken mixture into 2 equal mounds.

◦ Place a piece of parchment paper on the counter and lightly spray it with coconut oil. Put a mound of chicken in the middle of the paper and, with wet hands, mold it into a flat rectangle. Spray the rectangle with coconut oil, cover it with another sheet of parchment, and use a rolling pin to roll it out. You want it to be almost the size of the sheet of parchment paper, 17 by 12 inches, and no thicker than ⅛ inch. (The thinner the chips, the crispier they will be.)

◦ Just to make sure it won't stick, grab both pieces of parchment paper and flip the entire thing over onto a sheet pan, then lift off the top sheet of parchment, leaving the bottom sheet between the pan and the chicken mixture. Repeat this process with a second sheet pan and the remaining parchment paper and chicken mixture.

◦ Place both sheet pans in the oven, one in the middle rack and the other on the bottom rack, and bake for 30 minutes. After 30 minutes, remove the sheet pans from the oven and increase the temperature to 425°F.

◦ Transfer one of the chicken flatbreads to a cutting board. If it won't slide off the paper, flip it over and peel the paper back. Cut the flatbread into 2-inch-wide strips, then cut each strip into triangles. Transfer the chips to the sheet pan and spread them out in a single layer. Repeat with the second flatbread.

Per serving: Calories **394** · Fat **26.9g** · Total Carbs **3.7g** · Fiber **1.7g** · Protein **35.8g**

modifications: *To make these chips AIP compliant, omit the black pepper. If you can't do nutritional yeast, you may omit it and add 1 tablespoon fish sauce. To make the chips coconut-free, use flaxseed meal in place of the coconut flour and olive oil spray in place of the coconut oil spray.*

∘ Bake for 10 to 15 minutes, until the chips reach your desired crispiness. Use a spatula to remove the chips from the sheet pan and place them in a bowl. Toss with the remaining ½ teaspoon of salt before serving.

∘ Store leftover chips in an airtight container in the fridge for up to 5 days. To recrisp, bake on a sheet pan in a preheated 350°F oven for 5 minutes.

notes: *These chips are perfect with Blender Guac (page 110), Roasted Garlic "Hummus" (page 324), or Berry Much Like Caprese Salad (page 334).*

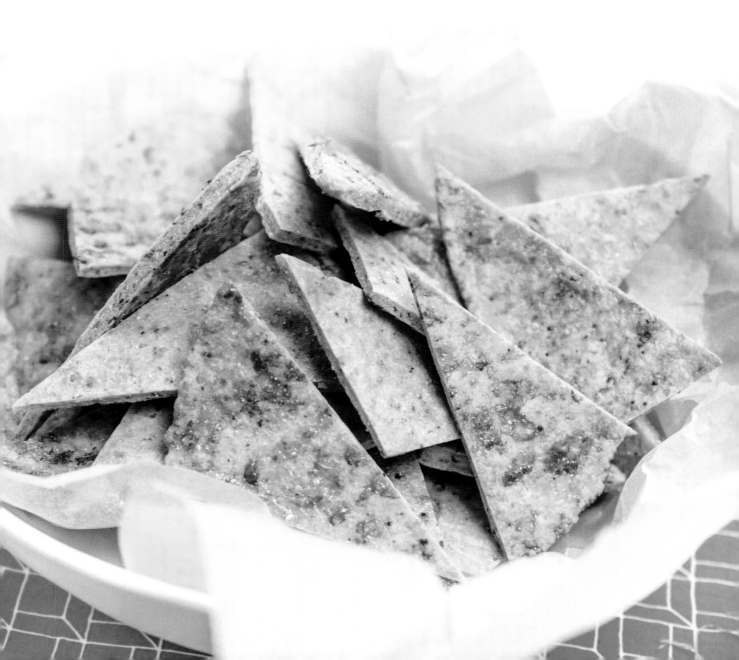

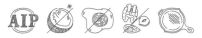

Lamb Lollipops

Serves 7 ◦ Prep Time: 8 minutes, plus 10 minutes to marinate ◦ Cook Time: 15 minutes

These meaty lollipops could double as an entrée, but I find that this protein finger food works better as an appetizer, snack, or alternative entrée at a large feast. It has all the traditional flavors of Mediterranean lamb and cooks up in minutes, so the extra time it takes to marinate the lamb is worth the wait.

14 lamb lollipops (aka rib chops)

1½ teaspoons fine salt, divided

½ cup dairy-free unsweetened plain yogurt (see note), plus more for serving

Juice of 1 lemon

4 cloves garlic, minced

Needles from 2 sprigs fresh rosemary, minced

2 tablespoons extra-virgin olive oil, for the pan

Lemon wedges, for serving

∘ Salt the chops with 1 teaspoon of the salt and set them aside.

∘ In a small bowl, whisk together the yogurt, lemon juice, garlic, rosemary, and remaining ½ teaspoon of salt. Coat the lamb chops in the yogurt mixture and set them in the refrigerator to marinate for at least 10 minutes.

∘ Heat a large skillet over medium heat. When it's hot, drizzle in the olive oil. Working in batches to avoid overcrowding the pan, sear the chops for 3 to 4 minutes on each side, until well browned and cooked to medium-rare.

∘ Serve on a platter with lemon wedges and extra yogurt for dipping. Store leftovers in the fridge for up to 4 days. To reheat, bake the chops in a preheated 350°F oven for 10 minutes.

note: *I prefer coconut milk yogurt, either homemade or a clean brand like Anita's. If you do well with dairy, unsweetened full-fat Greek yogurt would work well here too.*

Per serving (2 chops): Calories **255** · Fat **20g** · Total Carbs **2.7g** · Fiber **0.1g** · Protein **15.1g**

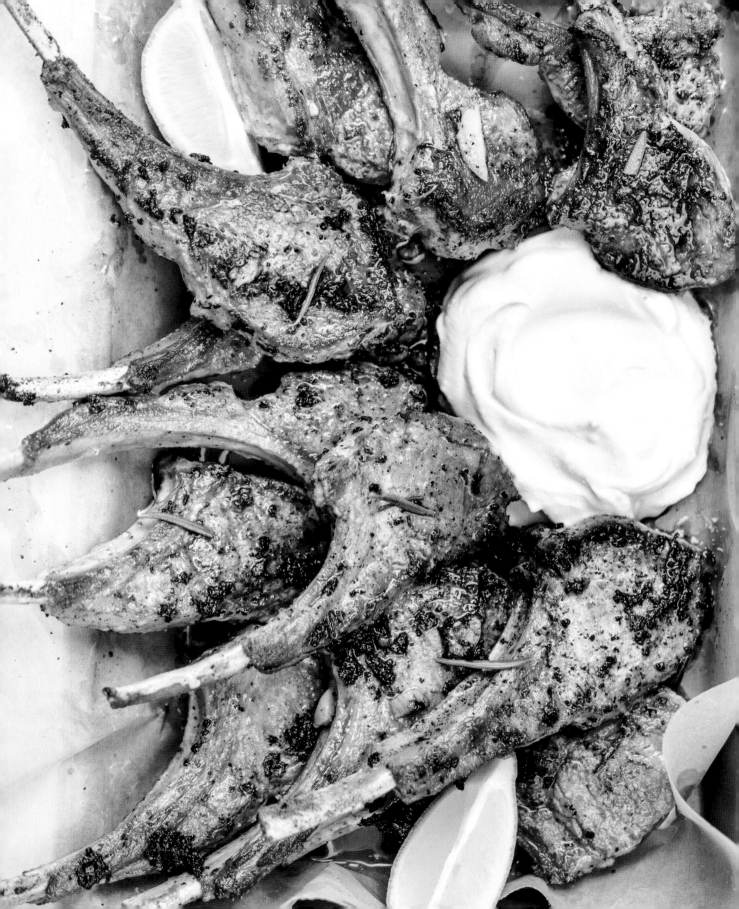

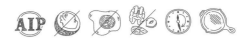

Loving Liver Mousse

Serves 4 ◦ Prep Time: 10 minutes ◦ Cook Time: 12 minutes

Don't let the fancy name fool you. This nutrient-dense spread comes together super quick. Cooked with bacon, green onions, and sage, liver mousse (aka pâté) is my favorite way to eat liver. On pork rinds, grain-free crackers, or celery sticks, it's a great snack that is great for you!

4 slices bacon, diced

4 cloves garlic, minced

4 green onions, white parts only, roughly chopped

Leaves from 2 sprigs fresh sage, plus more for garnish

¾ teaspoon fine salt

12 ounces beef liver, cut into 2-inch chunks

2 tablespoons aged balsamic vinegar (see notes, page 90)

1 tablespoon ghee or lard

◦ Heat a large skillet over medium heat. Put the bacon in the skillet and cook until it's lightly browned. Add the garlic, white parts of the green onions, and sage. Sauté for 6 minutes, or until the onions are tender.

◦ Stir in the salt and add the liver. Sauté for 3 minutes, or until the chunks of liver are browned. Stir in the vinegar and immediately remove the skillet from the heat.

◦ Transfer the liver mixture to a high-powered blender or food processor. Add the ghee and blend until smooth.

◦ Use a rubber spatula to transfer the mousse to four 4-ounce jars and garnish each with a sage leaf. (Note: If you plan to freeze the mousse, use freezer-safe jars with lids.)

◦ Store leftovers in the fridge for up to 4 days or in the freezer for up to 3 months. Put frozen mousse in the fridge to thaw overnight before eating.

Per serving: Calories **226** · Fat **10.1g** · Total Carbs **6.6g** · Fiber **0.3g** · Protein **25.7g**

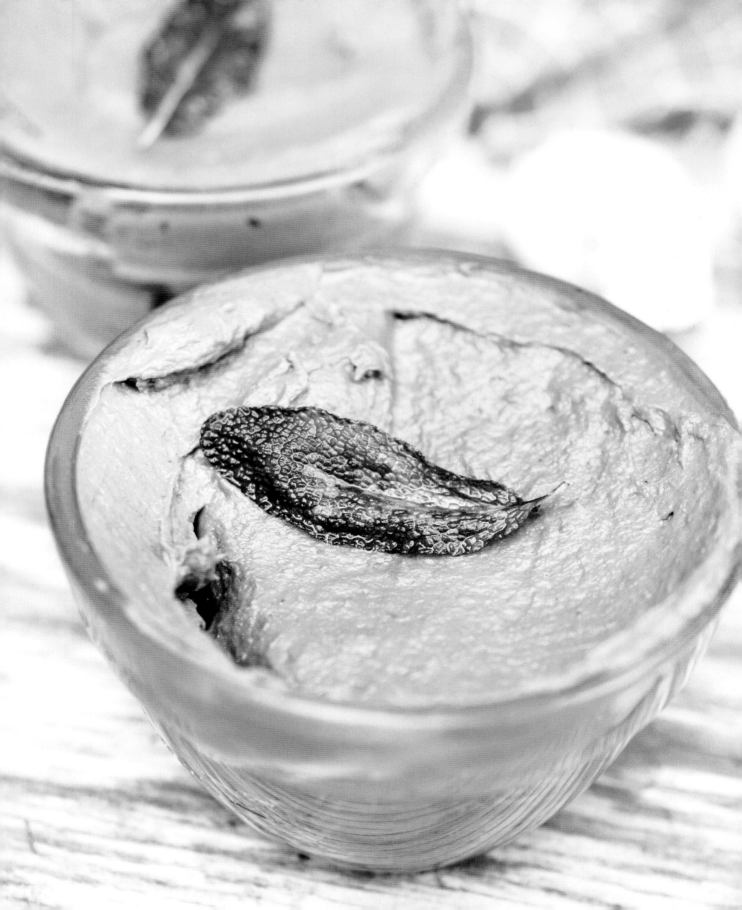

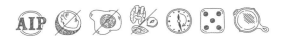

Herby Skillet Mushrooms

Serves 2 ◦ Prep Time: 5 minutes ◦ Cook Time: 10 minutes

Mushrooms are magical and oh-so-good for you. Herbs too. So here is a skillet full of both!
It's the perfect side dish for a steak dinner.

3 Frozen Herb Blocks (page 109)

5 ounces whole cremini mushrooms

1 teaspoon fine salt

2 tablespoons white wine vinegar

◦ Heat a 15-inch skillet over medium heat. When it's hot, put the herb blocks in the skillet. While they begin to melt, wipe the mushroom caps with a paper towel and remove the stems.

◦ Place the mushrooms cap side up in the skillet and sear for 4 to 5 minutes, then use tongs to flip them over. Sprinkle with the salt and sear for another 4 to 5 minutes, until very tender. Use a spoon to baste the mushrooms with the melted herb blocks.

◦ Add the vinegar to the skillet, stir well, and spoon the mushrooms into a serving dish. Serve hot.

◦ Store leftovers in the fridge for up to 3 days. Enjoy cold or sauté over medium heat to reheat.

Per serving: Calories **262** · Fat **27.1g** · Total Carbs **3.6g** · Fiber **0.7g** · Protein **2g**

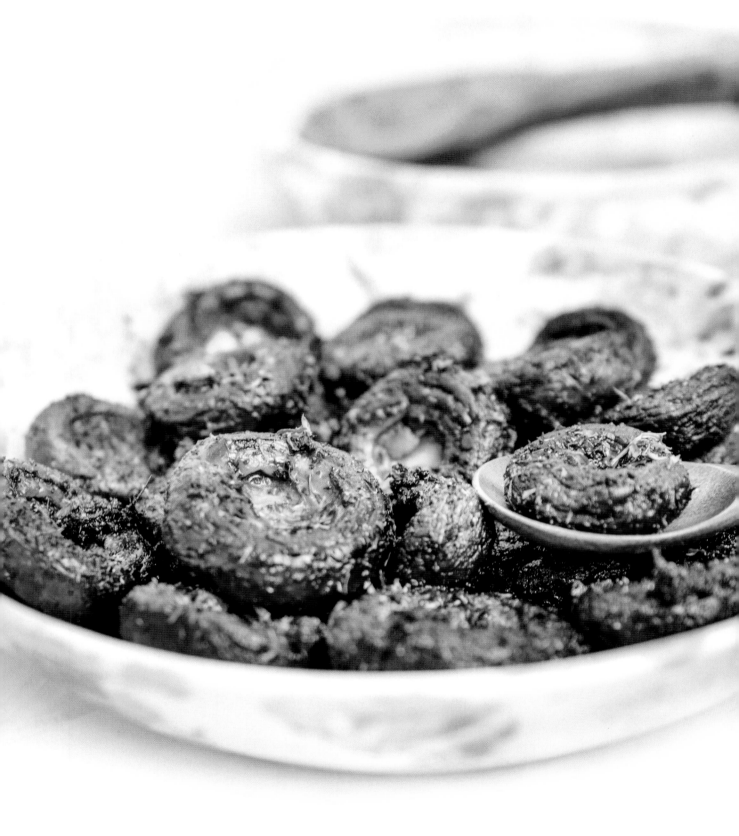

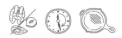

Fiber-Rich Naan

Serves 6 ◦ Prep Time: 15 minutes ◦ Cook Time: 15 minutes

Fiber is known for its ability to keep elimination regular and improve insulin sensitivity, but my favorite function of fiber is blocking estrogen from being reabsorbed in the colon. Yes, we eliminate excess hormones via the gut, but sometimes they are not eliminated properly, and that may cause imbalances. Today, many women face estrogen dominance, and I believe fiber to be useful for this. Bonus, this naan is so good—it makes a great dough that has a pull and chew to it. This is a wonderful nut-free and dairy-free bread that cooks up in a skillet and reheats perfectly!

½ cup whole psyllium husks

⅓ cup coconut flour

½ teaspoon fine salt

3 egg whites, whisked

2 tablespoons apple cider vinegar

¾ cup very warm filtered water

3 tablespoons extra-virgin olive oil, divided

◦ Whisk together the psyllium husks, coconut flour, and salt in a large bowl. Add the egg whites and vinegar and mix well.

◦ Add the warm water and mix until a dough forms. Then, using a rubber spatula, fold the dough several times as you slowly drizzle in 1 tablespoon of the olive oil.

◦ Let the dough rest for 2 to 3 minutes, then shape it into 6 evenly sized balls.

◦ Heat a large skillet over medium-high heat. When it's hot, drizzle the remaining 2 tablespoons of oil into the skillet.

◦ Use your fingers to flatten the balls until they're about the size of your palm and ¼ inch thick. Use a spatula to transfer 3 pieces at a time to the skillet. Cook for 3 to 4 minutes per side, flipping once. They will puff up as they cook. When done, they should have a nice browned crust and look cooked through, not doughy. Remove the naan from the pan and cook the remaining 3 pieces.

◦ To store, wrap the naan in paper towels to absorb moisture and store in an airtight container in the fridge for up to 4 days. Reheat in a skillet over medium heat or in a toaster for 3 to 5 minutes.

Per serving: Calories **109** · Fat **7.7g** · Total Carbs **6.8g** · Fiber **4.9g** · Protein **2.7g**

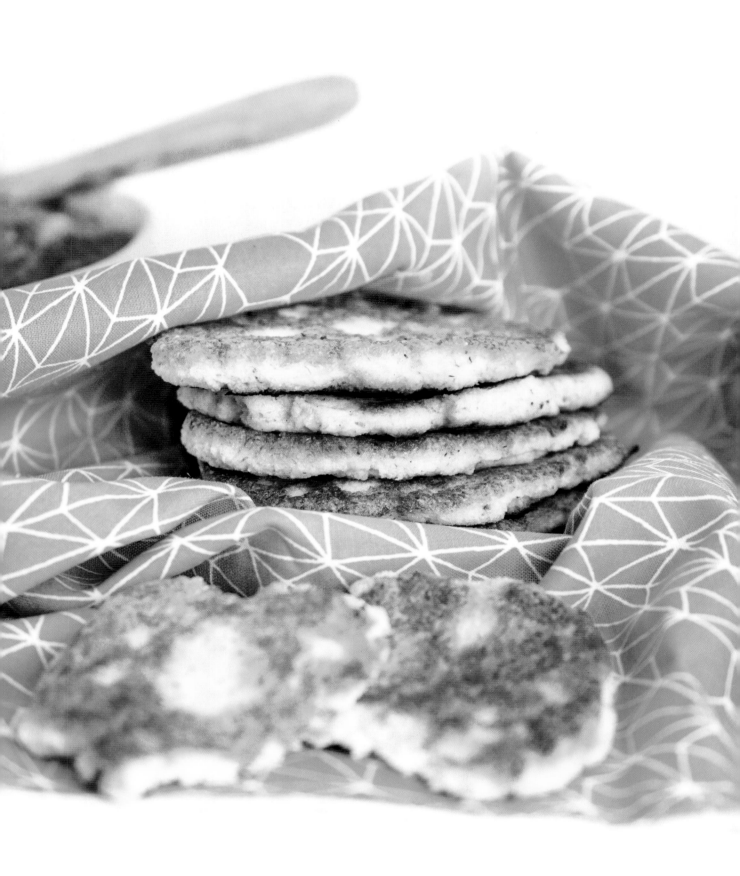

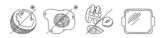

Cauliflower "Fried" Rice

Serves 4 ◦ Prep Time: 15 minutes ◦ Cook Time: 30 minutes

This recipe also lives on my blog; I've tweaked it a bit for this book, but the amazing flavor and texture are still there. This is a recipe that people fall in love with and call "the best thing I've eaten." It's also going to forever change the way you make cauliflower rice. What I love about this hearty side dish is that simply adding some shrimp or shredded chicken makes it an entrée!

2 (10-ounce) bags frozen riced cauliflower (about 4 cups)

½ cup chopped broccoli florets

¼ cup finely diced carrots

¼ cup finely diced onions

¼ cup shelled hemp seeds (aka hemp hearts)

1 teaspoon fine salt

1 teaspoon garlic powder

1 teaspoon ginger powder

½ teaspoon ground black pepper

3 tablespoons melted lard or bacon fat

3 tablespoons coconut aminos, divided

2 cooked scrambled eggs

1 tablespoon sesame seeds

1 tablespoon toasted sesame oil

1 green onion, thinly sliced

◦ Place an oven rack in the middle position. Preheat the oven to 400°F.

◦ Toss the riced cauliflower, broccoli, carrots, onions, hemp seeds, and dried seasonings together on a sheet pan.

◦ Drizzle everything with the lard. Toss again to mix well, then spread the mixture evenly over the sheet pan in a thin layer.

◦ Drizzle 2 tablespoons of the coconut aminos over everything. Roast on the middle rack of the oven for 25 to 30 minutes, until parts of the cauliflower are browned and toasty, practically burnt.

◦ Remove the pan from the oven and use a thin spatula to scrape up and mix together the toasty rice. Add the remaining tablespoon of coconut aminos, the eggs, sesame seeds, and sesame oil and mix well. Garnish with the sliced green onions and dig in!

◦ Store leftovers in the fridge for up to 4 days. To reheat, sauté in a skillet over medium heat for 5 minutes.

note: *If you do well with white rice and like to consume it on occasion, you can use half the amount of riced cauliflower and mix in 2 cups of leftover rice—perfect for a carb-up meal. Cooled and reheated rice becomes resistant starch, which benefits your gut microbiome and is less likely than regular white rice to spike your blood sugar. See pages 23 to 27 for more on blood sugar regulation.*

modifications: *To make this dish coconut-free, use low-sodium gluten-free tamari or liquid aminos instead of the coconut aminos. To make it egg-free, just leave them out.*

Per serving: Calories **294** · Fat **21.8g** · Total Carbs **16.3g** · Fiber **5.5g** · Protein **8.5g**

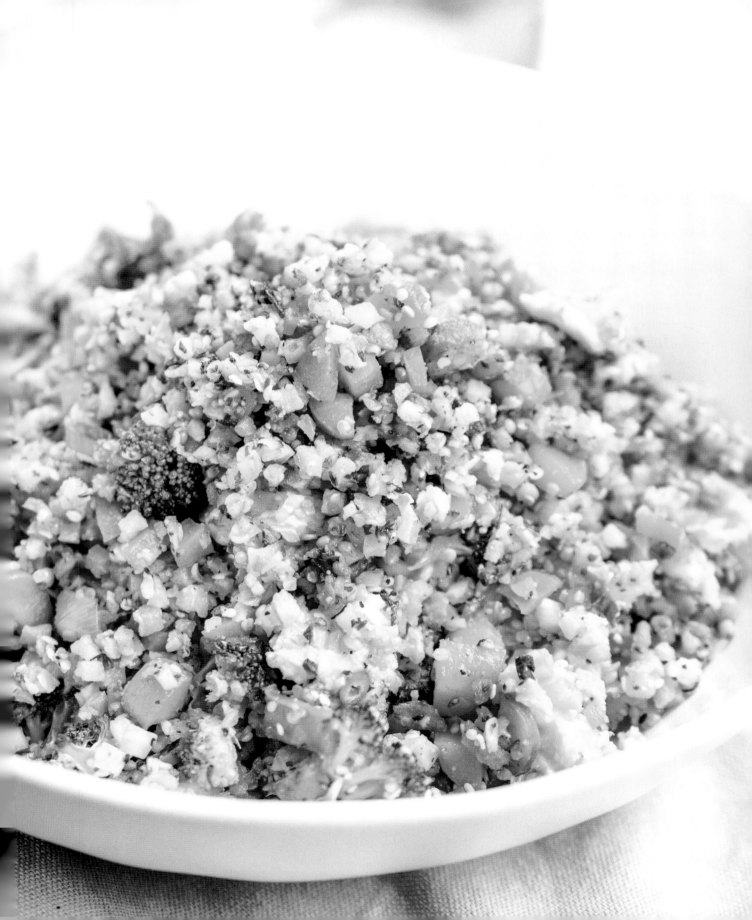

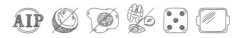

Crispy Garlic Rice

Serves 4 ◦ Prep Time: 5 minutes ◦ Cook Time: 30 minutes

I rarely do plain anything, and plain cauliflower rice makes me sad. Most of us who have left grains behind have done so for health reasons, to improve blood sugar regulation or gut health, but we often miss them. Plain cauliflower rice is a lame excuse for a replacement—but seasoning and roasting it magically turns it into a side dish worth craving! This super garlicky recipe uses both fresh garlic and garlic powder for a flavor kick you won't soon forget. With packaged riced cauliflower available everywhere now, there is no excuse not to get in on this trend!

1 pound frozen riced cauliflower

1 teaspoon fine salt

1 teaspoon garlic powder

8 cloves garlic, minced

2 tablespoons extra-virgin olive oil

◦ Place an oven rack in the middle position. Preheat the oven to 400°F.

◦ Toss all of the ingredients together on a sheet pan and spread the mixture evenly over the sheet pan in a thin layer.

◦ Roast on the middle rack of the oven for 25 to 30 minutes, until parts of the cauliflower are browned and toasty, practically burnt.

◦ Remove the pan from the oven and use a spatula to scrape up and mix together the toasty rice. Serve hot!

◦ Store leftovers in the fridge for up to 4 days. To reheat, sauté in a skillet over medium heat for 5 minutes.

Per serving: Calories **105** · Fat **7.5g** · Total Carbs **7.9g** · Fiber **2.9g** · Protein **3.2g**

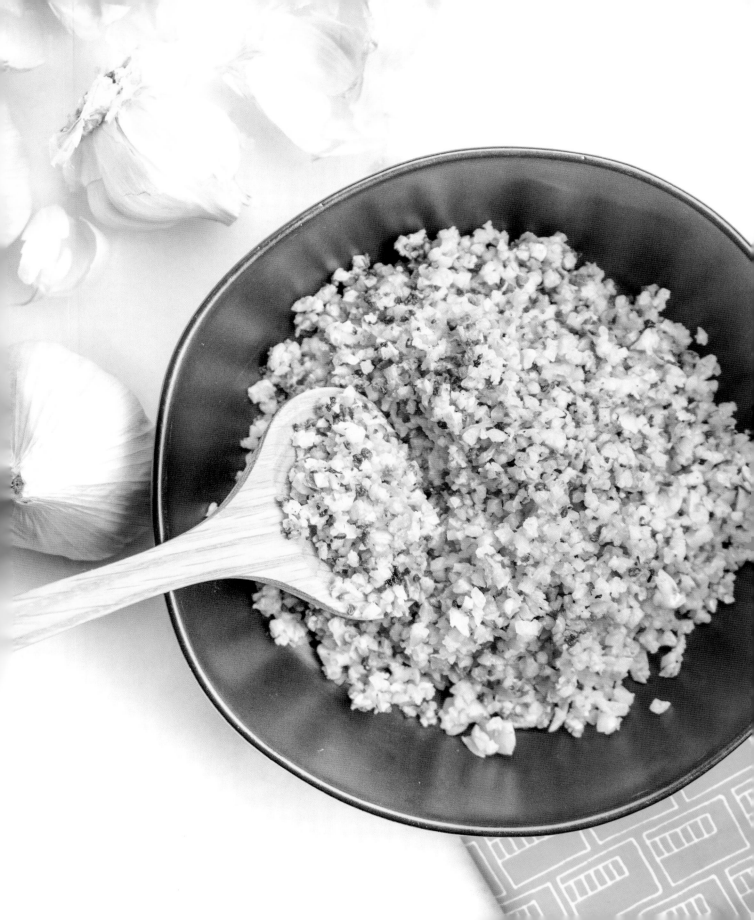

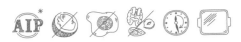

Spicy Yellow Rice

Serves 4 ○ Prep Time: 5 minutes ○ Cook Time: 25 minutes

For lovers of Latin American food, here's a low-carb arroz amarillo with a little added heat! It's perfect for taco bowls with Hail Mary Chicken (page 258) or Tasty Mojo Pork (page 204). *¡Buen provecho!*

1 pound frozen riced cauliflower

2 teaspoons garlic powder

1 teaspoon dried oregano leaves

1 teaspoon fine salt

1 teaspoon ground cumin

1 teaspoon ground white pepper

1 teaspoon turmeric powder

2 tablespoons extra-virgin olive oil

1 tablespoon melted ghee

modifications: *To make this dish AIP compliant, omit the cumin and white pepper and double the garlic powder.*

○ Place an oven rack in the middle position. Preheat the oven to 400°F.

○ Toss all of the ingredients together on a sheet pan and spread the mixture evenly over the sheet pan in a thin layer.

○ Roast on the middle rack for 25 minutes, or until parts of the cauliflower are browned and toasty, practically burnt.

○ Remove the pan from the oven and use a spatula to scrape up and mix together the toasty rice. Serve hot!

○ Store leftovers in the fridge for up to 4 days. To reheat, sauté in a skillet over medium heat for 5 minutes.

Per serving: Calories **166** · Fat **13.3g** · Total Carbs **10.1g** · Fiber **4.2g** · Protein **4.1g**

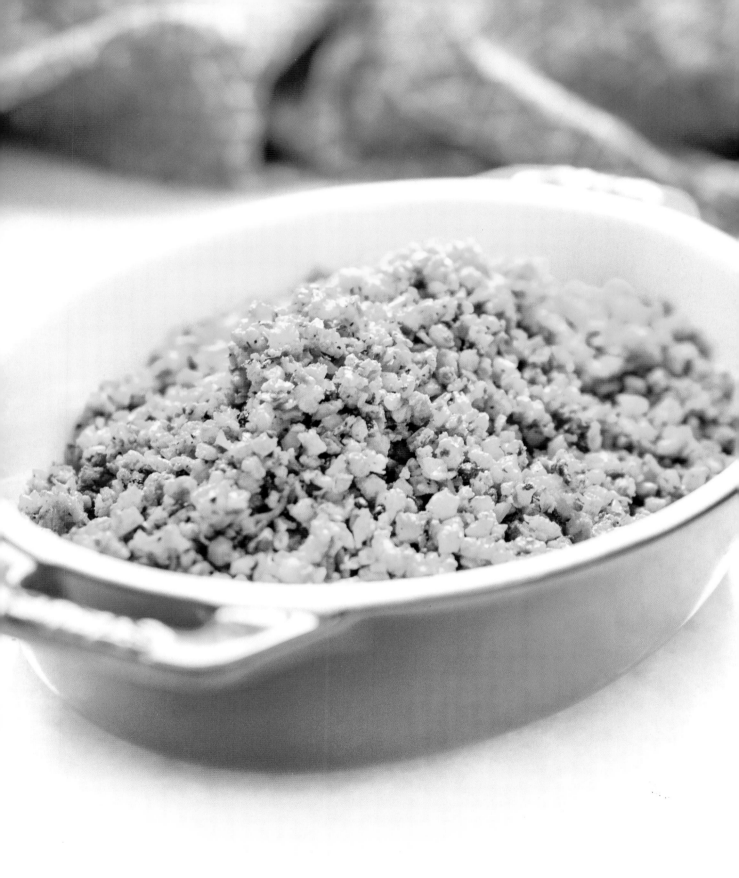

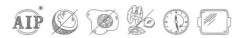

Rustic Roasted Summer Squash

Serves 4 ○ Prep Time: 8 minutes ○ Cook Time: 22 minutes

There comes a time each summer when zucchini is everywhere. Your CSA box is packed with it, or your garden is overrun, maybe your neighbor keeps leaving baskets at your door, or your grocery store has piles of it on sale. Zucchini noodles are great, but this roasted summer squash with a heavily seasoned crust is such an ode to this summer veg!

4 large zucchini and/or yellow squash (about 3 pounds), sliced on the bias

2 teaspoons fine salt

1 teaspoon garlic powder

1 teaspoon ground cumin

½ teaspoon ground black pepper

½ teaspoon ground sumac or grated lemon zest

2 tablespoons extra-virgin olive oil

modifications: To make this dish AIP compliant, replace the cumin and black pepper with 1 teaspoon onion powder and 1 teaspoon turmeric powder, and use lemon zest instead of sumac.

○ Place an oven rack in the middle position. Preheat the oven to 425°F.

○ Place the squash slices on a sheet pan and toss with the dried seasonings and olive oil until evenly coated. Arrange the slices so that they are lying flat on the pan and not overlapping.

○ Roast on the middle rack of the oven for 22 minutes, or until tender and well browned. Remove from the oven and serve hot.

○ Store leftovers in the fridge for up to 4 days. Reheat in a preheated 350°F oven for 5 minutes.

Per serving: Calories **120** · Fat **8g** · Total Carbs **10.8g** · Fiber **3.4g** · Protein **4.2g**

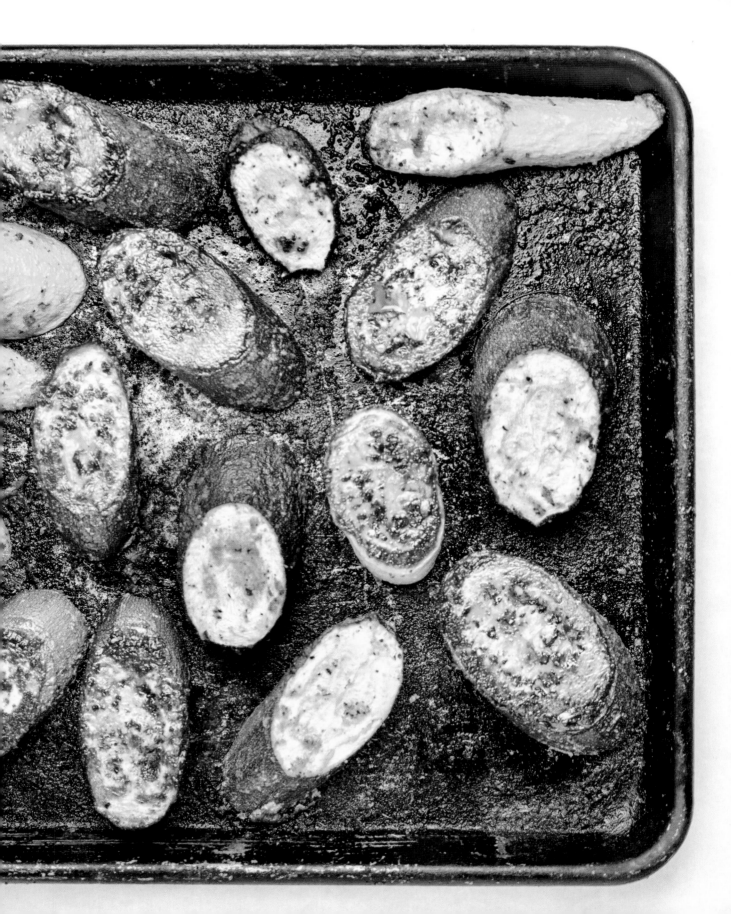

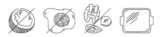

Roasted Garlic "Hummus"

Serves 8 ⊙ Prep Time: 15 minutes ⊙ Cook Time: 25 minutes

I made the hummus at my mom's restaurant for many years, and it was killer. This cauliflower-based hummus tastes just like the real thing. Roasting the cauliflower gives it the same slight nuttiness that chickpeas have and takes the texture from watery to starchy. Add plenty of tahini, lemon, and garlic, and boom! You've got a super convincing hummus that is easy to digest, lower in carbs, and packed with vitamin C and healthy fats. Remember, kids, if cauliflower can grow up to be pizza, rice, and hummus, you can be anything you want to be!

1 medium head cauliflower

10 cloves garlic, peeled

⅓ cup extra-virgin olive oil, divided, plus more for drizzling if desired

¾ teaspoon fine salt

⅓ cup tahini

Juice of 2 lemons

½ teaspoon ground black pepper

½ teaspoon ground cumin

⊙ Preheat the oven to 375°F.

⊙ Core the cauliflower and break the head into florets. On a sheet pan, toss the florets with the garlic cloves, 2 tablespoons of the olive oil, and the salt. Roast for 25 minutes, or until the cauliflower is tender and lightly browned.

⊙ Transfer the roasted cauliflower and garlic to a food processor. Pulse until broken down into crumbles and cooled off a bit.

⊙ Add the tahini, lemon juice, black pepper, cumin, and remaining olive oil and puree until smooth.

⊙ Use a rubber spatula to transfer the hummus to a glass bowl with a tight-fitting lid. Store in the fridge for up to a week. You can drizzle a little olive oil on top as a garnish before serving!

awesome additions: *As you can see in the photo, I like to use this hummus in a grazing platter with deli meats, grain-free crackers, Marcona almonds, broccoli florets, and celery sticks. It's also great with Crispy Chicken Chips (page 306): a balanced meal disguised as hummus and pita!*

Per serving: Calories **165** · Fat **13.8g** · Total Carbs **9.3g** · Fiber **3.1g** · Protein **3.9g**

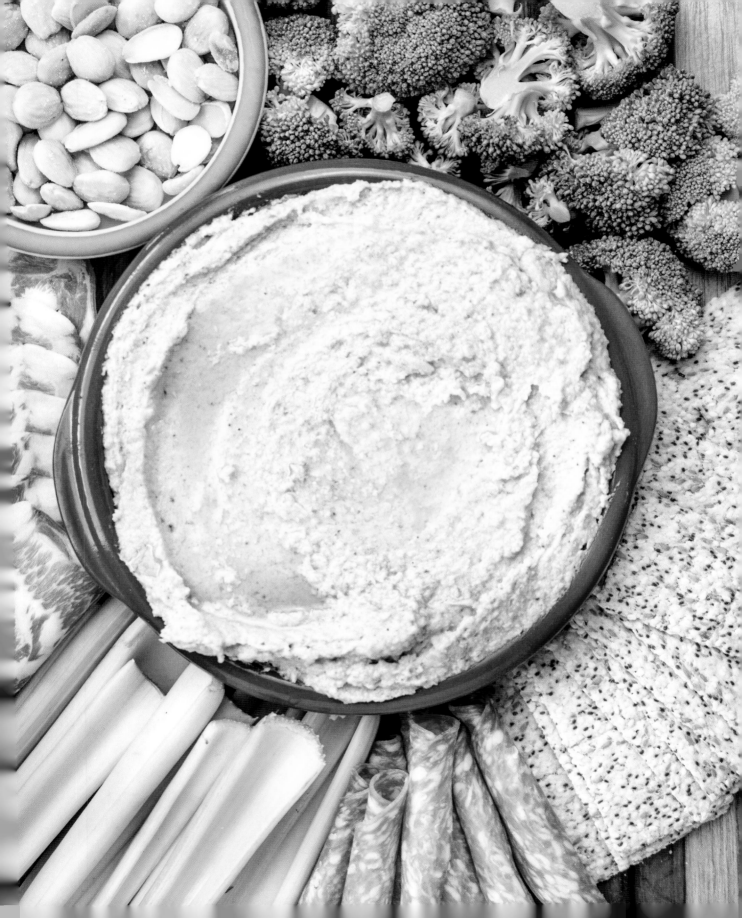

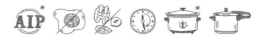

Pressure Cooker Saag

Serves 6 ○ Prep Time: 10 minutes ○ Cook Time: 20 minutes

I would not have attempted a nightshade-free saag (a creamed leafy green dish made in India) had it not been for my friend Amanda Workman. Amanda grew up all over the world and spent a lot of time in India, where she learned to cook the local cuisine from her surrogate family. She loves the Crispy Ginger Lime Chicken Wings recipe on my website, and she took that sauce and transformed it into a nightshade-free umami base for nightshade-free Indian cooking. Saag normally uses tomato paste, which is a hard-no food for me, so this substitute is genius, and Amanda was nice enough to share her secrets with me. This dish packs not only amazing vitamin and mineral content but a ton of healing spices too!

2 pounds frozen spinach

2 tablespoons ghee or coconut oil, plus more for serving

1 cup diced onions (about 2 small onions)

4 cloves garlic, minced

1 teaspoon dried dill weed

2 teaspoons ground cumin

1 teaspoon garlic powder

1 teaspoon ginger powder

1 teaspoon turmeric powder

1 tablespoon apple cider vinegar

¼ cup bone broth

2 tablespoons coconut aminos

1 tablespoon nutritional yeast

1 teaspoon fish sauce

1 teaspoon fine salt

modifications: *To make this dish AIP compliant, omit the cumin and use coconut oil, not ghee.*

○ Put the frozen spinach in a large colander in the sink. Run warm water over the spinach for 2 minutes, moving it around with your hands to break up the pieces, then leave it there to drain and thaw.

○ Put a pressure cooker in sauté mode. When it's hot, put the ghee in the cooker, followed by the onions. Sauté for about 4 minutes, until tender, then add the garlic, dill, and spices. Cook for another 5 minutes, or until you have an aromatic paste.

○ Add the vinegar and deglaze the pot, scraping up the browned bits from the bottom. Stir in the broth, coconut aminos, nutritional yeast, and fish sauce.

○ Use your hands to press down firmly on the spinach in the colander to remove as much water as possible. Transfer the spinach to the pressure cooker, add the salt, and stir to combine all the ingredients.

○ Cancel the sauté function, then seal the lid and cook on low pressure for 7 minutes. Release the pressure manually. Open the lid and use an immersion blender to cream the mixture for 1 to 2 minutes, until creamy.

○ If there is a lot of fluid in the pot, the spinach had too much water left in it, but it's an easy fix: just simmer on sauté mode until the excess fluid is gone.

○ Transfer the saag to a serving bowl and top with a spoonful of ghee.

○ Store leftovers in the fridge for up to 5 days. To reheat, sauté in a skillet over medium heat for 5 minutes.

Slow Cooker Method: Follow the recipe as written, but instead of pressure cooking for 7 minutes, cook in a slow cooker on high for 2 hours. Then cream with the immersion blender and serve.

Per serving: Calories **105** · Fat **5.4g** · Total Carbs **11g** · Fiber **5.1g** · Protein **6.4g**

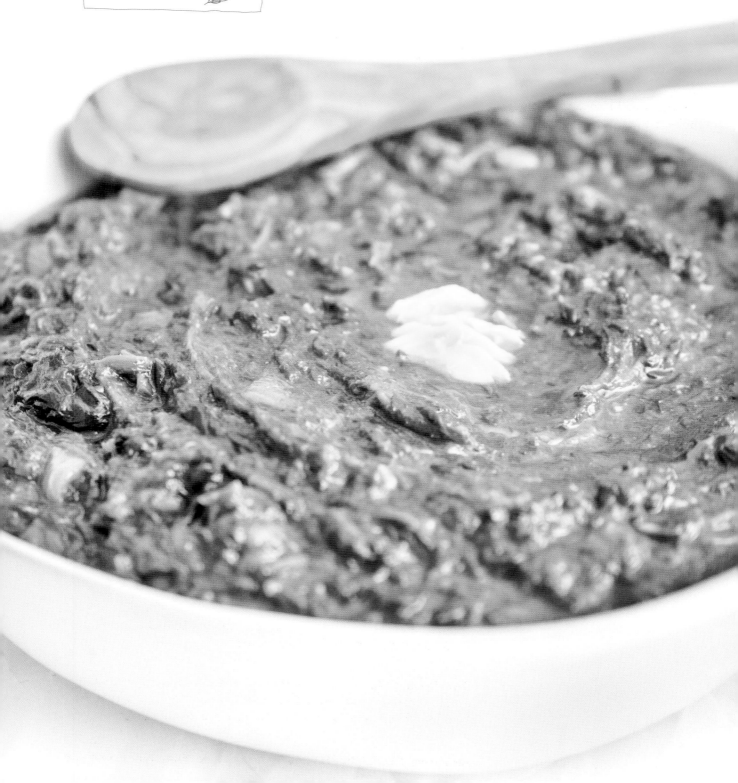

Get some stress support
with this delicious dose
of magnesium
and vitamin C.

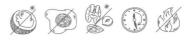

Cold Veggie Noodle Salad

Serves 2 ○ Prep Time: 15 minutes

With the exception of arugula and broccoli, there aren't many vegetables that I really enjoy raw. Yup, I said it. If you do see me eating raw veggies, you can count on them being covered in a delicious sauce. Case in point: this recipe. I could eat this salad all day! Use a vegetable peeler to make the ribbons.

½ large carrot, shaved into ribbons

1 medium zucchini, shaved into ribbons

1 green onion, sliced on the bias

1 clove garlic, minced

1 teaspoon sesame seeds, plus more for garnish

For the sauce:

2 tablespoons unsweetened, unsalted sunflower seed butter or cashew butter

1 tablespoon Dijon mustard

1 tablespoon toasted sesame oil

2 teaspoons coconut aminos

○ In a medium-sized bowl, toss the carrot and zucchini ribbons with the green onion, garlic, and sesame seeds.

○ In a small bowl, whisk together all of the sauce ingredients, then pour the sauce over the veggies and toss to mix. Garnish with sesame seeds and serve right away.

○ Store the sauce and veggies separately (so the veggie noodles don't become soggy) in the fridge for up to 3 days. Mix and serve when you want!

modifications: *To make this salad coconut-free, use low-sodium gluten-free tamari or liquid aminos instead of the coconut aminos.*

Per serving: Calories **213** · Fat **17.6g** · Total Carbs **9.2g** · Fiber **3.4g** · Protein **5.6g**

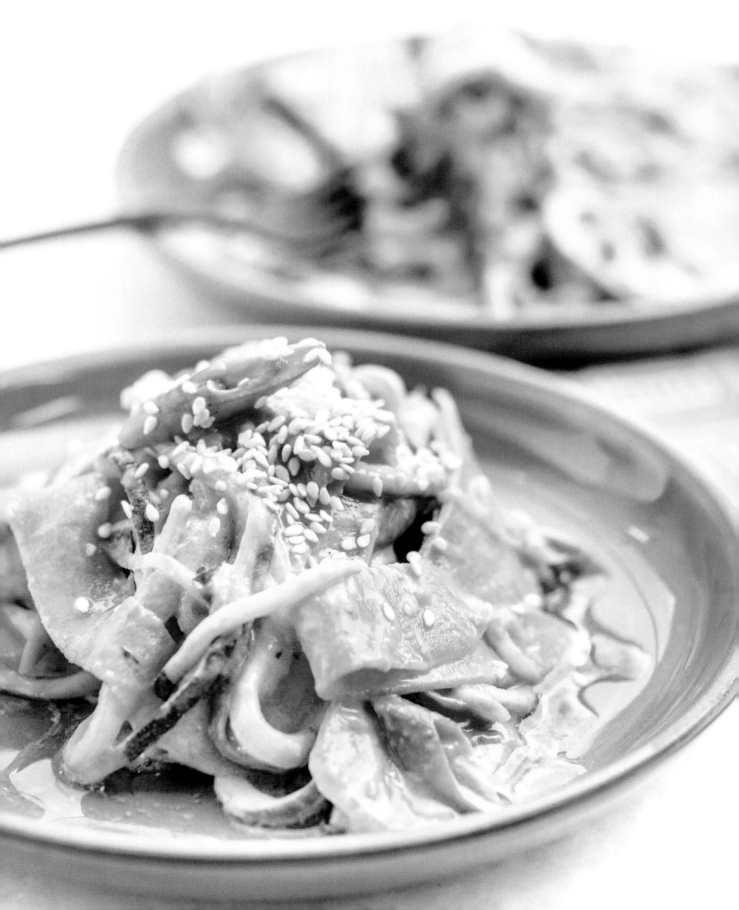

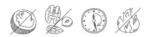

Not Yo' Momma's Coleslaw

Serves 6 ○ Prep Time: 10 minutes

Coleslaw is a dish that had amazing potential to be good for you, but took a wrong turn with added sugar and hydrogenated seed-based oils. Here I have given this potluck, barbecue, and picnic classic a makeover. Not only does it look and taste good, but it's also impressively good for you!

10 ounces coleslaw mix

1 cup sliced green onions (about 6 green onions)

1 cup sprouted pumpkin seeds (see notes, page 178)

½ cup chopped fresh parsley

½ cup Horseradish Mayo (page 94)

1 teaspoon fine salt

- Put all of the ingredients in a large bowl and mix well. Serve chilled.

- Store leftovers in the fridge for up to 4 days.

Per serving: Calories **223** · Fat **19.2g** · Total Carbs **7.2g** · Fiber **3.3g** · Protein **7.2g**

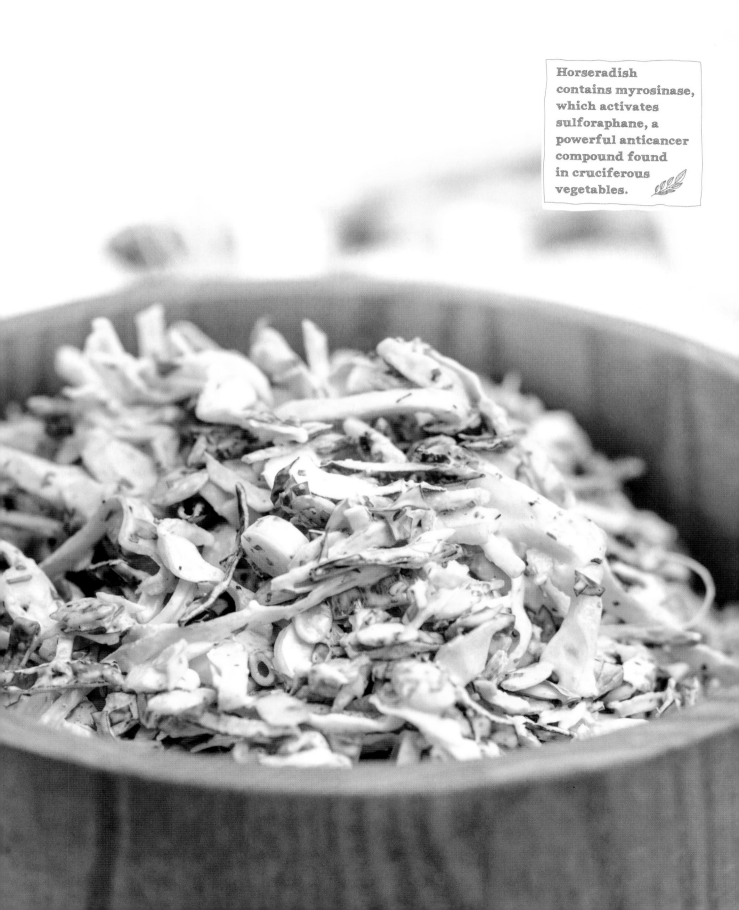

Horseradish contains myrosinase, which activates sulforaphane, a powerful anticancer compound found in cruciferous vegetables.

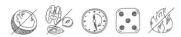

Ceci's Salad

Serves 4 ● Prep Time: 10 minutes

Holistic nutritional theories conclude that raw carrots are particularly good at clearing excess estrogen out of the gut. The fiber acts as a little internal scrub, not feeding the bacteria in our gut but cleaning house. One problem: I don't like raw carrots...unless I'm having this salad, created by my tia Ceci. I hope she doesn't mind that I'm sharing her recipe with all of you. I've added phytochemical-rich radishes because I love their peppery flavor!

8 ounces carrots

8 ounces radishes

5 cloves garlic, minced

¼ cup plus 2 tablespoons avocado oil mayonnaise

Pinch of fine salt

● Use a grater or the grater attachment of a food processor to shred the carrots and radishes.

● Put the carrots and radishes in a large bowl and mix with the garlic, mayonnaise, and salt. Taste and add more salt if needed.

● Store leftovers in the fridge for up to 3 days.

Per serving: Calories **162** · Fat **15.2g** · Total Carbs **8.4g** · Fiber **2.6g** · Protein **1.1g**

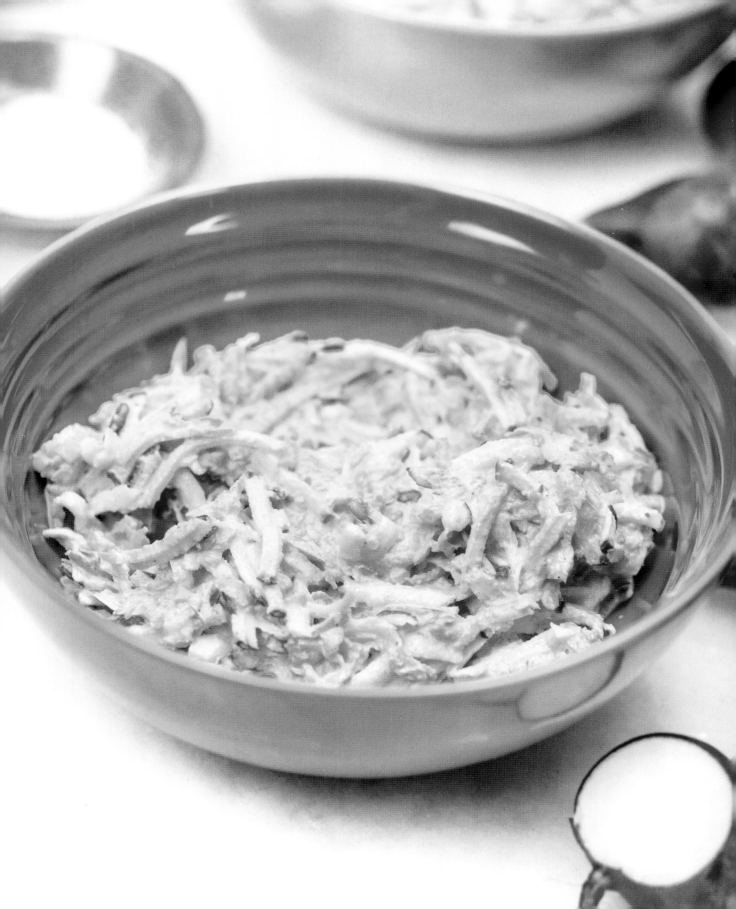

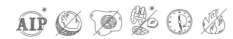

Berry Much Like Caprese Salad

Serves 5 ○ Prep Time: 15 minutes

Every cookbook needs at least one cheesy food pun. This caprese copycat recipe uses strawberries, zucchini, and our very own dairy-free mozzarella for an Italian-style salad that is perfect for those who can't do dairy or nightshades—like yours truly!

4 Mozz Blocks (page 104), cut into bite-sized pieces

12 ounces strawberries, quartered (about 2 cups)

4 ounces zucchini, finely diced (about ½ cup)

1 tablespoon fresh thyme leaves, minced

1 tablespoon aged balsamic vinegar (see notes, page 90)

1 tablespoon extra-virgin olive oil

1 teaspoon garlic powder

⅛ teaspoon fine salt

⅛ teaspoon ground black pepper

○ Place all of the ingredients in a large bowl and, using a large spoon, gently toss to combine. Serve chilled.

○ Store leftovers in the fridge for up to 3 days.

modifications: *To make this salad AIP compliant, make the AIP version of the Mozz Blocks and omit the black pepper. To make it nut-free, use the nut-free version of the Mozz Blocks.*

Per serving: Calories **145** · Fat **9.9g** · Total Carbs **10.4g** · Fiber **1.8g** · Protein **4.7g**

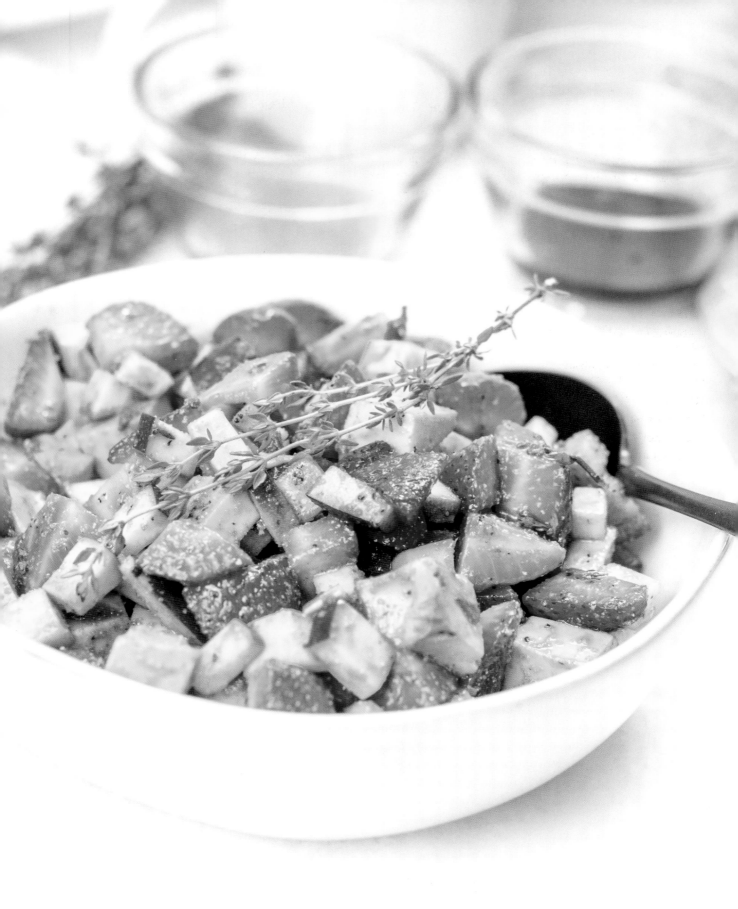

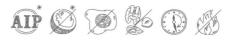

Smoked Salmon Dip

Serves 12 ◦ Prep Time: 10 minutes

This delicious dip has a favorable ratio of omega-3 to omega-6 fats—2:1! Keep a batch in the fridge for a quick no-cook snack. Smear this dip on your favorite grain-free crackers or roll it up in lettuce wraps. The flavor profile was inspired by Hawaiian poke—yum!

8 ounces smoked salmon

1 small red onion, minced

½ cup coconut cream

¼ cup fresh cilantro leaves

2 tablespoons toasted sesame oil

2 teaspoons apple cider vinegar

2 teaspoons coconut aminos

2 tablespoons sesame seeds, for garnish

modifications: *To make this dip AIP compliant, omit the sesame oil and sesame seeds. To make it coconut-free, use ½ cup shelled hemp seeds (aka hemp hearts) and 1 tablespoon unsweetened dairy-free milk instead of the coconut cream.*

◦ Place all of the ingredients except the sesame seeds in a food processor. Pulse until it becomes a creamy, mostly smooth dip.

◦ Use a rubber spatula to transfer the dip to a 16-ounce glass jar and sprinkle it with the sesame seeds. Store in the fridge for up to 10 days. Always use a clean spoon to scoop out the dip.

Per serving: Calories **154** · Fat **10.9g** · Total Carbs **1.5g** · Fiber **1g** · Protein **12.4g**

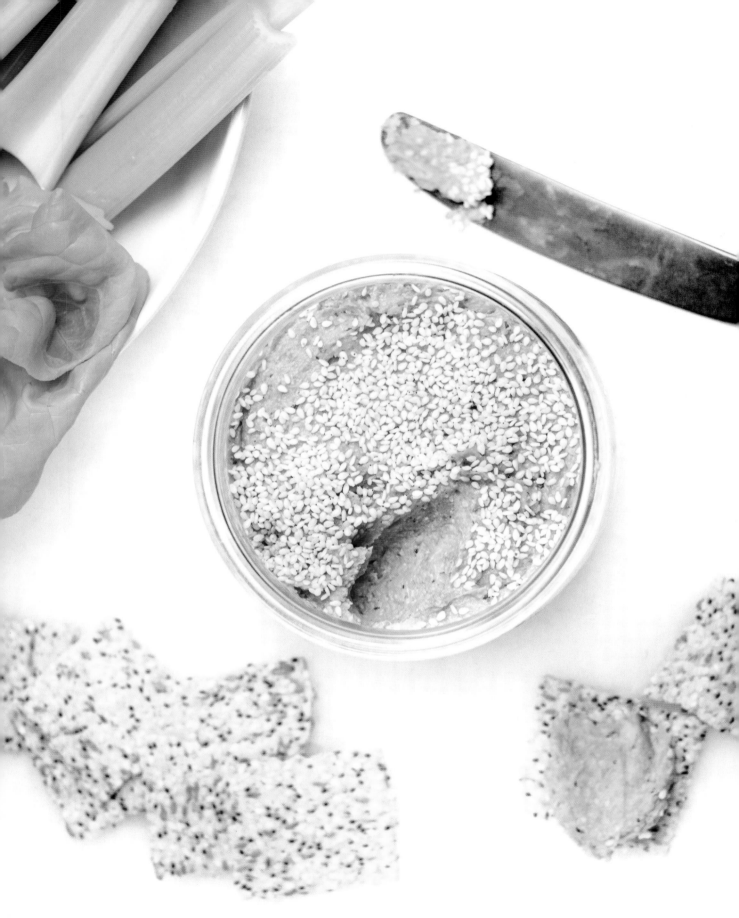

SWEETS + BEVERAGES

"Quality over quantity" is my motto when it comes to sweets. This chapter delivers just that: amazing treats that use only natural sweeteners and won't spike your blood sugar. I've mostly stuck to yacón syrup, which is made from the yacón root. It's like molasses but much sweeter. Used in small amounts, yacón syrup is delicious and easy to digest. I also use stevia glycerite, which is my preferred form of stevia because it does not have an aftertaste. It's not as strong as regular liquid stevia, so if you're using another type of stevia, be sure to adjust the amount. I've also added options for nutritive sweeteners like raw honey in the notes.

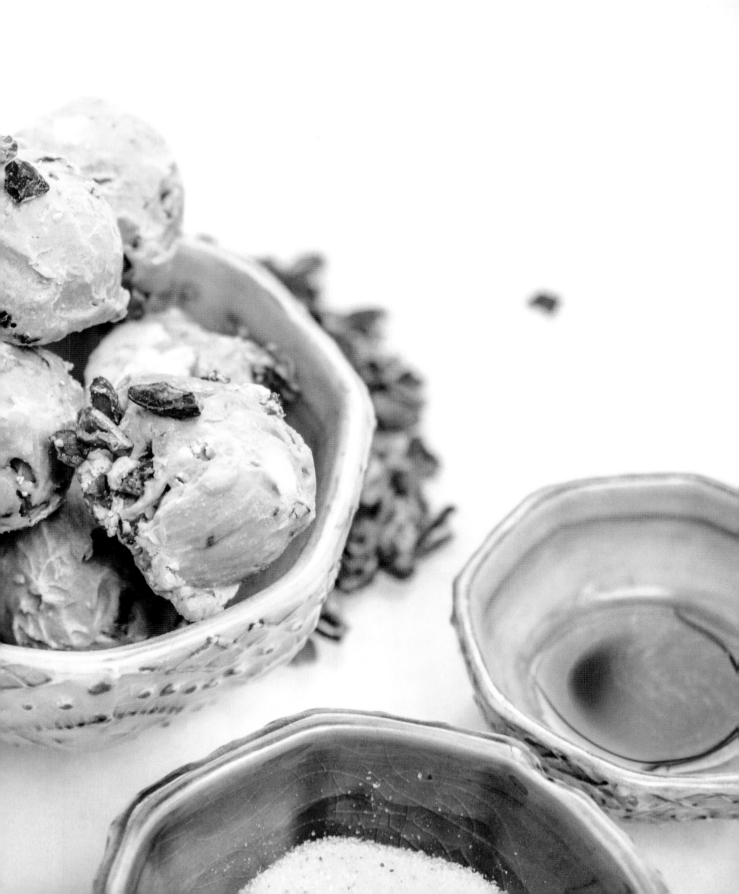

Low-Carb Blueberry Muffins

Makes 1 dozen muffins (1 per serving) ◦ Prep Time: 20 minutes ◦ Cook Time: 30 minutes

Moist blueberry muffins without cream cheese? Can it be? Yes, it can! These muffins are oh so delicious. High in fiber and lightly sweetened, they are perfect for a snack or treat.

½ cup sifted coconut flour

¼ cup whole psyllium husks

1 teaspoon baking powder (see note, page 148)

½ teaspoon fine salt

½ cup unsweetened, unsalted sunflower seed butter or cashew butter

½ cup canned unsweetened full-fat coconut milk

¼ cup melted (but not hot) coconut oil, ghee, or tallow

4 large eggs, room temperature

3 tablespoons yacón syrup (see notes)

1 teaspoon vanilla extract

1 cup fresh blueberries

2 teaspoons grated lemon zest

• Place an oven rack in the middle position. Preheat the oven to 350°F. Line a standard-size 12-cup muffin tin with cupcake liners.

• In a large bowl, whisk together the coconut flour, psyllium husks, baking powder, and salt.

• In a separate bowl, beat the sunflower seed butter, coconut milk, coconut oil, eggs, yacón syrup, and vanilla extract with an electric mixer until well combined and creamy. Add the wet mixture to the dry mixture and beat until a thick batter forms. Using a rubber spatula, fold in the blueberries and lemon zest.

• Using a ¼-cup scoop, evenly distribute the batter among the lined muffin wells. Bake on the middle rack of the oven for 25 to 30 minutes, until the muffins have risen and are round and golden on top.

• Remove the muffins from the oven and let them cool for 15 minutes, then unpan.

• Store in an airtight container in the fridge for up to 5 days.

notes: *You may use an equal amount of flaxseed meal in place of the psyllium husks.*

You may substitute stevia glycerite for the yacón syrup: use 2 teaspoons and add 1 tablespoon of fat. If you do well with raw honey, you can use ¼ cup of honey in place of the yacón syrup.

Per serving: Calories **176** · Fat **12.7g** · Total Carbs **10.3g** · Fiber **4.3g** · Protein **5.2g**

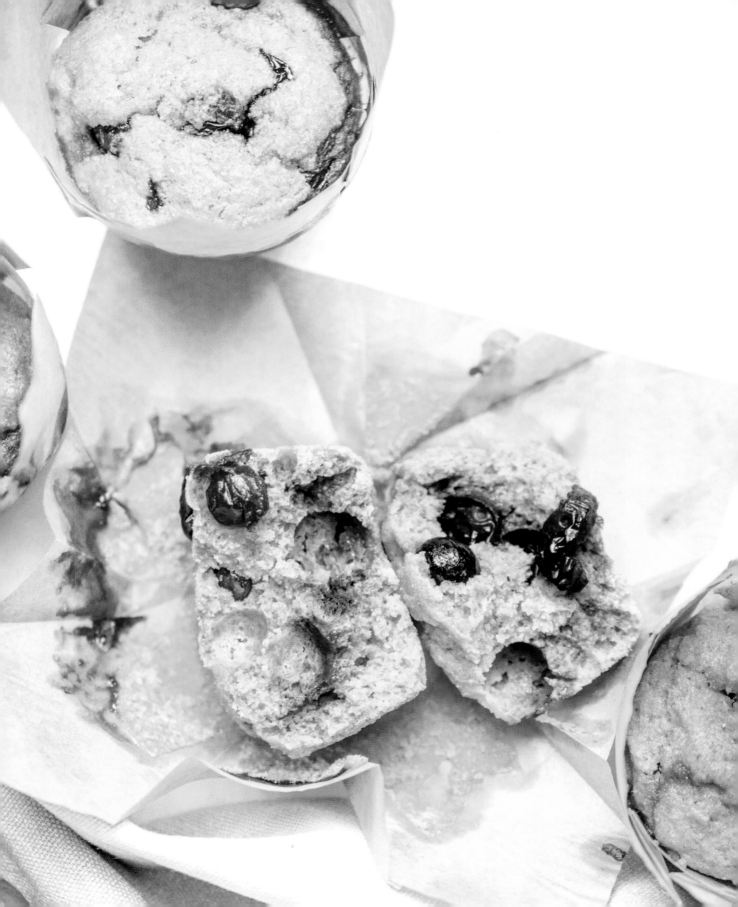

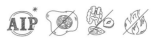

Chocolate Avocado Ice Cream

Serves 3 ◦ Prep Time: 10 minutes, plus 45 minutes to freeze avocados

Yes, it is delicious. No, it does not taste like avocado! This no-churn frozen treat is packed with potassium, fiber, and antioxidants. The possibilities are endless here. You can add nuts or seeds, swap the vanilla extract for peppermint, or go with chocolate chips for a more decadent treat. Make it your way—you can't go wrong with this avocado ice cream.

2 ripe Hass avocados, peeled, pitted, and finely diced

¼ to ½ cup canned unsweetened full-fat coconut milk

1 teaspoon stevia glycerite, or 2 tablespoons yacón syrup

1 teaspoon vanilla extract

¼ cup cacao powder

¼ teaspoon fine salt

1 tablespoon cacao nibs, for garnish

◦ Spread the diced avocados on a plate or tray. Set the tray in the freezer until the avocados are completely frozen, about 45 minutes.

◦ Transfer the avocados to a food processor. Turn it on and slowly pour in the coconut milk, adding just enough to create a smooth, creamy mixture. Hold the food processor while you do this; the frozen avocados are hard to mix and might make your appliance jump around.

◦ Add the remaining ingredients, except the cacao nibs, and process until well combined and completely smooth and creamy. Taste and add more sweetener or salt as needed. Scoop into bowls, sprinkle with the cacao nibs, and enjoy!

◦ If you're making this ice cream for later, use a rubber spatula to scrape the ice cream into a freezer-safe container and store it in the freezer for up to a month. Let it sit at room temperature for 10 to 20 minutes to soften before serving.

modifications: *To make this ice cream AIP compliant, use yacón syrup rather than stevia, replace the cacao powder with carob powder, and omit the vanilla extract and cacao nibs.*

Per serving: Calories **197** · Fat **15.9g** · Total Carbs **11.9g** · Fiber **7.4g** · Protein **3.1g**

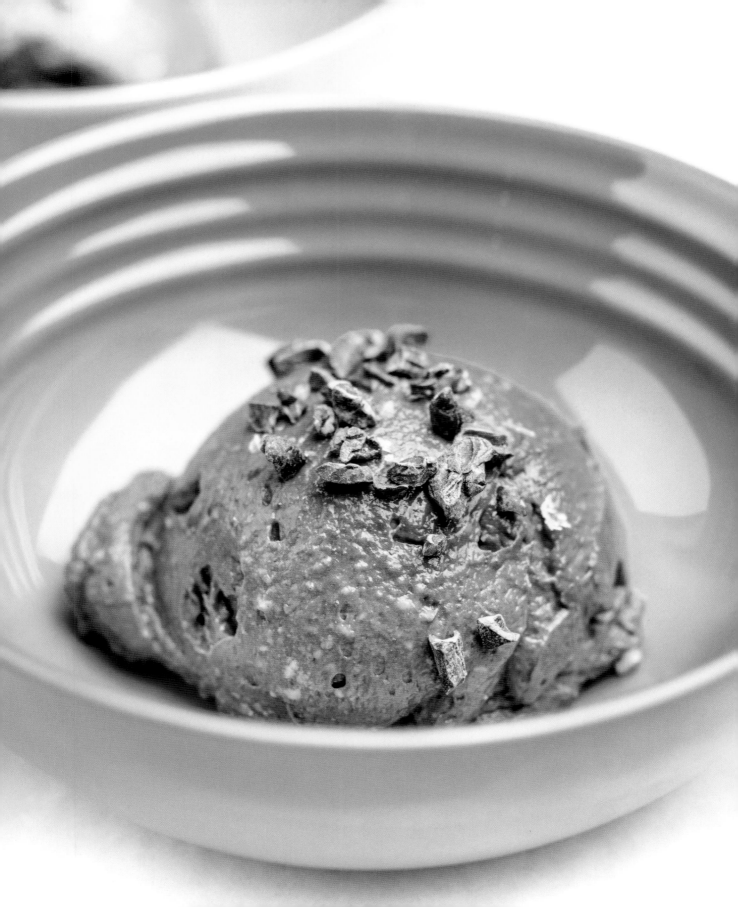

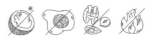

Tahini Cookie Cream Bites

Makes 9 fat bombs (1 per serving) ◦ Prep Time: 15 minutes, plus 20 minutes to freeze

Tahini has been around for over four thousand years. This rich sesame seed butter, a staple in Middle Eastern cuisine, was once served to royalty and thought of as food for the gods! It's exceptionally high in fat and protein, and it's an essential part of these no-bake fat bombs. They also include antioxidant-rich and sugar-free cacao nibs in lieu of chocolate chips for a bite-sized treat that packs some serious benefits.

½ cup coconut cream

2 tablespoons cacao nibs, plus more for garnish if desired

2 tablespoons tahini

1 teaspoon vanilla extract

5 drops stevia glycerite, or more if desired

¼ teaspoon fine salt

- Place all of the ingredients in a large bowl and whisk until well combined. Taste the mixture and add up to 5 drops more stevia glycerite, if desired. Freeze the mixture for 20 minutes, or until it is firm enough to hold a shape.

- Use a spoon or 2-teaspoon scoop to shape the mixture into 9 small balls. Set them in the freezer until hard, like frozen ice cream. Garnish with additional cacao nibs before serving, if desired.

- Store in an airtight container in the freezer for up to 2 months.

notes: *Use 1 teaspoon yacón syrup or raw honey instead of stevia if you prefer. You can also use peppermint instead of vanilla extract for a mint chip flavor.*

modifications: *To make these treats coconut-free, use cashew butter or cream cheese instead of the coconut cream. If you can't do tahini, any unsweetened nut or seed butter will do.*

awesome additions: *For a great anti-inflammatory treat, add some CBD oil.*

Per serving: Calories **85** · Fat **7.7g** · Total Carbs **2.2g** · Fiber **1.4g** · Protein **1.3g**

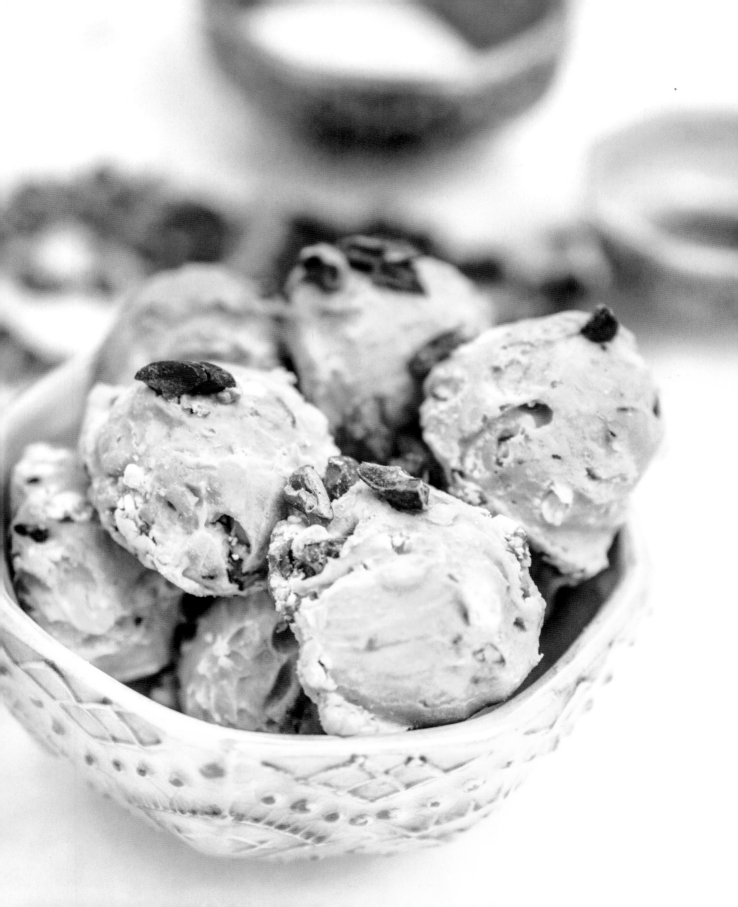

Flourless Chocolate Cake

Makes one 8-inch round cake (12 servings) ○ Prep Time: 20 minutes, plus 1 hour to cool ○ Cook Time: 35 minutes

This intensely dark and rich dessert, which has no added sweetener, originated with the 3-Ingredient Mug Cake that lives on my blog. I wanted to make it for my mom, who doesn't own a microwave—key for making the mug cake—so I mixed up the ingredients in a ramekin and baked it instead. The result was an elegant cake that was also sort of like a soufflé, and so delicious that I had to make a bigger one! When it's warm, it's melty and magical. When it's cold, it's dense and creamy, like fudge. Win-win!

2 tablespoons cacao powder, for dusting the pan

2 cups dark (85% cacao) chocolate chips (see notes)

1½ cups coconut cream, room temperature (see notes)

1 teaspoon vanilla extract

⅛ teaspoon fine salt

6 large eggs, whisked

Special equipment:

8-inch springform pan

○ Place an oven rack in the middle position. Preheat the oven to 350°F. Grease an 8-inch springform pan and dust it with the cacao powder.

○ Melt the chocolate in a double boiler, or place the chips in a microwave-safe container and microwave on medium power in 20-second increments until melted, stirring between increments.

○ Transfer the melted chocolate to a large mixing bowl and, while the chocolate is still hot, quickly whisk in the coconut cream, vanilla extract, and salt until a thick ganache forms. Whisk in the eggs until the ganache thickens further to become like pudding and lightens in color.

○ Pour the batter into the prepared pan. Bake on the middle rack of the oven until it rises and cracks slightly, about 30 minutes. It should look solid and not wet in the center. Remove the cake from the oven and let cool for 1 hour before unmolding. Slice and serve.

○ Store in an airtight container in the fridge for up to 5 days.

notes: *In place of the chocolate chips, you can use 12 ounces dark (85% cacao) chocolate, chopped. For the quantity of coconut cream used in this recipe, you will need 3 (13.5-ounce) cans of full-fat coconut milk. It's generally easier to extract coconut cream from cans of coconut milk after the cans have been chilled. If you chill your cans, be sure to allow the cream to come to room temperature before using it in this recipe.*

modifications: *To make this cake coconut-free, replace the coconut cream with heavy cream or Salted Cashew Cream (page 76)—both work very well.*

Per serving: Calories **285** · Fat **19.6g** · Total Carbs **12.5g** · Fiber **2.3g** · Protein **7.8g**

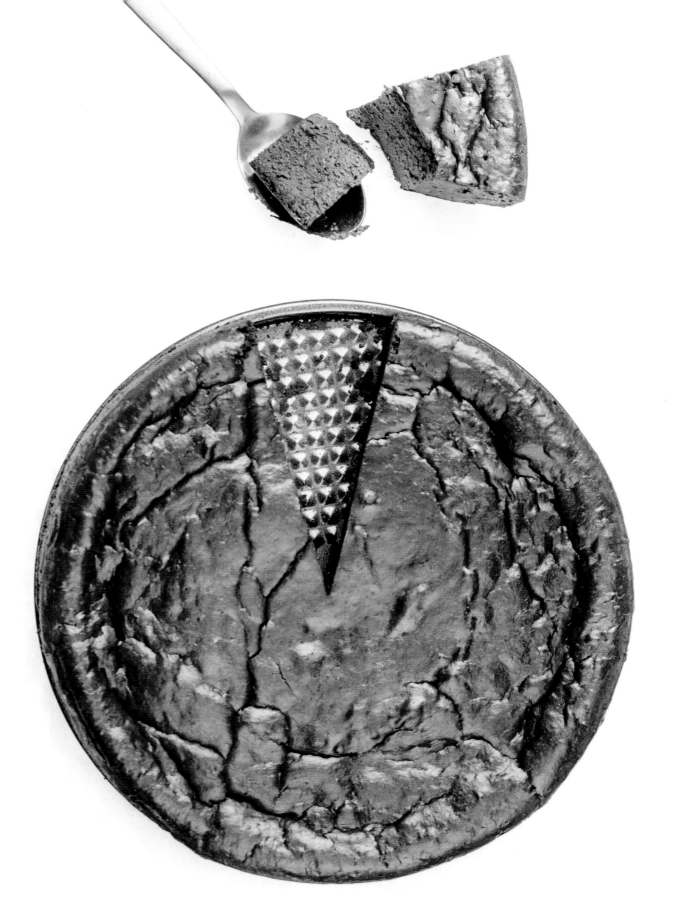

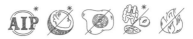

Pumpkin Pie Squares

Makes 8 squares (1 per serving) ⊚ Prep Time: 10 minutes, plus 1 hour to set

Gut-healing gelatin and frozen butternut squash make up these creamy squares that taste like pumpkin pie filling but are also a little bit like fudge.

10 ounces frozen cubed butternut squash

¼ cup canned unsweetened full-fat coconut milk

¼ cup unsweetened, unsalted sunflower seed butter or cashew butter

1 tablespoon melted coconut oil

2 teaspoons unflavored grass-fed beef gelatin

2 teaspoons vanilla extract

1 teaspoon ground cinnamon

¼ teaspoon ground nutmeg

⅛ teaspoon fine salt

10 to 15 drops stevia glycerite

• If your butternut squash comes in a steamable package, follow the package instructions to steam it until tender. If not, fill a saucepan with an inch of water and place the squash in the water. Bring to a boil, cover, and turn the heat down to medium. Steam until tender, 15 to 20 minutes.

• Transfer the hot squash to a blender and add the remaining ingredients, starting with 10 drops of stevia, then blend everything until smooth. Taste and add up to 5 drops more stevia, if desired.

• Pour the squash mixture into an 8½ by 4½-inch loaf pan lined with parchment paper or into silicone molds. Place in the fridge for 1 hour, or until completely set and firm.

• Use the parchment paper to lift the squash mixture out of the pan and cut it into eight 1-inch squares, or simply pop them out of the silicone molds.

• Store in the fridge for up to a week.

note: *Yes, you can use diced pumpkin instead of butternut squash!*

modifications: *To make these treats AIP compliant, use coconut cream instead of the sunflower seed butter or cashew butter, use 1 teaspoon yacón syrup instead of the stevia, and omit the vanilla extract and nutmeg. To make them coconut-free, use Salted Cashew Cream (page 76) instead of the coconut milk and melted ghee instead of the coconut oil.*

Per serving: Calories **90** · Fat **5.5g** · Total Carbs **7.2g** · Fiber **1.6g** · Protein **4.4g**

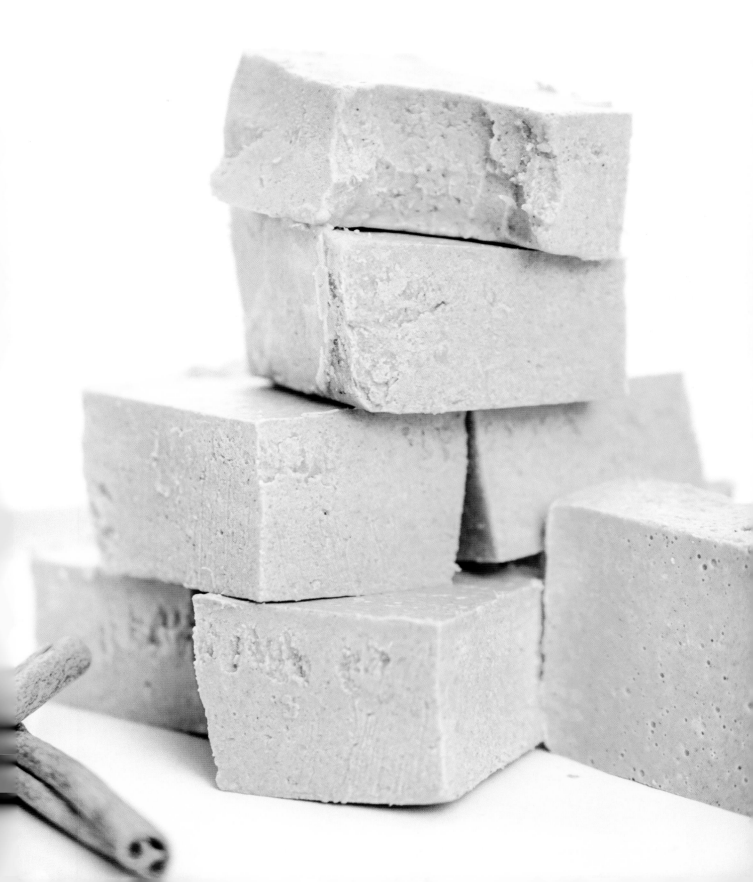

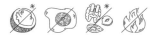

Chia Seed Pudding Five Ways

Serves 1 ○ Prep Time: 10 minutes, plus 1 hour to set

Chia seeds are a great source of fiber and have a decent amount of protein, so they serve as a satiating base for no-cook meals. They get a little gelatinous when wet, which makes them perfect for a quick egg-free pudding. Here's a base recipe and five ways to flavor it. Chia seed pudding options are oh so extra!

Base

3 tablespoons chia seeds

1 cup unsweetened dairy-free milk of choice

¼ teaspoon vanilla extract

2 to 5 drops stevia glycerite, according to taste, or ½ teaspoon yacón syrup

Pinch of fine salt

○ Whisk together all of the base ingredients in a small jar or container for 2 minutes. Let it sit for 2 minutes, then whisk again for another 2 minutes. Repeat until the mixture begins to thicken, then cover it and set it in the fridge until it firms to pudding consistency, about 1 hour.

○ For a flavored pudding, add the ingredients for the flavor of your choice (excluding garnishes) to the base recipe before it sets up in the fridge.

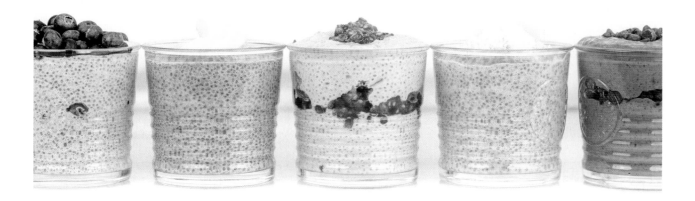

Per serving: Calories **325** · Fat **24.1g** · Total Carbs **20.1g** · Fiber **14.9g** · Protein **14.5g**

Blueberry Muffin

½ cup fresh blueberries, plus more for garnish

½ teaspoon grated lemon zest

½ teaspoon ground cinnamon

Calories **329** · Fat **24.2g** · Total Carbs **26.5g** · Fiber **16.4g** · Protein **14.8g**

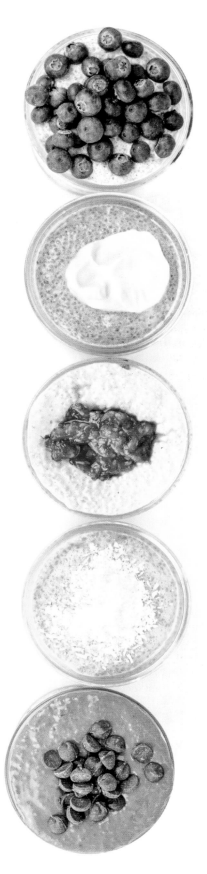

Boosted Latte

2 tablespoons cooled espresso or cold brew concentrate

1 tablespoon collagen peptides

1 tablespoon MCT oil

½ teaspoon ground cinnamon

1 teaspoon coconut cream, for garnish (optional)

With coconut cream:
Calories **476** · Fat **38.5g** · Total Carbs **21.2g** · Fiber **15.5g** · Protein **20.7g**

PB+J

2 tablespoons unsweetened, unsalted sunflower seed butter

2 tablespoons mashed fresh raspberries (do not mix with the rest of the ingredients; spoon them on top or swirl them in after the pudding has set up in the fridge)

Calories **541** · Fat **40.3g** · Total Carbs **30.9g** · Fiber **20.9g** · Protein **21.8g**

note: *If you tolerate nuts, you may swap out the sunflower seed butter for the nut butter of your choice.*

Golden Milk

½ teaspoon ground cinnamon

½ teaspoon turmeric powder

¼ teaspoon ginger powder

Pinch of ground black pepper

1 teaspoon shredded coconut, for garnish (optional)

Calories **351** · Fat **24.3g** · Total Carbs **22.3g** · Fiber **17.3g** · Protein **14.8g**

Chocolate Chip Protein

2 tablespoons chopped dark (85 to 90% cacao) chocolate or cacao nibs, plus more for garnish

1 scoop chocolate protein powder

1 teaspoon cacao powder

Calories **501** · Fat **29.6g** · Total Carbs **24.3g** · Fiber **17.2g** · Protein **41.4g**

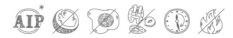

Anti-Inflammatory Tonic

Makes 24 ounces (6 servings) ○ Prep Time: 10 minutes

This is a blend of collagen-rich bone broth, which supports a healthy gut and joints, and a heavy dose of fresh cilantro. Cilantro isn't just delicious; it's a pretty cool herb that can lower blood pressure and protect against oxidative stress, and it's packed with electrolytes. Lemon juice and zest bring in immune-boosting antioxidant vitamin C, and turmeric is a popular anti-inflammatory root. The cool thing about this concoction is that it actually tastes really good! Blend it up and keep it in the fridge for a few days when you're feeling stiff or swollen, and drink a cup or two daily.

3 cups bone broth

2 cups chopped fresh cilantro

Juice of 1 lemon

1 teaspoon grated lemon zest

½ teaspoon turmeric powder

Pinch of ground black pepper

modifications: *To make this drink AIP compliant, omit the black pepper.*

○ Place all of the ingredients in a blender and blend until smooth. Drink at room temperature or chilled.

○ Store the tonic in a quart-sized jar in the fridge for up to a week. Shake before serving.

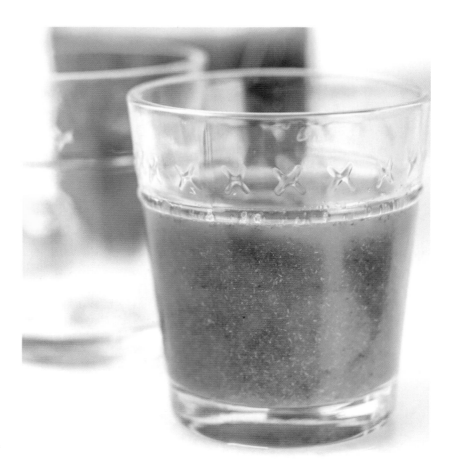

Per serving: Calories **29** · Fat **0.6g** · Total Carbs **1g** · Fiber **0.3g** · Protein **5.2g**

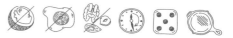

Tummy Tea

Makes 8 ounces (1 serving) ◦ Prep Time: 5 minutes ◦ Cook Time: 5 minutes, plus 10 minutes to steep

Our family's midwife suggested I drink this tea when our babies were colicky. This digestive tea got to the babies through the breast milk, but we learned that it was also very soothing for Mama. It's now our go-to remedy for indigestion.

1 cup filtered water

1 (1-inch) knob fresh ginger, peeled

1 tablespoon fennel seeds

2 bay leaves

◦ Bring everything to a simmer in a small saucepan. Remove from the heat and let the tea steep for 10 minutes. Strain through a fine-mesh sieve and discard the solids. Drink warm.

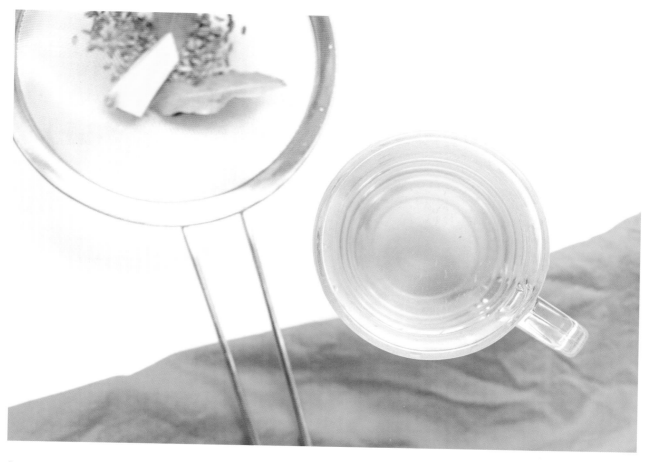

Per serving: Calories **0** · Fat **0g** · Total Carbs **0g** · Fiber **0g** · Protein **0g**

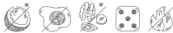

Antioxidant Iced Latte

Makes 32 ounces (2 servings) ◦ Prep Time: 5 minutes, plus 12 hours to cold brew

I love coffee, truly! When I was growing up, my mom made stovetop espresso regularly. I would beg her to give me a lick of the spoon when she made the *espumita,* or foam, which began with a simple syrup of whisked sugar and hot coffee. I had a taste for the stuff at a young age. While I think drinking too much coffee can exacerbate adrenal fatigue, in moderation it's quite good for you! Did you know that coffee is a major source of antioxidants in the American diet? To boost its antioxidant content, I included cacao powder, cinnamon, and turmeric in this easy cold brew. I chose the cold-brew method because it is less acidic and won't oxidize the oils in the coffee beans. I prefer light-roast beans for this reason as well.

¼ cup coarsely ground coffee

1 tablespoon cacao powder

2 teaspoons ground cinnamon

1 teaspoon turmeric powder

4 cups filtered water

For serving:

Ice cubes

¼ cup Stir-In Coffee Creamer
(page 107) (optional)

Special equipment:

4-cup French press

notes: *Adding creamer is optional; this smooth brew is lovely on its own.*

If you want to add creamer, I recommend my Stir-In Coffee Creamer for a dairy-free option with added collagen, but you can use any creamer you like. If you're avoiding nuts, you may use coconut cream; if you prefer dairy, raw milk or heavy cream is a good choice.

modifications: *My Stir-In Coffee Creamer can be made coconut-free or nut-free; see page 107 for those modifications.*

◦ In a 4-cup French press, combine the ground coffee, cacao powder, cinnamon, and turmeric. Pour in the water and gently stir with a wooden spoon. Put the top on, but do not press. Place in the fridge for 12 hours or overnight.

◦ In the morning, press the coffee; this will filter out the grounds.

◦ Fill 2 pint glasses with ice cubes. Pour the coffee over the ice cubes, then stir in the creamer, if desired. Enjoy!

Per serving (with creamer):
Calories **157** · Fat **12.8g** · Total Carbs **5.2g** · Fiber **2.7g** · Protein **8.5g**

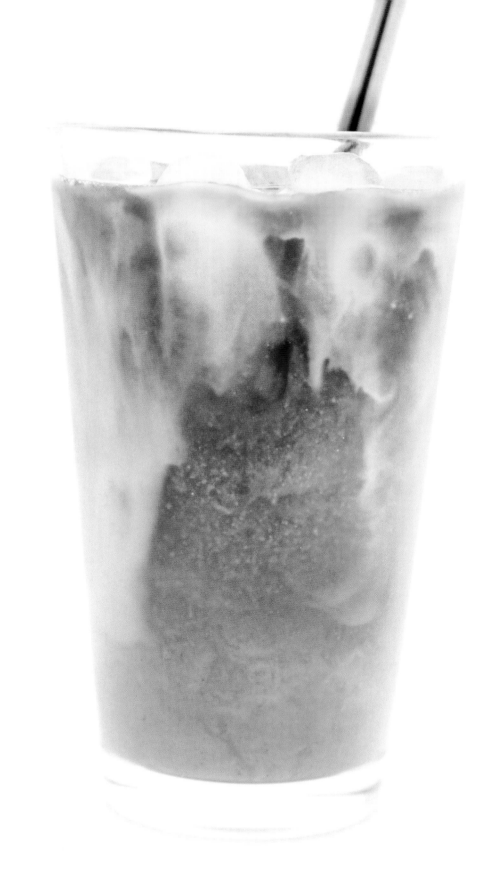

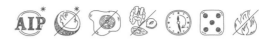

Berry Smart Smoothie

Makes 24 ounces (2 servings) ○ Prep Time: 5 minutes

What makes this smoothie so smart? It's loaded with probiotics, antioxidants, collagen, and healthy fats! Bonus: it's wonderfully creamy and thick. Frozen organic berries are picked at the height of the season and frozen, which means that they retain all of their nutritional goodness and you can enjoy them year-round. I like mixes of blackberries, raspberries, and strawberries, but you can use any kind you like.

1½ cups frozen berries

⅔ cup filtered water

½ cup dairy-free unsweetened plain yogurt (see notes)

¼ cup full-fat coconut cream

2 tablespoons grass-fed collagen

1 teaspoon ground cinnamon

○ Put all of the ingredients in a blender and blend until smooth. Serve right away.

notes: *I like using coconut milk yogurt for this smoothie, either the Anita's brand or my homemade version (you can find the recipe in my first book, Made Whole). There are several dairy-free yogurt alternatives on the market; I always look for an option with as few ingredients as possible and no added sugars. Full-fat dairy yogurts like Skyr are a good option for those who tolerate dairy.*

modifications: *To make this smoothie AIP compliant, use coconut milk yogurt (see notes). To make it coconut-free, use Salted Cashew Cream (page 76) instead of the coconut cream.*

Per serving: Calories **246** · Fat **13.1g** · Total Carbs **17.1g** · Fiber **3.6g** · Protein **13.3g**

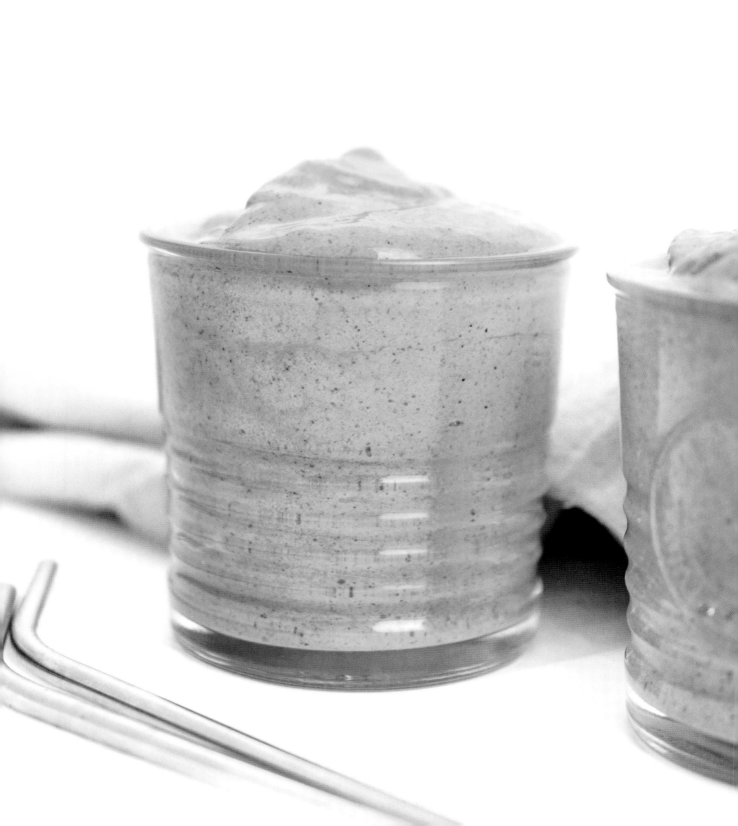

Acknowledgments

A BIG, HUGE THANK-YOU:

To my amazing husband, Justin. I truly appreciate everything you do for me and our son. You're selfless and funny and just the right amount of pain in the butt.

To my son, Jack, who's too smart for his own good and the sweetest boy who ever lived. Thank you for being my number one fan!

To my mom, for being my teacher and one-woman hype team. To my sister Laura, for being an amazing podcast cohost. Recording *Body Wise Podcast* with you brings me so much joy. To my little sister, Anavictoria, for loving my food and always inspiring me to be more me.

To Dana from *Real Food with Dana*, Michele from *Back Porch Paleo*, Frank from *Culinary Lion*, Jallyn de Leon, Tia Silvy, and Tia Yoyi, for helping me test the recipes when I had the manuscript crisis.

To my clients, readers, and followers, for being supportive and committed to healing. You all teach me more than I could ever teach you.

To the instructors at the Nutritional Therapy Association and my classmates, for all that you taught me and continue to teach me.

To pioneers in the food-as-medicine space like Ali Miller, Shawn Wells, Dr. Amy Meyers, Dr. Will Cole, Chris Kresser, Chris Masterjohn, Robb Wolf, Mark Sisson, Dr. Sarah Ballantyne, and so many more. You are changing the world!

Recommended Brands

Ingredients

Animal proteins: ButcherBox, US Wellness Meats, Five Mary's Farm, local farmers

Bacon: ButcherBox, Pederson's Natural Farms, Niman Ranch

Bone broth: Bonafide Provisions

Bratwursts and sausages: Niman Ranch, Pederson's Natural Farms

Coconut aminos: Thrive Market, The New Primal Noble Made

Coffee, teas, salts, spices, bone broth: Wild Foods

Dark chocolate for baking and treats: Alter Eco Blackout Organic Chocolate, Pascha Organic

Dried herbs and spices: Simply Organic, McCormick Organics, Primal Palate, Balanced Bites

Extra-virgin olive oil: Kasandrinos

Ghee: 4th and Heart with Himalayan Salt

Mayonnaise and other condiments: Primal Kitchen

Pastured collagen and gelatin: Vital Proteins

Pork panko: Bacon's Heir

Protein powder: PaleoPro, Naked Nutrition

Salt: Redmond Real Salt

Sprouted pumpkin seeds: Go Raw

Stevia glycerite: Now Foods

Sugar-free fish sauce: Red Boat 40°N

Unsweetened full-fat coconut milk: 365 Brand, Thai Kitchen Organic, Aroy-D

Unsweetened nut milk: Elmhurst

Yacón syrup: Alovitox

Tools

Cast-iron cookware: Lodge

Enameled cast-iron cookware: Le Creuset

Water filter: Berkey

References

Chapter 1: The House Won't Fall If the Bones Are Good

[1] Qinghui Mu, Jay Kirby, Christopher M. Reilly, and Xin M. Luo, "Leaky Gut as a Danger Signal for Autoimmune Diseases," *Frontiers in Immunology* 8 (May 2017), article 598, doi: 10.3389/fimmu.2017.00598.

[2] Shaun K. Riebl and Brenda M. Davy, "The Hydration Equation: Update on Water Balance and Cognitive Performance," *ACSM's Health and Fitness Journal* 17, no. 6 (2013): 21–28.

[3] National Research Council, *Diet and Health: Implications for Reducing Chronic Disease Risk* (Washington, DC: National Academies Press, 1989), https://doi.org/10.17226/1222.

[4] Jerzy Z. Nowak, "Oxidative Stress, Polyunsaturated Fatty Acids–Derived Oxidation Products and Bisretinoids as Potential Inducers of CNS Diseases: Focus on Age-Related Macular Degeneration," *Pharmacological Reports* 65, no. 2 (2013): 288–304.

[5] Elaine Patterson et al., "Health Implications of High Dietary Omega-6 Polyunsaturated Fatty Acids," *Journal of Nutrition and Metabolism* 2012 (2012), article 539426.

[6] James DiNicolantonio and James H. O'Keefe, "Importance of Maintaining Low Omega-6/Omega-3 Ratio for Reducing Inflammation," *Open Heart* 5, no. 2 (2018), http://dx.doi.org/10.1136/openhrt-2018-000946.

[7] Panayoula C. Tsiotra et al., "High Insulin and Leptin Increase Resistin and Inflammatory Cytokine Production from Human Mononuclear Cells," *BioMed Research International* 2013 (2013), article 487081, http://dx.doi.org/10.1155/2013/487081.

Chapter 2: Where We Get Our Fuel

[8] Clark Spencer Larsen, "Animal Source Foods and Human Health During Evolution," *Journal of Nutrition* 133, no. 11 (2003): 3893S–3897S, https://doi.org/10.1093/jn/133.11.3893S.

Ancient diets global map: Harriet V. Kuhnleini and Rula Soueida, "Use and Nutrient Composition of Traditional Baffin Inuit Foods," *Journal of Food Composition and Analysis* 5, no. 2 (1992): 112–126, https://doi.org/10.1016/0889-1575(92)90026-G; Joanita Kantet et al., "Contemporary Use of Wild Fruits by the Lakota in South Dakota and Implications for Cultural Identity," *Great Plains Research* 25, no. 1 (2015): 13–24, doi: 10.1353/gpr.2015.0011; I. P. Berezovikova and F. R. Mamleeva, "Traditional Foods in the Diet of Chukotka Natives," *International Journal of Circumpolar Health* 60, no. 2 (2001): 138–142, www.ncbi.nlm.nih.gov/pubmed/11507962; Christopher Masterjohn, "The Masai Part II: A Glimpse of the Masai Diet at the Turn of the 20th Century—A Land of Milk and Honey, Bananas from Afar," *Mother Nature Obeyed* (blog), Weston A. Price Foundation, September 13, 2011, www.westonaprice.org/the-masai-part-ii-a-glimpse-of-the-masai-diet-at-the-turn-of-the-20th-century-a-land-of-milk-and-honey-bananas-from-afar/; Donald E. Worcester, book review of *Gauchos and the Vanishing Frontier*, by Richard W. Slatta, Western Historical Quarterly 15, no. 4 (October 1984): 462–463, https://doi.org/10.2307/969473; Cherl-Ho Lee and Moonsil Lee Kim, "History of Fermented Food in Northeast Asia," in *Ethnic Fermented Foods and Alcoholic Beverages of Asia*, ed. Jyoti Prakash Tamang (Springer India, 2016), 1–17.

[9] William Leonard, Josh Snodgrass, and Marcia Robertson, "Evolutionary Perspectives on Fat Ingestion and Metabolism in Humans," in *Fat Detection: Taste, Texture, and Post Ingestive Effects*, ed. Jean-Pierre Montmayeur and Johannes le Coutre (Boca Raton, FL: CRC Press/Taylor & Francis, 2010), 3–18.

[10] Neil Mann, "Meat in the Human Diet: Anthropological Perspective," *Nutrition and Dietetics* 64, no. s4 (September 2007): S102–S107, https://doi.org/10.1111/j.1747-0080.2007.00194.x.

[11] Romily E. Hodges and Deanna M. Minich, "Modulation of Metabolic Detoxification Pathways Using Foods and Food-Derived Components: A Scientific Review with Clinical Application," *Journal of Nutrition and Metabolism* 2015, article 760689, doi: 10.1155/2015/760689.

Chapter 3: Eating for Healing

[12] J. Garcia-Leme and Sandra P. Farsky, "Hormonal Control of Inflammatory Responses," *Mediators of Inflammation* 2, no. 3 (1993): 181–198, doi: 10.1155/S0962935193000250.

[13] Qingui Mu et al., "Leaky Gut as a Danger Signal for Autoimmune Disease," *Frontiers in Immunology* 8 (March 2017): 598.

[14] Robert H. Howland, "Vagus Nerve Stimulation," *Current Behavioral Neuroscience Reports* 1, no. 2 (June 2014): 64–73, doi: 10.1007/s40473-014-0010-5.

[15] Shanta R. Dube et al., "Cumulative Childhood Stress and Autoimmune Diseases in Adults," *Psychosomatic Medicine* 71, no. 2 (2009): 243–250, doi: 10.1097/PSY.0b013e3181907888.

Meal Makers Index

My Meal Makers recipes are so versatile, and they really do make a meal! For easy references, here's a list of all the recipes in this book that make use of the Meal Makers, either in the ingredient lists directly or in serving suggestions that accompany the recipes.

Gut-Healing Teriyaki Sauce

Garlic Steak + Mushrooms (page 162; see notes)

Sesame Meatballs + Broccoli with Teriyaki Sauce (page 164)

Beef Curry Bowls (page 178; see notes)

Teriyaki Noodle Bowl (page 216)

Panko Turkey Meatballs with Bok Choy (page 226; see headnote)

Everything Sauce

Breakfast Rice Bowls (page 130; see additions)

Crispy Brats + Cabbage (page 198)

Curried Drumsticks with Burnt Cabbage (page 232)

Baked Chicken Tenders with Celery Fries (page 234)

Hasselback Sausage Boats (page 236; see additions)

Crispy Ranch Wings (page 242; see additions)

Cauliflower Sour Cream

Eggs Bianca (page 114)

Steakhouse Stir-Fry (page 150; see modifications)

Balsamic Braised Meatballs + Kale (page 152; see modifications)

Kitchen Sink Casserole (page 170)

Ground Pork Stroganoff (page 190)

Sumac Braised Pork Chops with Creamy Spinach + Noodles (page 192)

Spaghetti Squash Bratwurst Boats (page 200; see notes)

Cheesy Mushroom Meatzas (page 230; see modifications)

Hasselback Sausage Boats (page 236; see modifications)

Salmon Noodle Soup (page 272; see modifications)

Salted Cashew Cream

Green Basil Curry Sauce (page 106; see modifications)

Slow Cooker Fritatta (page 132; see note)

Steakhouse Stir-Fry (page 150)

Balsamic Braised Meatballs + Kale (page 152; see modifications)

Ground Pork Stroganoff (page 190; see note)

Spaghetti Squash Bratwurst Boats (page 200; see notes)

Chicken Scaloppine (page 218; see modifications)

Hasselback Sausage Boats (page 236; see modifications)

Salmon Noodle Soup (page 272; see modifications)

Flourless Chocolate Cake (page 346; see modifications)

Asian Garlic Compound Butter

Superhero Bowls (page 144)

Homemade Pork Panko

Burger Bar (page 136)

Crispy Chicken + Strawberry Balsamic Salad (page 222)

Panko Turkey Meatballs with Bok Choy (page 226)

Legit Fried Chicken Tenders (page 228)

Baked Chicken Tenders with Celery Fries (page 234)

Castaway Seed Blend

Pumpkin Bolognese (page 140)

Steakhouse Stir-Fry (page 150; see notes)

Balsamic Braised Meatballs + Kale (page 152)

Meatballs + Mushroom Gravy (page 160)

Kitchen Sink Casserole (page 170)

Hasselback Sausage Boats (page 236)

Pressure Cooker Ribs (page 206)

Allergen Index

* modification available

Recipe	Page	AIP										
Garlic Chicken over Zoodles	256	✓	✓	✓	✓					✓	*	
Hail Mary Chicken	258	*	*	✓	✓					*	✓	
Balsamic Cashew Chicken	260		✓	✓						*	✓	
Reina Pepiada	262		✓	✓		✓			✓			
Shrimp Curry with Broccoli	266	*	*	✓	✓	✓						✓
Crispy Salmon Wraps	268	*	✓	✓	✓							✓
Salmon Herb Skillet Cake	270		✓	✓	✓							✓
Salmon Noodle Soup	272	*	*	✓	✓							✓
Cumin-Dusted Mahi-Mahi	274		✓	✓	✓	✓						✓
Herbed Yellowfin Tuna Steaks	276	✓	✓	✓	✓	✓	✓					✓
Butternut Sage Smoked Oyster Chowder	278	*	*	✓	*							✓
Sardine Cake Boats	280			✓		✓						✓
Quick Citrus Salmon	282	✓	*	✓	✓		✓					
Mustard Salmon + Bok Choy	284		*	✓	✓	✓	✓					
Tuna-Stuffed Mushrooms	286		✓		✓		✓					
Shrimp + Sausage Sheet Pan	288	*	✓	✓	✓	✓	✓					
Balsamic Salmon with Toasty Vegetables	290	*	✓	✓	✓	✓	✓					
Presque Gumbo	292		*	✓	✓						✓	
Crispy Tuna Salad	294		✓		✓	✓			✓			
Warm Garlic Herb Radish Salad	298	✓	✓	✓	✓	✓	✓					✓
Charred Kale Soup	300	*	✓	✓	✓	✓						✓
Creamy Bacon Mushroom Noodles	302	*	✓	✓	*	✓						✓
Perfect Roasted Brussels Sprouts	304	✓	✓	✓	✓			✓				
Crispy Chicken Chips	306	*	*	✓	✓			✓				
Lamb Lollipops	308	✓	*	✓	✓							✓
Loving Liver Mousse	310	✓	✓	✓	✓	✓						
Herby Skillet Mushrooms	312	✓	✓	✓	✓	✓	✓					
Fiber-Rich Naan	314					✓						✓
Cauliflower "Fried" Rice	316		*	*	✓			✓				
Crispy Garlic Rice	318	✓	✓	✓	✓		✓	✓				
Spicy Yellow Rice	320	*	✓	✓	✓	✓		✓				
Rustic Roasted Summer Squash	322	*	✓	✓	✓	✓		✓				
Roasted Garlic "Hummus"	324		✓	✓	✓			✓				
Pressure Cooker Saag	326	*		✓	✓	✓				*	✓	
Cold Veggie Noodle Salad	328		*	✓	*	✓			✓			
Not Yo' Momma's Coleslaw	330		✓		✓	✓			✓			
Ceci's Salad	332		✓		✓	✓	✓		✓			
Berry Much Like Caprese Salad	334	*	✓	✓	*	✓			✓			
Smoked Salmon Dip	336	*	*	✓	✓	✓			✓			
Low-Carb Blueberry Muffins	340				*							
Chocolate Avocado Ice Cream	342	*		✓	✓				✓			
Tahini Cookie Cream Bites	344		*	✓	✓				✓			
Flourless Chocolate Cake	346		*		✓		✓					
Pumpkin Pie Squares	348	*	*	✓	*				✓			
Chia Seed Pudding Five Ways	350		*	✓	*				✓			
Anti-Inflammatory Tonic	352	*	✓	✓	✓	✓			✓			
Tummy Tea	353		✓	✓	✓	✓	✓					✓
Antioxidant Iced Latte	354		*	✓	*	✓			✓			
Berry Smart Smoothie	356	*	*	✓	✓	✓	✓		✓			

* modification available

Recipe Index

Meal Makers

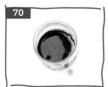
70
Gut-Healing Teriyaki Sauce

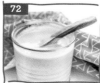
72
Everything Sauce

74
Cauliflower Sour Cream

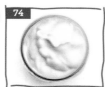
76
Salted Cashew Cream

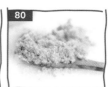
78
Asian Garlic Compound Butter

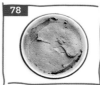
80
Homemade Pork Panko

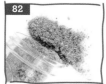
82
Castaway Seed Blend

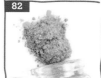
82
Citrus Curry Powder

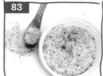
83
Cuban Sazón

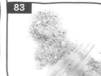
83
Turn Up the Heat Spice Blend

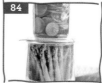
84
Pickled Asparagus + Pickled Radishes

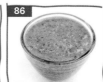
86
Gremolata with Olive Oil

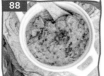
88
Onion + Bacon Spread

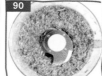
90
Briny Arugula Pesto

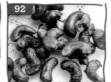
92
Balsamic Roasted Cashews

94
Horseradish Mayo

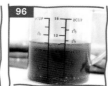
96
Balsamic Mustard Vinaigrette

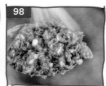
98
Green Onion Relish

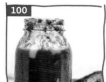
100
Slow Cooker Blueberry BBQ Sauce

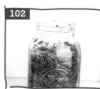
102
Homemade Kraut

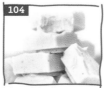
104
Mozz Blocks

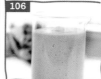
106
Green Basil Curry Sauce

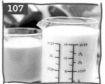
107
Stir-In Coffee Creamer

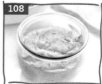
108
Cilantro Aioli

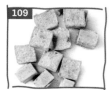
109
Frozen Herb Blocks

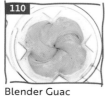
110
Blender Guac

Breakfast

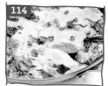
114
Eggs Bianca

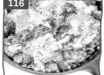
116
Broccoli Noodle Egg Skillet

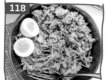
118
Sweet Onion Breakfast Bowls

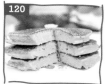
120
Pumpkin Pancakes

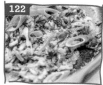
122
Radish + Pork Belly Hash Browns

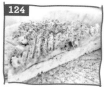
124
Protein Avocado Toast

126
Protein Waffles

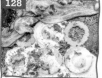
128
Sheet Pan Breakfast

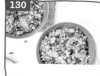
130
Breakfast Rice Bowls

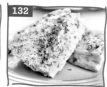
132
Slow Cooker Frittata

Beef

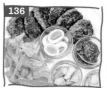
136
Burger Bar

138
Sweet Osso Buco

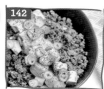
140
Pumpkin Bolognese

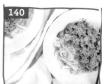
142
Perfect Ground Beef with Avocado

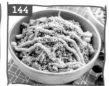
144
Superhero Bowls

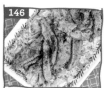
146
Marinated Steak + Buttery Cabbage

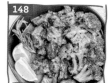
148
Lemon Herb Beef + Broccoli

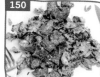
150
Steakhouse Stir-Fry

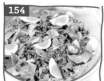
152
Balsamic Braised Meatballs + Kale

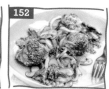
154
Hamburger Salad

156
Beef + Broccoli Skillet Casserole

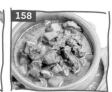
158
Rich Slow-Cooked Stew

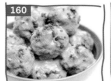
160

Meatballs +
Mushroom Gravy

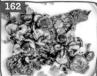
162

Garlic Steak +
Mushrooms

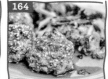
164

Sesame Meatballs
+ Broccoli with
Teriyaki Sauce

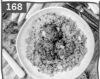
166

Ginger Cilantro
Steak + Tangy
Cauliflower

168

Carne Asada
Meatballs

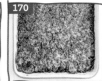
170

Kitchen Sink
Casserole

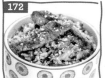
172

Mustard Beef +
Broccoli Rice
Sheet Pan Stir-Fry

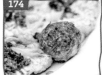
174

Mushroom Herb
Meatballs with
Cauliflower Steaks

176

Creamy Beef +
Bacon Soup

178

Beef Curry Bowls

180

Savory Short Ribs

Pork

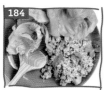
184

Anti-Inflammatory
Pork Wraps

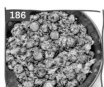
186

Glazed Sausage
Skillet

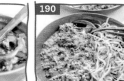
188

Breakfast Sausage
Soup

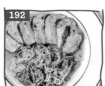
190

Ground Pork
Stroganoff

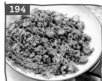
192

Sumac Braised Pork
Chops with Creamy
Spinach + Noodles

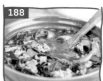
194

South Florida
Stir-Fry

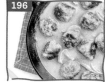
196

Coconut Lime
Spiced Meatballs

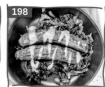
198

Crispy Brats +
Cabbage

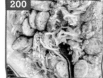
200

Spaghetti Squash
Bratwurst Boats

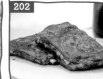
202

BBQ Spare Ribs

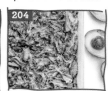
204

Tasty Mojo Pork

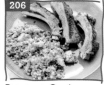
206

Pressure Cooker
Ribs

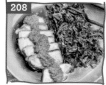
208

Curried Pork Chops
with Cabbage

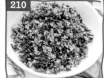
210

Pork + Kale in an
Instant

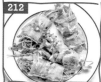
212

Prosciutto Wraps

Poultry

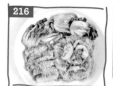
216
Teriyaki Noodle Bowl

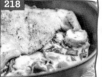
218
Chicken Scaloppine with Creamy Spinach + Artichokes

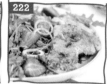
220
Turkey Burger Bowls

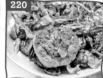
222
Crispy Chicken + Strawberry Balsamic Salad

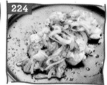
224
Victoria's Pollo Encebollado

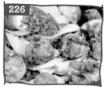
226
Panko Turkey Meatballs with Bok Choy

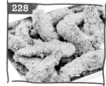
228
Legit Fried Chicken Tenders

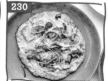
230
"Cheesy" Mushroom Meatzas

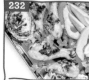
232
Curried Drumsticks with Burnt Cabbage

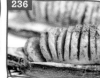
234
Baked Chicken Tenders with Celery Fries

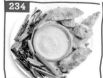
236
Hasselback Sausage Boats

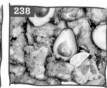
238
Crispy Curry Chicken Thighs

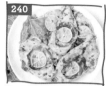
240
Spring Chicken with Baby Zucchini

242
Crispy Ranch Wings

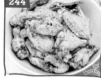
244
Tarragon + Spice Chicken Wings

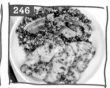
246
Triple Green Chicken

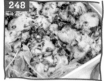
248
Sweet Sage Chicken Thighs

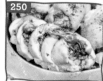
250
Stuffed Chicken Thighs

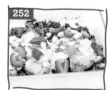
252
Strawberry Balsamic Baked Chicken with Kale

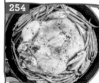
254
Perfect Roast Chicken with Green Beans

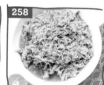
256
Garlic Chicken over Zoodles

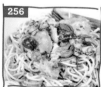
258
Hail Mary Chicken

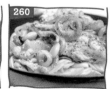
260
Balsamic Cashew Chicken

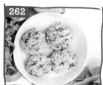
262
Reina Pepiada

Fish + Seafood

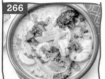 266
Shrimp Curry with Broccoli

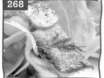 268
Crispy Salmon Wraps

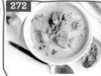 270
Salmon Herb Skillet Cake

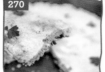 272
Salmon Noodle Soup

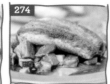 274
Cumin-Dusted Mahi-Mahi

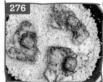 276
Herbed Yellowfin Tuna Steaks

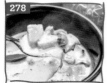 278
Butternut Sage Smoked Oyster Chowder

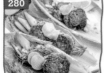 280
Sardine Cake Boats

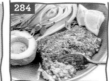 282
Quick Citrus Salmon

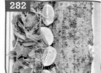 284
Mustard Salmon + Bok Choy

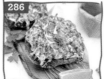 286
Tuna-Stuffed Mushrooms

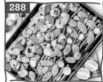 288
Shrimp + Sausage Sheet Pan

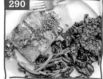 290
Balsamic Salmon with Toasty Vegetables

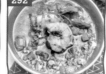 292
Presque Gumbo

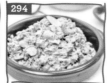 294
Crispy Tuna Salad

Sides + Snacks

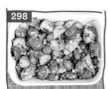 298
Warm Garlic Herb Radish Salad

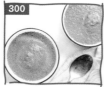 300
Charred Kale Soup

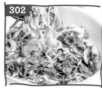 302
Creamy Bacon Mushroom Noodles

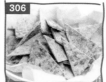 304
Perfect Roasted Brussels Sprouts

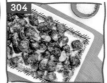 306
Crispy Chicken Chips

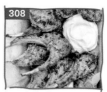 308
Lamb Lollipops

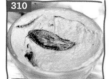 310
Loving Liver Mousse

 312
Herby Skillet Mushrooms

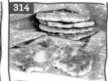 314
Fiber-Rich Naan

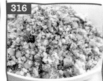 316
Cauliflower "Fried" Rice

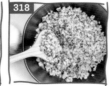 318
Crispy Garlic Rice

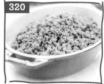 320
Spicy Yellow Rice

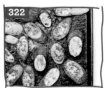
322

Rustic Roasted
Summer Squash

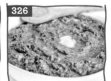
324

Roasted Garlic
"Hummus"

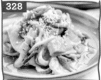
326

Pressure Cooker
Saag

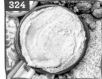
328

Cold Veggie Noodle
Salad

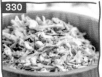
330

Not Yo' Momma's
Coleslaw

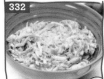
332

Ceci's Salad

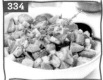
334

Berry Much Like
Caprese Salad

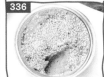
336

Smoked Salmon Dip

Sweets + Beverages

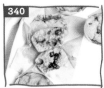
340

Low-Carb Blueberry
Muffins

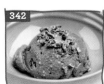
342

Chocolate Avocado
Ice Cream

344

Tahini Cookie
Cream Bites

346

Flourless Chocolate
Cake

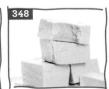
348

Pumpkin Pie
Squares

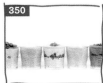
350

Chia Seed Pudding
Five Ways

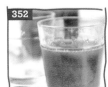
352

Anti-Inflammatory
Tonic

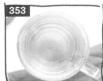
353

Tummy Tea

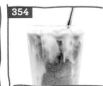
354

Antioxidant
Iced Latte

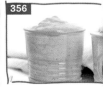
356

Berry Smart
Smoothie

General Index